T0263067

Emergency General Surgery

Editors

VIREN PREMNATH PUNJA
PAUL J. SCHENARTS

SURGICAL CLINICS
OF NORTH AMERICA

www.surgical.theclinics.com

Consulting Editor
RONALD F. MARTIN

December 2023 • Volume 103 • Number 6

ELSEVIER

1600 John F. Kennedy Boulevard • Suite 1800 • Philadelphia, Pennsylvania, 19103-2899

http://www.surgical.theclinics.com

SURGICAL CLINICS OF NORTH AMERICA Volume 103, Number 6
December 2023 ISSN 0039–6109, ISBN-13: 978-0-443-18254-9

Editor: John Vassallo (j.vassallo@elsevier.com)
Developmental Editor: Anita Chamoli

Surgical Clinics of North America (ISSN 0039–6109) is published bimonthly by Elsevier Inc., 360 Park Avenue South, New York, NY 10010-1710. Months of publication are February, April, June, August, October, and December. Business and Editorial Offices: 1600 John F. Kennedy Blvd., Suite 1800, Philadelphia, PA 19103-2899. Periodicals postage paid at New York, NY and additional mailing offices. Subscription prices are $479.00 per year for US individuals, $1045.00 per year for US institutions, $100.00 per year for US & Canadian students and residents, $575.00 per year for Canadian individuals, $1327.00 per year for Canadian institutions, $580.00 for international individuals, $1327.00 per year for international institutions and $250.00 per year for foreign students/residents. To receive student/resident rate, orders must be accompanied by name of affiliated institution, date of term, and the *signature* of program/residency coordinator on institution letterhead. Orders will be billed at individual rate until proof of status is received. Foreign air speed delivery is included in all *Clinics* subscription prices. All prices are subject to change without notice. POSTMASTER: Send address changes to *Surgical Clinics*, Elsevier Health Sciences Division, Subscription Customer Service, 3251 Riverport Lane, Maryland Heights, MO 63043. **Customer Service (orders, claims, online, change of address): Telephone: 1-800-654-2452 (U.S. and Canada); 314-447-8871 (outside U.S. and Canada). Fax: 314-447-8029. E-mail: journalscustomerservice-usa@elsevier.com (for print support); journalsonlinesupport-usa@elsevier.com (for online support).**

Reprints. For copies of 100 or more, of articles in this publication, please contact the Commercial Reprints Department, Elsevier Inc., 360 Park Avenue South, New York, New York 10010-1710. Tel. 212-633-3874, Fax: 212-633-3820, E-mail: reprints@elsevier.com.

Surgical Clinics of North America is also published in Spanish by McGraw-Hill Interamericana Editores S.A., P.O. Box 5-237 06500 Mexico D.F. Mexico; and in Portuguese by Interlivros Edicoes Ltda., Rua Comandante Coelho 1085, CEP 21250, Rio de Janeiro, Brazil; and in Greek by Paschalidis Medical Publications, Athens Greece.

Surgical Clinics of North America is covered in *MEDLINE/PubMed (Index Medicus), EMBASE/Excerpta Medica, Current Contents/Clinical Medicine, Current Contents/Life Sciences, Science Citation Index*, and *ISI/BIOMED.*

Contributors

CONSULTING EDITOR

RONALD F. MARTIN, MD, FACS
Colonel (Retired), United States Army Reserve, Department of General Surgery, Pullman Regional Hospital and Clinic Network, Pullman, Washington

EDITORS

VIREN PREMNATH PUNJA, MB, BS, FACS
Associate Professor, Department of Surgery, Creighton University, School of Medicine, Omaha, Nebraska

PAUL J. SCHENARTS, MD, FACS, MAMSE
Professor, Department of Surgery, Creighton University School of Medicine, Omaha, Nebraska

AUTHORS

ZANA ALATTAR, MD
General Surgery Resident, University of Arizona College of Medicine–Phoenix, Phoenix, Arizona

ELLIOT BISHOP, MD
Assistant Professor, Department of Surgery Atlanta, Georgia

JACQUELINE BLANK, MD
Fellow, Department of Surgery, Division of Trauma, Surgical Critical Care and Emergency Surgery, Fellow-In-Exception, Perelman School of Medicine, University of Pennsylvania, Philadelphia, Pennsylvania

KRISTIN C. BREMER, MD
General Surgery Resident, Department of Surgery, Creighton University School of Medicine, Omaha, Nebraska

CHRISTINE CASTATER, MD, MBA
Morehouse School of Medicine, Grady Memorial Hospital, Atlanta, Georgia

CHRISTOPHER DECKER, MD
Clinical Assistant Professor, Department of Surgery, Temple University Hospital, Philadelphia, Pennsylvania

DESMOND M. D'SOUZA, MD
Associate Professor, Division of Thoracic Surgery, Department of Surgery, The Ohio State Wexner Medical Center, Columbus, Ohio

MELISSA K. DREZDZON, MD
Colorectal Research Fellow, Division of Colorectal Surgery, Department of Surgery, Medical College of Wisconsin, Milwaukee, Wisconsin

CARLOS A. FERNANDEZ, MD, FACS
Assistant Professor of Surgery, Trauma ICU Director, Department of Surgery, Creighton University Medical Center, Omaha, Nebraska

MARI FREEDBERG, MD
Associate, Department of Surgery, University, Atlanta, Georgia

CHAD GRIESBACH, MD
Resident Physician, Department of General Surgery, & White Medical Center, Temple, Texas

CHAD HALL, MD
Department of General Surgery, & White Medical Center, Temple, Texas

BRETT HARDEN WAIBEL, MD
Associate Professor of Surgery, Division of Acute Care Surgery, Department of Surgery, University of Nebraska Medical Center, Omaha, Nebraska

TERESA A. HUYNH, MD
Surgery Resident, Riverside Community Hospital, Riverside, California

NADIA IWANYSHYN, PharmD, BCPS
Clinical Associate Professor of Pharmacy, University of Florida College of Pharmacy, Jacksonville, Florida

DONALD JOHNSON, PharmD, BCPS, BCCP
Clinical Associate Professor of Pharmacy, University of Florida College of Pharmacy, Jacksonville, Florida

ANDREW JAMES KAMIEN, MD
Assistant Professor of Surgery, Division of Acute Care Surgery, Department of Surgery, University of Nebraska Medical Center, Omaha, Nebraska

LEWIS J. KAPLAN, MD, FACS, FCCP, FCCM
Professor of Surgery, Perelman School of Medicine, University of Pennsylvania; Professor, Division of Trauma, Department of Surgery; Section Chief, Surgical Critical Care and Emergency Surgery, Surgical Services, Section of Surgical Critical Care and Emergency General Surgery, Corporal Michael J. Crescenz VA Medical Center, Philadelphia, Pennsylvania

NATASHA KERIC, MD, FACS
Associate Professor of Surgery, University of Arizona College of Medicine–Phoenix, Banner–University Medical Center Phoenix, Phoenix, Arizona

PHILLIP KIM, MD
Associate, Department of Surgery, Atlanta, Georgia

DOROTHY LIU, MD
Surgical Critical Care Fellow, Temple University Hospital, Philadelphia, Pennsylvania

AHMED MAHMOUD, MD, FACS, FRCS
Associate Professor of Clinical Surgery, University of California Riverside, Program Director of General Surgery Residency, Surgery Clerkship Director, General and Thoracic Surgeon, Riverside Community Hospital, Riverside, California

KALYANA C. NANDIPATI, MBBS, MD
Professor of Surgery, Division of Clinical Research, Department of Surgery, Creighton University School of Medicine; Director of Esophageal Center, Minimally Invasive Surgery, Omaha, Nebraska

HADDON PANTEL, MD
Assistant Professor of Surgery, Department of Colon and Rectal Surgery, Rectal Surgery, Yale School of Medicine, New Haven, Connecticut

CARRIE Y. PETERSON, MD, MS, FACS, FASCRS
Associate Professor, Division of Colorectal Surgery, Department of Surgery, Medical College of Wisconsin, Milwaukee, Wisconsin

VIVY PHAN, MD
General Surgery Resident, & White Medical Center, Temple, Texas

VIKRAM B. REDDY, MD, PHD, MBA
Chief of Colon and Rectal Surgery, Department of Surgery, Yale School of Medicine, New Haven, Connecticut

DANIEL REGIER, MD
Resident, of Surgery, West Virginia University, Morgantown, West Virginia

ADORA SANTOS, DO
Trauma, Acute Care and Surgical Critical Care Fellow, Department of Surgery Atlanta, Georgia

GREGORY SCHAEFER, DO, FACS
Professor of Surgery, Division of Trauma, Surgical Critical Care, and Acute Care Surgery, West Virginia University, Medical Director, Surgical Critical Care, J.W. Ruby Memorial Hospital, West Virginia University, Morgantown, West Virginia

CHRISTOPHER SCIARRETTA, MD
Resident, University of Tennessee College of Medicine, University of Tennessee, Chattanooga, Tennessee

ADAM M. SHIROFF, MD, FACS
Professor of Clinical Surgery, Division of Trauma, Department of Surgery, Surgical Critical Care and Emergency Surgery, Perelman School of Medicine, University of Pennsylvania, Surgical Services, Section of Surgical Critical Care and Emergency General Surgery, Corporal Michael J. Crescenz VA Medical Center, Philadelphia, Pennsylvania

DAVID J. SKARUPA, MD, FACS, FCCM
Associate Professor, Department of Surgery, University of Florida College of Medicine, Jacksonville, Florida

CONLEY STOUT, MD
Resident of Surgery, West Virginia University, Morgantown, West Virginia

RAYMOND TRAWEEK, MD
Resident Physician, & White Medical Center, Temple, Texas

RACHEL LYNNE WARNER, DO
Assistant Professor, Department of Surgery, University of Florida College of Medicine, Jacksonville, Florida

BRIANNA S. WILLIAMS, MD
Surgery Resident, Riverside Community Hospital, Riverside, California

JANE ZHAO, MD, MS
Medical Resident, Department of Surgery, The Ohio State Wexner Medical Center, Columbus, Ohio

Contents

 Video content accompanies this article at http://www.surgical. theclinics.com.

> Early primary assessment and abdominal examination can often be enough to triage the patient with abdominal pain into those with less severe underlying pathologic condition from those with more acute findings. A focused history of the patient can then allow the clinician to develop their differential diagnosis. Once the differential diagnoses are determined, diagnostic imaging and laboratory findings can help confirm the diagnosis and allow for expeditious treatment and intervention.

> Traditionally, the workflow surrounding a general surgery patient allows for a period of evaluation and optimization of underlying medical issues to allow for risk modification; however, in the emergency, this optimization period is largely condensed because of its time-dependent nature. Because the lack of optimization can lead to complications, the ability to rapidly resuscitate the patient, proceed to procedural intervention to control the situation, and manage common medical comorbidities is paramount. This article provides an overview on these subjects.

> In this review article, we aim to provide an overview of common and uncommon general surgery thoracic emergencies as well as basic thoracic anatomy, common diagnostic tests, and operative positioning and access considerations. We also describe specific thoracic procedures. We hope that this article simplifies some of the challenges associated with the management of thoracic emergencies.

jaundice, coagulopathy, and in some instances, encephalopathy. The differential can be broad and may include infectious, inflammatory, and even iatrogenic etiologies. Workup with appropriate lab and imaging studies can help discern between different pathologies and thus guide their management. Interventions can range broadly from conservative management with medical therapy to endoscopic options or surgery. This article explores the diagnostic workup and evaluation as well as the current therapeutic interventions for a variety of these nontraumatic hepatobiliary emergencies based on the most current literature.

Diabetes is a systemic illness that can cause a broad range of physiologic effects. Infection rates and wound healing are both affected through multiple mechanisms. Other physiologic changes increase risk for wounds as well as complex soft tissue infections ranging from simple cellulitis to necrotizing soft tissue infections. Clinicians and surgeons need to have a low index of suspicion for severe infection in a patient presenting with diabetes, and even more so in patients with uncontrolled diabetes.

Nonobstetrical surgical emergencies can occur throughout pregnancy but are often difficult to diagnose due to the physiologic and anatomical changes that occur during pregnancy. Medical providers should have insight into these changes and be familiar with options for the diagnosis and management of common nonobstetrical surgical emergencies, such as appendicitis, cholecystitis, and small bowel obstruction. Surgeons should also be aware of obstetrical emergencies, such as ectopic pregnancy and severe vaginal bleeding, which may be life threatening to mother and the fetus. Intraoperatively, surgeons should be familiar with minimally invasive approaches for surgical diseases and special anesthetic considerations for pregnant patients.

Emergency surgery in patients with significant comorbidities benefits from a structured approach to preoperative evaluation, intra-operative intervention, and postoperative management. Providing goal concordant care is ideal using shared decision-making. When operation cannot achieve the patient's goal, non-operative therapy including Comfort Care is appropriate. When surgical therapy is offered, preoperative physiology-improving interventions are far fewer than in other phases. Reevaluation of clinical care progress helps define trajectory and inform goals of care. Palliative Care Medicine may be critical in supporting loved ones during a patient's critical illness. Outcome evaluation defines successful strategies and outline opportunities for improvement.

Geriatric patients undergoing emergency surgery are at significantly higher risk for complications and death when compared with younger patients. Optimizing care for these patients requires a multidisciplinary team, special attention to physiologic changes and medication use, as well as targeted intervention to mitigate complications such as delirium, which can worsen overall outcomes. Frailty can be assessed preoperatively to identify patients at the highest risk for complications. Shared decision-making with both the family and patient during the consent process is integral to defining patient's goals of care in these high-risk situations.

Selective non traumatic emergency surgery patients are targets for damage control surgery (DCS) to prevent or treat abdominal compartment syndrome and the lethal triad. However, DCS is still a subject of controversy. As a concept, DCS describes a series of abbreviated surgical procedures to allow rapid source control of hemorrhage and contamination in patients with circulatory shock to allow resuscitation and stabilization in the intensive care unit followed by delayed return to the operating room for definitive surgical management once the patient becomes physiologic stable. If appropriately applied, the DCS morbidity and mortality can be significantly reduced.

Acute care surgeons encounter patients experiencing surgical emergencies related to advanced malignancy, catastrophic vascular events, or associated with multisystem organ failure. The acute nature is a factor in establishing a relationship between surgeon, patient, and family. Surgeons must use effective communication skills, empathy, and a knowledge of legal and ethical foundations. Training in palliative care principles is limited in many medical school and residency curricula. We offer examples of clinical situations facing acute care surgeons and discuss evidence-based recommendations to facilitate successful treatment and outcomes.

SURGICAL CLINICS
OF NORTH AMERICA

SERIES OF RELATED INTEREST

Advances in Surgery
https://www.advancessurgery.com/
Surgical Oncology Clinics
https://www.surgonc.theclinics.com/
Thoracic Surgery Clinics
https://www.thoracic.theclinics.com/

THE CLINICS ARE AVAILABLE ONLINE!
Access your subscription at:
www.theclinics.com

Foreword

General Surgical Emergencies

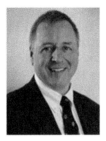

Ronald F. Martin, MD, FACS
Consulting Editor

Patients would like to believe that hospitals are capable of helping 24/7/365. Patients also tend to believe (if you believe in polling and focus group responses) that "Quality" is assumed. In other words, most people in the United States are of the belief that in an emergency they can go to any facility and get the care they need—right now. Of course, every locality has its collections of local citizens who hold strong opinions of which hospital they may or may not choose, but beyond their local sense of resources, they do not really think much about hospital capabilities.

Sadly, most of our fellow citizens are woefully underinformed if not misinformed.

Perhaps the only time when health care was homogenously distributed in the United States was when it was equally primitive and hard to find everywhere. The rise of medical centers that developed largely from charities and the development of collective groups with shared goals quickly changed the landscape through the 1800s to the mid to late 1900s. What has had greater impact since the very late 1900s up to now has been the transformation of the medical work force. For the sake of this discussion, I will confine my remarks to Surgery, although they could easily apply to other fields, especially those that are procedural in nature.

In this series, we have discussed many times the tensions that arose from the generalist-specialist divide. In fact, we have discussed the tensions that arose from the specialist-hyperspecialist divide. These concerns are not new. Specialties have been peeled off from general surgery for nearly a century. The change of the last 25 to 30 years has been more driven from the extremely high percentage of general surgery residents who have chosen fellowship training. And more specifically, the overall redistribution of the surgical workforce capability that created.

Some of these changes, as alluded to in this excellent issue by Drs Punja and Schenarts, are educational choices by trainees. Some changes stem from the somewhat responsive curriculum changes by our collective educational establishment. The net effect has been a greater challenge to train surgeons to work in *any* work environment

Surg Clin N Am 103 (2023) xiii–xv
https://doi.org/10.1016/j.suc.2023.07.011
0039-6109/23/© 2023 Published by Elsevier Inc.
surgical.theclinics.com

she or he may encounter. Training choices are not the only causes of this misalignment (or malalignment) of patient need to patient care. Some of forces derive from economic choices as well as population-density constraints. Even within well-to-do, densely populated areas, there are wide diversities in capability within and between facilities based on time of day or day of week.

No matter how well trained a general surgeon is, there are likely to be aspects of care that will be beyond the scope of what she or he can offer. For example, I can't think of any general surgeons who perform interventional cardiology for a postop STEMI. In reality, we surgeons are all quite dependent on other specialties and the benefits they bring to the table. For some lucky few, many of those subspecialty partners are readily available around the clock. I was one of those people for most of my career. Others have those resources either not at all or only sometimes. When I was deployed to Iraq or Afghanistan, we had as much capability as we did personnel in our unit. We were self-reliant to a very large degree. Honestly, that worked quite well by local standards. Having no laparoscopy, endoscopy, or interventional radiology available was just a way of life. To be fair, for those persons who met the Medical Rules of Eligibility (MROE), we had arguably the best patient transfer and transport system in the world. For those who did not meet MROE criteria, we would be the best hospital their local population had ever seen. However, if we were to apply those austere environment standards of care here in the United States, we would be practicing in a way that is either bordering on negligent or just plain negligent. While our transport system in the States is generally quite good, it really can't quite compare to our military model, in capability or cost to the patient. As regards the transfer piece, since the pandemic, an across-the-board loss of *staffed* beds—particularly at referral centers—has profoundly exacerbated our weaknesses.

The solutions to these problems are not simple given our current health care configuration. Many facilities, usually smaller ones, have chosen to simply not staff their hospitals with surgical coverage on nights or weekends or when someone is on vacation. This leaves their emergency room providers or hospitalists spending hours calling around for anyone who can help. Inpatient dialysis care is hard to find in many hospitals. Diagnostic radiology can usually be acquired remotely but not so for interventional services. Complex endoscopy is completely hit-or-miss in many places, and general surgeons have had to pick up the slack for screening or diagnostic endoscopy but don't always have the training or support for interventional endoscopy.

There are many ways one could approach solving any and all the problems described above. I don't think our current political climate suggests that government input is likely soon. From a corporate standpoint, there is little incentive for for-profit or not-for-profit entities to tackle the demands. Small facilities don't have the cash; large facilities *may* have the cash in some limited cases but (a) can't/won't risk investment on something that may be a financial loser (it is getting harder and harder to explain to boards about bad quarterly returns); and (b) cannot necessarily acquire reliable staffing to make a financially viable model.

If government won't help and the corporations (that most of us now work for) cannot or will not help, then it would seem, dear reader, that it is up to you for now—especially if you are a surgeon, modern medicine's equivalent of a Swiss Army Knife. Even within surgery, this is going to fall to the true general surgeon disproportionately. As many of our surgical specialty colleagues are quite happy to declare themselves experts during the sunny hours of weekdays—holidays excluded, naturally—they are also happy to confer the blessings of nocturnal or weekend excellence of skill to those surgeons who are willing to take emergency call in order that our daytime experts may not take call.

This collection of articles prepared for us by Drs Punja and Schenarts, along with their colleagues, is an excellent source to guide the interested reader through how to deal with myriad complex situations as well as find a way to identify *early* in the process if the patient's needs are not best met by you or your facility. Paramount in good surgical care is that one does not always have to know exactly what is going wrong for the patient, but one does always need to know what exactly must be done for the patient. For some of us, we will be able to do that in our own facilities 24/7. For others, some problems will evade our grasp at our facility all the time, and for others yet, we may have capabilities sometimes but not other times. Knowing which of these situations you find yourself in is every bit as important to good patient care as being able to diagnose well and operate.

As always, we hope this series provides a basis for self-growth as well as a basis to work with our medical colleagues and community partners to improve our ability to be part of the solution. We are indebted deeply to those who contribute to this series. I am personally deeply grateful to Dr Schenarts for all the support, guidance, and friendship he has given me over the years. We are also very grateful to the readership of the *Surgical Clinics*, who has supported this effort for over a century.

Ronald F. Martin, MD, FACS
Colonel (retired), United States Army Reserve
Department of General Surgery
Pullman Surgical Associates
Pullman Regional Hospital and Clinic Network
825 Southeast Bishop Boulevard, Suite 130
Pullman, WA 99163, USA

E-mail address:
rfmcescna@gmail.com

Preface

The Tides of Change: Emergencies in General Surgery

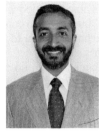 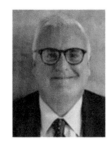

Viren Premnath Punja,
MB, BS, FACS

Paul J. Schenarts,
MD, FACS, MAMSE

Editors

Historically general surgeons took care of patients across a breadth of surgical problems. Over time this has changed due to a variety of different reasons: a shift in preference in certain practice settings, changes in the curriculum, and more focused training in current general surgery programs. Surgical education has been restructured with the emergence of more fellowship training programs and with the changes made to the ACGME work hours.[1] As a result, the practice patterns of general surgeons have evolved during this period.

A 5-year residency in general surgery provides exposure and training across a wide array of surgical specialties, such as bariatrics, thoracic surgery, hepatobiliary surgery, and many other areas, and surgical pathologies involving the entire gastrointestinal tract. Over the past decade we have witnessed an upward trend whereby nearly 85% of graduating general surgery residents pursue fellowship training.[2] In addition, we are facing a shortage in the general surgical workforce, especially in rural areas where the existing population of general surgeons is aging.[3,4] During this timeframe it was observed that general surgeons performed less subspecialty procedures compared with general surgeons in the past. This is partially due to a lack of comfort with these procedures and to patients seeking more specialized care. Hence trainees are increasingly pursuing specialized fellowship training, leading to a redefinition of the role of the general surgeon but also creating a void in the field of general surgery, especially in rural areas.

Despite these trends it remains important for general surgeons in the community to be able to identify, diagnose, temporize, and treat general surgical emergencies. This is dependent on time sensitivity, proximity to a tertiary care center, complexity of the problem, critical care capabilities, and availability of subspecialty coverage at that hospital.

As in other areas of medicine, the management of surgical disease processes have undergone modifications and continues to change based on new emerging evidence;

Surg Clin N Am 103 (2023) xvii–xviii
https://doi.org/10.1016/j.suc.2023.07.010
0039-6109/23/© 2023 Published by Elsevier Inc.

surgical.theclinics.com

this can sometimes be difficult for general surgeons with a limited scope of practice to stay abreast of new guidelines and more current management strategies regardless of whether they are in an academic or community practice setting.

The purpose of this issue of *Surgical Clinics* is to discuss the most common and important surgical emergencies within different areas of general surgery and within other surgical subspecialties. It focuses on a variety of surgical disease processes that most general surgeons are likely to encounter in practice over the course of their careers. It is our goal that this will serve as a guide to manage these conditions either in their entirety, depending on one's level of comfort, or in part, whereby one is able to temporize the situation prior to transfer and most importantly to recognize at the outset which conditions are outside their scope and will benefit from early and expeditious transfer to a higher level of care to be managed by the appropriate experts in that field.

It has been a pleasure to identify, recruit, and work with this distinguished group of surgeons with expertise in their respective fields. This blend of early to mid-career surgeons and experienced surgeons with their unique perspectives allows the reader to appreciate how nuance and innovation help question established dogma, while being ushered through changes in this field.

A huge thank you to all the authors for their valuable time and contribution to this issue, which we are confident you will find stimulating and educational. This project would not have been possible without the support of the entire Elsevier publishing team and last but not least the vision and drive of Dr Ronald F. Martin, who continues to dedicate his efforts toward surgical education.

Viren Premnath Punja, MB, BS, FACS
Department of Surgery
Creighton University, School of Medicine
Omaha, NE 68124, USA

Paul J. Schenarts, MD, FACS, MAMSE
Department of Surgery
Creighton University, School of Medicine
Omaha, NE 68124, USA

E-mail addresses:
virenpremnath.punja@commonspirit.org (V.P. Punja)
PJSchenartsMD@gmail.com (P.J. Schenarts)

REFERENCES

1. Potts JR. General surgery residency: past, present, and future. Curr Probl Surg 2019;56(5):170–2. https://doi.org/10.1067/j.cpsurg.2019.01.006.
2. Quinn M, Burns B Jr, Taylor M. Early autonomy may contribute to an increase in the general surgical workforce. Curēus (Palo Alto, CA) 2020;12(2):e7108. https://doi.org/10.7759/cureus.7108.
3. Larson EH, Andrilla CHA, Kearney J, et al. The distribution of the general surgery workforce in rural and Urban America in 2019. March 2021. WWAMI RHRC. Available at: https://familymedicine.uw.edu/rhrc/publications/the-distribution-of-the-general-surgery-workforce-in-rural-and-urban-america-in-2019/. Accessed.
4. Shelton J, MacDowell M. The aging general surgeon of rural America. J Rural health 2021;37(4):762–8. https://doi.org/10.1111/jrh.12577.

Evaluation of Abdominal Emergencies

Zana Alattar, MD[a], Natasha Keric, MD[b],*

KEYWORDS

- Abdominal emergencies • Acute abdomen • Peritonitis • Shock
- Pneumoperitoneum

KEY POINTS

- Early recognition of an abdominal emergency can be crucial to preventing catastrophic outcomes.
- Formulating accurate differential diagnoses of abdominal pain relies strongly on a thorough history and physical examination, along with the clinical acumen of the physician.
- Diagnostic imaging and laboratory testing can be an excellent adjunct to the clinician's initial evaluation, in the appropriate patient.

 Video content accompanies this article at http://www.surgical.theclinics.com.

INTRODUCTION

Accounting for 8.4% of all emergency department visits in 2020, abdominal pain has consistently been one of the most common chief complaints of patients presenting to the emergency department in the United States. [6–8] The underlying cause of this presenting complaint can range from inconsequential pathologic condition to devastating causes (**Table 1**).[9] Deciphering between the differential diagnoses requires a thorough initial assessment to identify pertinent findings that can help delineate the abdominal emergencies—those that require immediate surgical intervention.

Abdominal pain is a universal chief complaint, which can present in differing patient populations such as pediatric, geriatric, pregnant, immunosuppressed, and healthy adults.[10–13] Patients can also present in a variety of clinical settings such as emergency, ambulatory, or inpatient, which broadens the differential diagnosis. Clinicians must rely on an astute and vast clinical acumen because they work up patients who present with abdominal pain.

---

[a] University of Arizona College of Medicine-Phoenix, 1441 North 12th Street, First Floor, Phoenix, AZ 85006, USA; [b] University of Arizona College of Medicine-Phoenix, Banner-University Medical Center Phoenix, 1441 North 12th Street, First Floor, Phoenix, AZ 85006, USA
* Corresponding author.
E-mail address: Natasha.Keric@bannerhealth.com

Surg Clin N Am 103 (2023) 1043–1059
https://doi.org/10.1016/j.suc.2023.05.010
0039-6109/23/© 2023 Elsevier Inc. All rights reserved.

surgical.theclinics.com

Table 1	
Risk factors for common surgical emergencies	
Common Abdominal Emergencies	**Corresponding Risk Factors**
Acute mesenteric ischemia	• Atrial fibrillation • Atherosclerotic disease • Earlier myocardial infarction • Earlier embolic event • Hypercoagulable disorder • Connective tissue disorder • Portal hypertension • Use of vasopressors
Perforated ulcer	• Nonsteroidal anti-inflammatory use • Tobacco use • *Helicobacter pylori* infection • Prolonged periods of fasting • Cocaine and methamphetamine use • Excessive alcohol consumption • Zollinger-Ellison syndrome • Corticosteroid use
Small bowel obstruction	• Earlier surgery • Crohn disease • Neoplasia • Hernia
Volvulus	• Chronic constipation • High-fiber diet • Frequent use of laxatives • Earlier laparotomy
Acute appendicitis	• Age 10–20 years • Male age

Although not comprehensive of all the possible abdominal emergencies, here, we list common diagnoses and their risk factors.[1,2,3–5]

HISTORY AND PHYSICAL EXAMINATION

The relevance of a pertinent history and physical examination in assessing the patient with abdominal pain cannot be overemphasized. A thorough workup leads to a focused diagnosis and expeditious treatment.

THE HISTORY OF PRESENT ILLNESS
Patient Demographics

Basic demographic information such as age and gender can help categorize patients' risk factors and remove certain differential diagnoses from the list of possibilities.

For example, in the pediatric population further delineating age can help provide more common causes of acute abdominal pain. In infants aged younger than 1 year, incarcerated inguinal hernia is a common underlying cause that warrants surgical intervention. Whereas in children aged older than 1 year, the most common surgical cause of acute abdominal pain is acute appendicitis.[14]

One must always pay close attention to the women of childbearing age. Although common surgical causes of acute abdominal pain such as appendicitis should be considered, gynecologic causes must also be factored in, especially those which also require emergent intervention such as ectopic pregnancy or ovarian torsion.[12,15,16]

Elderly patients present an even more challenging clinical picture. These patients often have many coexisting diseases that provide difficulties in management. Dire diagnoses such as ruptured abdominal aortic aneurysm and acute mesenteric ischemia become more common in this population. In addition, more common causes of surgical abdominal pain such as perforated viscus, bowel obstruction, or acute appendicitis become more consequential at their age.[17]

Patient Risk Factors

Similar to all patients, the assessment of patients presenting with abdominal pain requires a complete history including medical history and medications, surgical history, family history, and social history. This allows for a clear understanding of patients' risk factors, as well as their current anatomy and physiology. Do patients have underlying comorbidities that increase their risk for certain pathologic conditions? Although patients with a history of atrial fibrillation and atherosclerosis have an increased risk for mesenteric ischemia, the immunocompromised patients may have an increased risk for perforated viscus.[1,18] Knowledge of patients' prescribed medications and their compliance with these medications can also be crucial in understanding possible underlying pathologic condition. Just as the patient with daily Nonsteroidal Anti-Inflammatory Drug (NSAID) use is at higher risk for peptic ulcer disease, so is the chronic corticosteroid user, whose abdominal examination findings could seem benign and require a high clinical suspicion for accurate diagnosis.[2,18] Understanding the patient's surgical history is paramount to understanding of the patient's anatomy and possible diagnoses that may not have previously been considered. A patient with an earlier appendectomy likely does not have acute appendicitis, whereas a patient with a previous Roux-en-Y gastric bypass surgery might have an internal hernia that may not have been otherwise considered.[19]

Symptomatology

When evaluating a patient who presents with a complaint of abdominal pain, gaining a better understanding of the clinical symptoms is the foundation for narrowing the differential diagnosis. Questions that elucidate the time and acuity of onset, distribution, and character of the pain, exacerbating and relieving factors, and other associated symptoms such as history of earlier similar episodes are critical to focusing the next steps in the evaluation.[20]

In assessing patients who present with a neurologic stroke, we often hear family members being asked "when was their last known normal?" A question that, in neurology, receives response that tells clinicians whether patients meet the window for certain treatments. However, regarding abdominal pain, a similar question can also allow clinicians to establish the patient's symptoms chronologically and the progression from onset. Understanding what the patient was doing at the time of onset can often clarify certain diagnoses. Did something specific trigger the pain? Are there certain factors that make the pain better or worse? For example, while abdominal pain worsened with eating may allude to acute cholecystitis or mesenteric ischemia, pain relieved with eating may be concerning for a duodenal ulcer.[21–23] How did the pain change since its onset? Classically, generalized periumbilical pain that later localizes to the right lower quadrant, or more specifically the right iliac fossa, points to acute appendicitis.[24] These are all questions that, in the hands of a trained clinician, can sometimes be all that is needed to make a working diagnosis and begin targeted evaluation.

PHYSICAL EXAMINATION

As with all presenting complaints, the initial evaluation of a patient with abdominal pain should begin immediately with a primary assessment. Evaluating the patient's mental status, cardiopulmonary state, and performing a complete abdominal examination can often provide crucial information to identify rapidly life-threatening pathologic conditions.

Primary Assessment

The trained clinician should be able to identify quickly a patient who is in shock.

Shock is defined as a state of multisystem organ hypoperfusion. This can present as tachycardia, tachypnea, hypotension, diaphoresis, poorly perfused skin and extremities, altered mental status, and decreased urine output.[25] Almost all these findings can be identified by performing a primary assessment. In trauma, the primary assessment involves evaluation of the airway, breathing, and circulation. Similar principles apply to the emergency surgical patient: evaluation of the main organ systems and identification of organ failure or hypoperfusion. It is within the first few moments of evaluating the patient that the clinician should be able to assess their neurologic, cardiac, and respiratory systems. This can be done simply by visualizing the patient's demeanor, asking 1 to 2 basic questions, and assessing vital signs.

By evaluating whether the patient is conversational and protecting their airway, the physician can determine neurologic and respiratory status. The simple task of asking for the patient's name can often be enough to evaluate this. This is complemented by obtaining the patient's complete vital signs, which can demonstrate evidence of shock and indicate strain to the cardiac or respiratory systems. Simply inspecting the patient for a few moments to look for diaphoresis, pallor, skin turgor can be informative. Within seconds of entering the room, a skilled clinician can make their primary assessment of the patient and determine whether there is cause for concern.

The Abdominal Examination

A seasoned clinician can obtain several information from simply visualizing the abdomen. Earlier surgical scars on examination can help delineate the patient's earlier surgical history in situations where patients may be unsure of their own surgical history. Identifying masses that are concerning for a hernia or, in the thin patient, a possible abdominal aortic aneurysm can provide a quick diagnosis. Large volume distention of the abdomen can often be seen, before any percussion or palpation.

To elucidate the patient's subjective pain before performing an examination, it can be quite helpful to ask the patient themselves to point to the location of maximal pain. This knowledge can help guide the next part of the abdominal examination: palpation and percussion. Palpation should be initiated at the part of the abdomen furthest from the point of maximal tenderness and culminated with the area of maximal tenderness. It should be noted that gentle palpation is key to a successful examination because it provides patient's trust and avoids confounding the examination with rough palpation in areas that otherwise would have been nontender. Percussion of the abdomen can also be performed to estimate the amount of distention that is seen on visualization and to identify areas of dullness consistent with fluid comparatively to the areas of hyperresonance consistent with air.[20]

The complete abdominal examination: the groin and rectal examination

Inspection, palpation, and percussion of the abdomen alone are not sufficient for the complete abdominal examination. A thorough examination includes evaluation of the groin, as well as a complete digital rectal examination. Assessing the spaces in which an inguinal or femoral hernia would exist should be included in every clinician's assessment of the abdominal emergency. More so, a digital rectal examination should be performed to assess for frank blood, obvious masses, or stricture.[20,26,27]

Special consideration: abdominal examination in the setting of corticosteroids
Cope's Early Diagnosis of the Acute Abdomen summarizes the evaluation of patients who are on steroid therapy the best: "The attenuation of abdominal pain in patients being treated by corticosteroids makes it imperative to consider even slight abdominal pain as serious. Neglecting this warning may have serious results."[20]

Definitions: peritonitis and the acute abdomen
Although the terms peritonitis and the acute abdomen seem to be used interchangeably in the medical field, they are not the same. Peritonitis is defined as inflammation of the peritoneum, or the lining of the inner wall of the abdomen. It can be caused by irritation from intra-abdominal spillage of bile, urine, blood, or enteric contents. This definition also differs from the colloquially used phrase "the peritonitic abdomen," which is used to refer to the presence of abdominal rigidity. Abdominal rigidity is due to the contraction of the abdominal muscles, which may be a response to underlying generalized peritonitis. However, it is important to note that this true rigidity is less frequent in the presence of underlying peritonitis than is perceived, especially in patients whose muscle tone is weak or difficult to identify as in the elderly, frail, obese, or in patients in a state of shock. Therefore, the absence of the classic "board-like" abdomen does not exclude an underlying abdominal emergency. The term "acute abdomen," however, refers to the presentation of sudden onset of acute abdominal pain, which can be caused by peritonitis, as well as other gastrointestinal diagnoses, vascular events, obstetric and gynecologic causes, or urologic conditions.[20,27]

DIAGNOSTIC TESTING AND IMAGING

Although the initial history and physical examination can often provide enough information to separate the abdominal emergencies from the more benign causes of abdominal pain, adjunct testing can be helpful in cinching the diagnosis and useful in guiding operative planning.

Imaging Modalities

First discovered in late 1895, x-rays have been used in the medical field long before many other medical innovations.[28,29] Today, x-rays are quick and can provide rapid information for the concerned physician. The portable nature of x-rays makes it safe and easy to obtain them because the patient can remain in their room with continued resuscitation while the radiograph is being taken. Although an x-ray cannot completely rule out an abdominal emergency, evidence of extraluminal air on an upright chest radiograph or abdominal radiograph is a cause for concern.[30] X-rays can also identify gas patterns in the stomach and bowel, including dilated loops of small bowel, which can quickly allude to small bowel obstruction. Large bowel obstruction can also be seen on simple plain film, with dilation of the cecum being of most concern because distention more than 8 cm accounts for a high risk of perforation. A massive stomach seen with a large gastric bubble can quickly signify a possible gastric outlet obstruction.[31]

Definitions: pneumoperitoneum
Pneumoperitoneum is the presence of air or gas in the peritoneal cavity. The presence of pneumoperitoneum is most commonly a sign of perforated viscus from peptic ulcer disease, diverticulitis, trauma, malignancy, bowel ischemia, appendicitis, or complications from endoscopy.[32,33] It should be noted, however, that pneumoperitoneum may also be a sign of recent surgical intervention, after which it is expected that air may be seen in the abdominal cavity (**Fig. 1**).

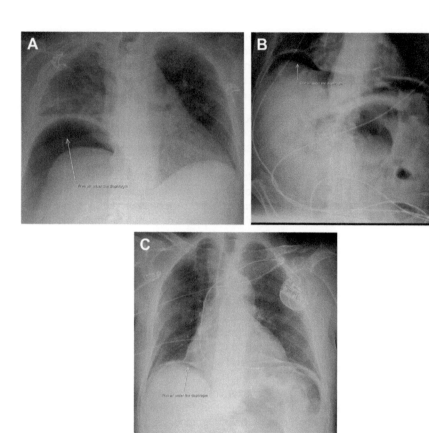

Fig. 1. Upright x-rays of the chest and diaphragm can easily identify free air under the diaphragm (*arrowhead*), pneumoperitoneum. As seen in these images, free air can be subtle or more obvious and it is crucial that care be taken to look for even the smallest signs of free air if there is concern for a possible underlying perforation. (*A*) Large amount of free air on chest x-ray. (*B*) Moderate amount of free air noted on abdominal x-ray. (*C*) Small amount of free air seen on chest x-ray.

Although x-ray made its debut in the nineteenth century, it was not until 1973 when the first whole body computerized tomography (CT) scan was introduced. Since then, advancements in CT technology have revolutionized how and when we can use this machine.[34] When used correctly, CT performed in the emergency department can help confirm diagnosis and lead to timelier surgical intervention. It can also reduce unnecessary hospital admissions and reduce unnecessary surgery in some patients. However, it must also be remembered that CT is an adjunct to the well-performed history and physical examinations. It can increase confidence in diagnoses that have already been delineated as a possibility by the experienced clinician.[35–38] Overutilization of CT scans can sometimes cause unnecessary delays in patient care and unnecessary cost for the patient in the health-care system.[39–41] Thus, the clinician should always consider the question, "how will this additional testing change my plan of care?"

One must also again review the differential diagnoses created based on the information already gathered to decide what type of CT imaging should be obtained, what type of contrast is needed, and what part of the body needs imaging. First, it should be stated that if obtaining a CT of the abdomen, the pelvis should almost always be included. Similar to the physical examination, where the groin and rectum are an important part of a complete abdominal examination, imaging of the pelvis is key to a complete diagnostic evaluation. The importance of intravenous contrast is also paramount. Often, CT imaging without contrast provides little beneficial information; although they are fast and involve minimal risk to the patient, they are difficult to interpret. Intravenous contrast is critical in delineating active pathologic condition such as inflammatory changes, neoplasms, abscesses, and infarcts. An additional angiography phase is helpful in diagnosing bowel ischemia, arterial thrombosis, and active arterial extravasation. There is no question that the CT with intravenous contrast is superior to that without contrast.[42] However, providers can sometimes hesitate in administering intravenous contrast due to concerns for nephrotoxicity. Patients who are thought to have risk of contrast-induced acute kidney injury and are not evaluated with a CT with intravenous contrast can be subject to delayed or missed diagnosis because of this misconception. This should not be the case. In a 2020 consensus statement made by the American College of Radiology and the National Kidney Foundation, it was stated, "The risk of acute kidney injury (AKI) developing in patients with reduced kidney function following exposure to intravenous iodinated contrast media has been overstated." Patients who are coming in with an acute abdominal emergency can often have signs of multisystem organ failure, as discussed, which can include acute kidney injury. This is not a contraindication to intravenous iodinated contrast. Moreover, even in the patients with chronic kidney disease (CKD), it is only in the patients with CKD stage 4 or 5 (glomerular filtration rate <30 mL/min/1.73 m^2) who are not undergoing maintenance hemodialysis who are at potential risk of contrast-induced nephropathy. In these patients, administration of intravenous iodinated contrast is relatively contraindicated but should not be withheld if contrast administration is required for a life-threatening diagnosis.[42–46] Obtaining imaging of the pelvis in addition to the abdomen, as well as administering intravenous iodinated contrast are quick modifications to the CT that provide invaluable information and assistance with confirming the diagnosis in an abdominal emergency. They are descriptors to the CT order that should be cause for little hesitation. However, the clinician can also consider the adjuncts of oral and rectal contrast in certain situations. These adjuncts should not be used routinely but may be useful in differentiating small bowel loops from abdominal and pelvic masses or abscesses and can be helpful in identifying the location of perforations in the small or large bowel. These studies can take time. Patients may not tolerate consumption of sufficient quantities of oral contrast. Ultimately, intraluminal contrast may not change the plan of care.[42]

In addition to identifying the correct imaging type to order, the clinician evaluating the abdominal emergency must also review the images obtained. Time is of the essence; therefore, having a systematic method to evaluate the images every time is critical. Images should be looked at in the axial, sagittal, and coronal planes as well as abdominal and lung windows, and finally in different arterial and venous phases. Each image plane, window, and protocol can provide information in a unique way than the other views. Free air can be best seen in the lung view (**Fig. 2**, Video 1).[47] An arterial embolus needs to be seen on the arterial phase, and a superior mesenteric artery occlusion can often most easily be seen on a sagittal view (Video 2).[48] Coronal views can allow for a better visualization of the foregut.[49] Even the scout image on the CT can provide valuable information; they may be a quick method to identify foreign bodies or see free air before even delving into the full CT images.[50] Finally, additional annotations such as the Hounsfield units (HU) can provide further information on the density of fluid in the abdomen and differentiating blood from simple fluid. Acute blood

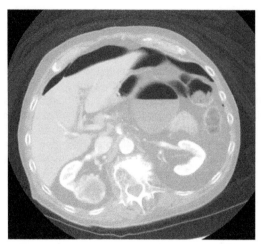

Fig. 2. Abdominal CT scan showing intra-abdominal free air between the liver and anterior abdominal wall with accentuation of the falciform ligament.

measures about 30 to 40 HU while clotted blood is between 40 and 70 HU with areas of high attenuation (the clot) being surrounded by areas of lower attenuation (serum).[51]

Clinical pearl

CT imaging is an invaluable tool when correctly used. Here are some big takeaways on the use of CT imaging when addressing abdominal emergencies.

1. Obtain imaging of the abdomen and pelvis. The additional few seconds it takes to scan the pelvis can be critical in diagnosis.

2. Do not be afraid to give intravenous contrast. CT imaging without contrast is often unhelpful and the benefit of useful imaging outweighs the risk of damage to the kidneys.

3. Review your own images as soon as they are available. Do not wait for the official interpretation before you look at your images, and do not hesitate to give the radiologist a call to discuss your concerns.

4. Make sure to look at all of the views available to you. Often, certain pathologic condition is seen better on the sagittal or coronal views, than the more commonly reviewed axial images. Lung windows and different phases can also provide excellent adjunct information.

Another quick, readily available imaging modality is the ultrasound. In the hands of a clinician with ultrasound experience, an ultrasound can help quickly identify the presence of free fluid in the abdomen, which can be useful in supporting certain differential diagnoses. In the trauma setting, it is reliably used to perform the focused assessment with sonography in trauma. In nontraumatic causes of abdominal pain, ultrasound can be especially helpful in children, in women of childbearing age, and in diagnosis of acute biliary disease in adults. Acute appendicitis and pyloric stenosis are the most frequent differential diagnoses in children that are commonly evaluated and identified on ultrasonography.[52-54]

Laboratory Findings

The fundamentals are critical to the evaluation of abdominal pain. Moreover, when it comes to the fundamentals of laboratory testing, a complete blood count (CBC) and a complete metabolic panel (CMP) are at the core. The CBC will provide information on the white blood cell count, hemoglobin, and platelet count, which are useful to both delineate possible infection and provide information on the patient's hematologic status. In considering the coagulation pathway and its possible derangements that may be contributing to pathologic condition, it is also useful to obtain an international normalized ratio (INR), prothrombin time, and partial thromboplastin time. These can also be helpful in the anticoagulated patient to determine their current coagulation physiology. In addition, while obtaining these coagulation studies, it is helpful to obtain enough blood samples for a type and screen, to allow the initiation of blood products being placed on hold for the patient in case of surgical intervention or bleeding, especially in the setting of coagulopathy. The CMP then looks at the patient's chemistry and can also be supplemented with additional chemistry testing, such as magnesium and phosphate levels.

Evidence of hypoperfusion and end organ damage can be clear when reviewing some of these laboratory results. Dysfunction of the coagulation pathway might present with elevated INR or platelet count less than 80,000 or half of what it was 24 hours earlier. Hyperbilirubinemia can be present with gastrointestinal dysfunction. Elevated creatinine is a marker of kidney injury. However, one laboratory test that is commonly relied on to evaluate for hypoperfusion is the lactic acid levels. Why are lactate levels so important? Because they can indicate a low oxygen state. In the absence of oxygen, cells cannot initiate the Krebs cycle to convert pyruvate into large amounts of energy, and instead, pyruvate is preferentially transformed into lactate. Moreover, lactate is metabolized by the liver (50%), the kidneys (20%), and by the skeletal muscle, heart, and brain. In times of physiologic stress, in addition to the over production of lactate, there is also reduced clearance by these organs, especially in extreme conditions of pH.[55] Increased plasma lactate concentration is therefore found in times of shock, sepsis, hepatic, and renal failure.[56]

DIFFERENTIAL DIAGNOSES
Acute Appendicitis

Acute appendicitis is the most common abdominal surgical emergency in the world. It can be seen in people of any age but is most common in pediatric patients and young adults aged between 10 and 30 years. There is a male predominance in prevalence of the disease.[57,58] The diagnosis of acute appendicitis is largely clinical. The pain associated with the diagnosis is often described as a colicky central, or periumbilical, abdominal pain, which migrates to the right iliac fossa. Loss of appetite is commonly seen, as well as nausea and constipation, and sometimes vomiting. Low-grade fever is often present. Pain may worsen with coughing and moving, which may indicate peritoneal involvement. A question that can often be asked is whether pain was worsened when driving over speed bumps and being suddenly jostled. There are also atypical presentations in patients with retrocecal appendices or those who are pregnant because they may present with right flank or costovertebral angle pain, or sometimes right testicular pain. Urinary frequency can also be seen in atypical presentations.[5,24,58–60] In addition to these patient demographics and patient symptomatology, the physical examination can be extremely revealing for the diagnosis of abdominal pain. Patients will often have tenderness in the right lower quadrant of the abdomen, a third of the distance along the line between the anterior superior iliac spine and the umbilicus, an anatomic landmark known as McBurney point. There are also several signs that can demonstrate inflammation of the peritoneum secondary to appendicitis. These include Psoas sign, Obturator sign, Rovsing sign, and Dunphy's sign, described in **Table 2**. Laboratory findings will demonstrate elevated white blood cell count with a neutrophil predominance, and in the case of greater than 12 hours of symptoms, an elevated c-reactive protein can be seen. In addition, a urinalysis will be abnormal in about a quarter of patients with appendicitis. Although x-ray does not provide much diagnostic value for acute appendicitis, ultrasound can be useful in children. CT with intravenous contrast is the leading imaging modality for the diagnosis of acute appendicitis in adult patients. CT imaging commonly demonstrates a dilated appendix with periappendiceal fat stranding and a possible appendicolith (Video 3). Other common changes include wall thickening and mural hyperenhancement. In pediatric patients for whom ultrasound is inconclusive or some pregnant patients, MRI can also be used for diagnosis. However, it should be stated that although MRI is accurate in the diagnosis of appendicitis, it can often be timely and cause delays, and therefore, CT remains a useful imaging modality in pregnant patients.[58–68]

SMALL BOWEL OBSTRUCTION

Small bowel obstruction remains a leading cause of emergency surgical admissions. Although not always requiring operative intervention, the diagnosis of small bowel obstruction is best managed by a surgical team. As always, patient risk factors are critical to identifying the patient at risk for small bowel obstruction. The leading causes of small bowel obstruction are adhesions from earlier surgical intervention, intraabdominal neoplasms, hernias (both internal and abdominal wall), and inflammatory bowel disease, such as Crohn disease. Classic symptoms include colicky abdominal pain, nausea and emesis, abdominal distention, and constipation. These symptoms can range in severity depending on the severity of the obstruction itself. For example, emesis may be bilious, nonbilious, or feculent. Feculent vomiting may be suggestive of a high-grade small bowel obstruction. In these patients, abdominal distention is often visualized on physical examination. In addition, inspection of the abdomen is critical to identifying earlier surgical scars and presence of ventral, inguinal, or femoral hernias. The location of tenderness on examination is variable. However, diagnostic imaging is often revealing of distended small bowel to a point, past which bowel is decompressed, known as the transition point. It should be noted that oral contrast, specifically water-soluble gastrografin, can be useful for the patient with small bowel obstruction, as both a diagnostic and therapeutic intervention. This should be used only in the patients with early small bowel obstruction or those without signs of clinical deterioration. Laboratory abnormalities are nonspecific for an obstruction alone. However, they may be helpful in detecting the feared complications of small bowel obstructions: bowel ischemia or bowel perforation. These complications can be seen with complete mechanical bowel obstruction or in closed loop obstruction, where a bowel segment is occluded at 2 points. In complete bowel obstruction, patients are

Table 2	
Signs of acute appendicitis[61–64]	
Psoas sign	Pain on passive extension of the right thigh while the patient is lying in the left lateral decubitus position
Obturator sign	Pain on passive internal rotation of the flexed thigh while the patient is in supine position
Rovsing sign	Pain in the right iliac fossa elicited by deep palpation on the left iliac fossa
Dunphy's sign	Pain elicited by asking the patient to cough before palpation

unable to pass flatus and often have severe vomiting, with air fluid levels seen on imaging; this is due to the complete inability of air and fluid to pass through. Closed loop obstruction often presents with pain out of proportion to examination, as seen with mesenteric ischemia, due to compromise of blood flow in a closed loop. The development of subsequent ischemia or perforation may be suggested by high fevers, systemic toxicity, or laboratory findings consistent with intra-abdominal sepsis or multiorgan failure.[4,69–75]

PERFORATED VISCUS

Perforation of the gastrointestinal tract includes perforation of the stomach, small bowel, or large bowel. Regardless of location, alimentary tract perforations represent a life-threatening abdominal emergency. Patient's symptomatology differs based on the underlying site of perforation but often includes acute pain, nausea, vomiting, and fevers.[76]

Perforated peptic ulcer, whether gastric or duodenal, is the most common perforated viscus and is classically noted to have sudden onset abdominal pain, tachycardia, and abdominal rigidity. Risk factors for peptic ulcer disease include chronic nonsteroidal anti-inflammatories or corticosteroids, H pylori, smoking, excessive alcohol consumption, and Zollinger-Ellison syndrome. An upright chest or abdominal x-ray will often reveal free air under the diaphragm.[77] In patients who can tolerate it, CT can provide more information on location of perforation and guide surgical intervention. CT can also be useful in the patient for whom perforated viscus is suspected but extraluminal air is not seen on radiograph.[78]

Perforation of the small bowel is relatively rare but can be seen secondary to closed loop small bowel obstruction, ischemia, tumors such as small bowel lymphoma, foreign bodies, Crohn disease, or Meckel diverticulum. There are also some infectious causes such as typhoid fever, human immunodeficiency virus, and tuberculosis. With small bowel perforation, the volume of free air is usually small and often will not be seen on radiograph. Even on CT imaging, findings can be subtle and may only include localized interloop collections of extraluminal gas and/or fluid. In some cases, small bowel wall thickening and mesenteric fat stranding may be the only findings seen and can be critical in patients for whom clinical suspicion for small bowel perforation is high.[79,80]

Large bowel perforation can be seen secondary to colorectal cancer or colonic diverticulitis.[81] Similar to perforations of the stomach or small bowel, perforations of the large intestine also present with complaints of abdominal pain, nausea, and vomiting. They will also have evidence of free air on upright x-ray and/or CT imaging. It is in these patients that one might consider pursuing a CT with rectal contrast, if the patient can tolerate it and is clinically stable to allow for the time necessary to conduct the CT.[82] However, these patients are more likely to present in septic shock and are often emergently taken to the operating room, leaving less time for additional diagnostic testing.[83,84]

MESENTERIC ISCHEMIA

Acute mesenteric ischemia is a potentially fatal, vascular intra-abdominal emergency, caused by an arterial embolism, arterial thrombus, nonocclusive disease, or venous thrombus. Typically, patients with arterial embolus or thrombus present with acute onset of severe abdominal pain with associated diarrhea, which may be bloody. Classically, these patients display pain out of proportion to their physical exam. Patients with nonocclusive mesenteric ischemia are typically critically ill and in a "low-flow" state. In these patients, as well as those with mesenteric vein thrombosis, symptoms typically present slowly. Patients with mesenteric vein thrombosis often have associated diarrhea and anorexia because they often have postprandial pain that results in "food fear." Regardless of cause, mesenteric ischemia can be rapidly fatal, and a high index of suspicion is necessary in diagnosis. The diagnosis should be carefully considered in patients aged older than 60 years, those with history of atrial fibrillation, myocardial infarction, congestive heart failure, or arterial emboli. Laboratory findings often demonstrate hemoconcentration, leukocytosis, metabolic acidosis with anion gap, and an elevated lactic acid. CT angiography is critical in identifying occlusion of the mesenteric vessels, especially with associated findings of thickened bowel wall, intramural hematoma, dilated fluid-filled bowel loops, pneumatosis, or mesenteric or portal venous gas (Video 4).[85–89]

VOLVULUS

Volvulus can be seen in the sigmoid colon, cecum, splenic flexure, and transverse colon. Volvulus occurs when bowel and its mesentery twist on a fixed point at the base and can result in a closed loop obstruction, which compromises the blood supply to the colon. Sigmoid volvulus is the most common colonic volvulus and typically presents with several days of abdominal pain with bloating, constipation, and sometimes inability to pass flatus.[90,91] Second in frequency to sigmoid volvulus is cecal volvulus. Regardless of location, concern for volvulus is due to its progression because it can lead to ischemia, gangrene, and perforation. Thus, it is essential to rapidly diagnose and treat these patients. Radiologic examination is key to diagnosis because CT imaging can demonstrate dilation of the affected portion of the colon with a single air fluid level and distal decompression, often with swirling of the mesentery.[92,93]

DISCUSSION

The patient with abdominal pain is a unique clinical quandary because it requires a thorough evaluation to delineate the abdominal emergencies from the less ominous causes of abdominal pain. The evaluation of these patients involves multiple approaches, at the core of which is a strong history and physical examination. In conjunction with these principles, adjunct blood testing and diagnostic imaging can provide critical information to decipher between differential diagnoses put together by the clinician. It is also important to remember that the evaluation of an abdominal emergency sometimes needs to occur simultaneously with the initial management and resuscitation. For example, the principles of resuscitation involve intravenous access, and this should be done while obtaining blood samples for laboratory testing. While considering intra-abdominal sepsis as the cause for a patient in shock, it should be remembered to obtain blood cultures and then immediately initiate antibiotics. If initial x-ray imaging demonstrates distended bowel gas patterns, especially with a large gastric bubble, concerning for small bowel obstruction, a nasogastric tube can be placed for decompression. This, of course, relies on multiple members of the medical team caring for the patient simultaneously, all providing critical aspects of the patient's care.

SUMMARY

Early primary assessment and abdominal examination can often be enough to triage the patient with abdominal pain into those with less severe underlying pathology from those with more acute findings. A focused history of the patient can then allow the clinician to develop their differential diagnosis. Once the differential diagnoses are determined, diagnostic imaging and laboratory findings can help confirm the diagnosis and allow for expeditious treatment and intervention.

CLINICS CARE POINTS

- Evaluation of the patient with abdominal pain requires astute clinical accumen.
- Patients with hemodynamic instability may require immediate surgical intervention.
- Radiologic studies such as ultrasound, x-ray, and computed tomography can be helpful in determining the underlying cause of an acute abdomen and planning surgical intervention.

DISCLOSURE

The authors have nothing to disclose.

SUPPLEMENTARY DATA

Supplementary data related to this article can be found online at https://doi.org/10.1016/j.suc.2023.05.010.

REFERENCES

1. Stone JR, Wilkins LR. Acute mesenteric ischemia. Tech Vasc Interv Radiol 2015; 18(1):24–30.
2. Søreide K, Thorsen K, Harrison EM, et al. Perforated peptic ulcer. Lancet 2015; 386(10000):1288–98.
3. Perrot L, Fohlen A, Alves A, et al. Management of the colonic volvulus in 2016. Journal of Visceral Surgery 2016;153(3):183–92.
4. Miller G, Boman J, Shrier I, et al. Etiology of small bowel obstruction. Am J Surg 2000;180(1):33–6.
5. Humes DJ, Simpson J. Acute appendicitis. BMJ 2006;333(7567):530–4.
6. Cairns C. and Kang K. National Hospital Ambulatory Medical Care Survey: 2020 Emergency Department Summary Tables. 2022, 121911, https://doi.org/10.15620/cdc.
7. Hooker EA, Mallow PJ, Oglesby MM. Characteristics and trends of emergency department visits in the United States (2010–2014). J Emerg Med 2019;56(3): 344–51.
8. Graff LG, Robinson D. Abdominal pain and emergency department evaluation. Emerg Med Clin 2001;19(1):123–36.
9. Brewer RJ, Golden GT, Hitch DC, et al. Abdominal pain. Am J Surg 1976;131(2): 219–23.
10. Tseng Y-C, Lee M-S, Chang Y-J, et al. Acute abdomen in pediatric patients admitted to the Pediatric Emergency Department. Pediatrics & Neonatology 2008;49(4):126–34.
11. Martinez JP, Mattu A. Abdominal pain in the elderly. Emerg Med Clin 2006;24(2): 371–88.
12. Augustin G, Majerovic M. Non-obstetrical acute abdomen during pregnancy. Eur J Obstet Gynecol Reprod Biol 2007;131(1):4–12.
13. McKean J, Ronan-Bentle S. Abdominal pain in the immunocompromised patient—human immunodeficiency virus, transplant, cancer. Emerg Med Clin 2016;34(2):377–86.

14. Hijaz N, Friesen C. Managing acute abdominal pain in pediatric patients: current perspectives. Pediatr Health Med Therapeut 2017;ume 8:83–91.

15. Jearwattanakanok K, Yamada S, Suntornlimsiri W, et al. Clinical indicators for differential diagnosis of acute lower abdominal pain in women of reproductive age. Journal of Current Surgery 2013. https://doi.org/10.4021/jcs179w.

16. McWilliams GDE, Hill MJ, Dietrich CS. Gynecologic emergencies. Surg Clin 2008; 88(2):265–83.

17. Hendrickson M, Naparst TR. Abdominal surgical emergencies in the elderly. Emerg Med Clin 2003;21(4):937–69.

18. Spencer SP, Power N. The acute abdomen in the immune compromised host. Cancer Imag 2008;8(1):93–101.

19. Higa KD, Ho T, Boone KB. Internal hernias after laparoscopic roux-en-Y gastric bypass: Incidence, treatment and prevention. Obes Surg 2003;13(3):350–4.

20. Cope Z, Silen W. Cope's early diagnosis of the acute abdomen. 22nd ed. Oxford, NY: Oxford Univ. Press; 2010.

21. Gallaher JR, Charles A. Acute cholecystitis. JAMA 2022;327(10):965.

22. Sreenarasimhaiah J. Chronic mesenteric ischemia. Best Pract Res Clin Gastroenterol 2005;19(2):283–95.

23. Malfertheiner P, Chan FKL, McColl KEL. Peptic ulcer disease. Lancet 2009; 374(9699):1449–61.

24. Stringer MD. Acute appendicitis. J Paediatr Child Health 2017;53(11):1071–6.

25. Hall J.B., Schmidt G.A. and Kress J.P., Chapter 113: Shock, In: Hall J.B., Schmidt G.A., Kress J.P., *Principles of critical care*, 2015, McGraw-Hill Education; New York.

26. Macaluso C, McNamara R. Evaluation and management of acute abdominal pain in the emergency department. Int J Gen Med 2012;5:789–97.

27. Langell JT, Mulvihill SJ. Gastrointestinal perforation and the acute abdomen. Med Clin 2008;92(3):599–625.

28. Hessenbruch A. A brief history of X-rays. Endeavour 2002;26(4):137–41.

29. Toledo-Pereyra LH. X-rays surgical revolution. J Invest Surg 2009;22(5):327–32.

30. Pinto A, Miele V, Laura Schillirò M, et al. Spectrum of signs of pneumoperitoneum. Seminars Ultrasound, CT MRI 2016;37(1):3–9.

31. Sureka B, Bansal K, Arora A. Pneumoperitoneum: What to look for in a radiograph? J Fam Med Prim Care 2015;4(3):477.

32. Kumar A, Muir MT, Cohn SM, et al. The etiology of pneumoperitoneum in the 21st Century. J Trauma Acute Care Surg 2012;73(3):542–8.

33. Sittig DF, Ash JS, Ledley RS. The story behind the development of the first whole-body computerized tomography scanner as told by Robert S. Ledley. J Am Med Inform Assoc 2006;13(5):465–9.

34. Rosen MP, Sands DZ, Longmaid HE, et al. Impact of abdominal CT on the management of patients presenting to the emergency department with acute abdominal pain. Am J Roentgenol 2000;174(5):1391–6.

35. Rosen MP, Siewert B, Sands DZ, et al. Value of abdominal CT in the emergency department for patients with abdominal pain. Eur Radiol 2003;13(2):418–24.

36. Kocher KE, Meurer WJ, Fazel R, et al. National trends in use of computed tomography in the emergency department. Ann Emerg Med 2011;58(5). https://doi.org/10.1016/j.annemergmed.2011.05.020.

37. Stoker J, van Randen A, Laméris W, et al. Imaging patients with acute abdominal pain. Radiology 2009;253(1):31–46.

38. Kanzaria HK, Hoffman JR, Probst MA, et al. Emergency physician perceptions of medically unnecessary advanced diagnostic imaging. Acad Emerg Med 2015; 22(4):390–8.
39. Tung M, Sharma R, Hinson JS, et al. Factors associated with imaging overuse in the emergency department: A systematic review. Am J Emerg Med 2018;36(2): 301–9.
40. Raja AS, Mortele KJ, Hanson R, et al. Abdominal imaging utilization in the Emergency Department: Trends over two decades. Int J Emerg Med 2011;4(1). https://doi.org/10.1186/1865-1380-4-19.
41. Gore RM, Miller FH, Pereles FS, et al. Helical CT in the evaluation of the acute abdomen. Am J Roentgenol 2000;174(4):901–13.
42. Davenport MS, Perazella MA, Yee J, et al. Use of intravenous iodinated contrast media in patients with kidney disease: Consensus statements from the American College of Radiology and the National Kidney Foundation. Radiology 2020; 294(3):660–8.
43. McDonald JS, McDonald RJ, Lieske JC, et al. Risk of acute kidney injury, dialysis, and mortality in patients with chronic kidney disease after intravenous contrast material exposure. Mayo Clin Proc 2015;90(8):1046–53.
44. McDonald JS, McDonald RJ, Comin J, et al. Frequency of acute kidney injury following intravenous contrast medium administration: A systematic review and meta-analysis. Radiology 2013;267(1):119–28.
45. McDonald RJ, McDonald JS, Bida JP, et al. Intravenous contrast material–induced nephropathy: Causal or coincident phenomenon? Radiology 2013; 267(1):106–18.
46. McDonald JS, McDonald RJ, Carter RE, et al. Risk of intravenous contrast material–mediated acute kidney injury: A propensity score–matched study stratified by baseline-estimated glomerular filtration rate. Radiology 2014;271(1): 65–73.
47. Reich H, Chou D, Melo N. Chapters 6-20: Perforated hollow viscus. In: Butler KL, Harisinghani M, editors. Acute care surgery: imaging essentials for rapid diagnosis. McGraw Hill; 2015.
48. Stangenberg L, Wyers M. Mesenteric ischemia. In: Butler KL, Harisinghani M, editors. Acute care surgery: imaging essentials for rapid diagnosis. McGraw Hill; 2015.
49. Sandrasegaran K, Rydberg J, Tann M, et al. Benefits of routine use of coronal and sagittal reformations in multi-slice CT examination of the abdomen and pelvis. Clin Radiol 2007;62(4):340–7.
50. Lee MH, Lubner MG, Mellnick VM, et al. The CT scout view: complementary value added to abdominal CT interpretation. Abdominal Radiology 2021;46(10): 5021–36.
51. Lucey BC, Varghese JC, Anderson SW, et al. Spontaneous hemoperitoneum: a bloody mess. Emerg Radiol 2007;14(2):65–75.
52. Chapter 8: Surgeon-performed ultrasound in acute care surgery. In: Feliciano DV, Mattox KL, Moore EE, editors. Trauma, 9e. McGraw Hill; 2020.
53. Toorenvliet BR, Wiersma F, Bakker RF, et al. Routine ultrasound and limited computed tomography for the diagnosis of acute appendicitis. World J Surg 2010;34(10):2278–85.
54. van Randen A, Laméris W, van Es HW, et al. A comparison of the accuracy of ultrasound and computed tomography in common diagnoses causing acute abdominal pain. Eur Radiol 2011;21(7):1535–45.
55. De Backer D. Lactic acidosis. Intensive Care Med 2003;29(5):699–702.

56. Verma I, Kaur S, Goyal S, et al. Diagnostic value of lactate levels in acute abdomen disorders. Indian J Clin Biochem 2013;29(3):382–5.

57. Baird DL, Simillis C, Kontovounisios C, et al. Acute appendicitis. BMJ 2017. https://doi.org/10.1136/bmj.j1703.

58. Petroianu A. Diagnosis of acute appendicitis. Int J Surg 2012;10(3):115–9.

59. Sellars H, Boorman P. Acute appendicitis. Surgery 2017;35(8):432–8.

60. Colvin JM, Bachur R, Kharbanda A. The presentation of appendicitis in preadolescent children. Pediatr Emerg Care 2007;23(12):849–55.

61. Bhangu A, Søreide K, Di Saverio S, et al. Acute appendicitis: modern understanding of pathogenesis, diagnosis, and Management. Lancet 2015; 386(10000):1278–87.

62. Yang H-R, Wang Y-C, Chung P-K, et al. Laboratory tests in patients with acute appendicitis. ANZ J Surg 2006;76(1–2):71–4.

63. Moris D, Paulson EK, Pappas TN. Diagnosis and management of acute appendicitis in adults. JAMA 2021;326(22):2299.

64. Chandrasekaran TV, Johnson N. Acute appendicitis. Surgery 2014;32(8):413–7.

65. Brown MA. Imaging acute appendicitis. Seminars Ultrasound, CT MRI 2008; 29(5):293–307.

66. Debnath J, George RA, Ravikumar R. Imaging in acute appendicitis: what, when, and why? Med J Armed Forces India 2017;73(1):74–9.

67. Burke LMB, Bashir MR, Miller FH, et al. Magnetic resonance imaging of acute appendicitis in pregnancy: a 5-year Multiinstitutional study. Am J Obstet Gynecol 2015;213(5). https://doi.org/10.1016/j.ajog.2015.07.026.

68. Castro MA, Shipp TD, Castro EE, et al. The use of helical computed tomography in pregnancy for the diagnosis of acute appendicitis. Am J Obstet Gynecol 2001; 184(5):954–7.

69. Aquina CT, Becerra AZ, Probst CP, et al. Patients with adhesive small bowel obstruction should be primarily managed by a surgical team. Ann Surg 2016; 264(3):437–47.

70. Rami Reddy SR, Cappell MS. A systematic review of the clinical presentation, diagnosis, and treatment of small bowel obstruction. Curr Gastroenterol Rep 2017;19(6). https://doi.org/10.1007/s11894-017-0566-9.

71. Maung AA, Johnson DC, Piper GL, et al. Evaluation and management of small-bowel obstruction. J Trauma Acute Care Surg 2012;73(5). https://doi.org/10.1097/ta.0b013e31827019de.

72. Cappell MS, Batke M. Mechanical obstruction of the small bowel and colon. Med Clin 2008;92(3):575–97.

73. Paulson EK, Thompson WM. Review of small-bowel obstruction: the diagnosis and when to worry. Radiology 2015;275(2):332–42.

74. Balthazar EJ, Birnbaum BA, Megibow AJ, et al. Closed-loop and strangulating intestinal obstruction: CT signs. Radiology 1992;185(3):769–75.

75. Silva AC, Pimenta M, Guimaraes LS. Small bowel obstruction: what to look for. Radiographics 2009;29(2):423–39.

76. Romano L, Pinto A, editors. Imaging of alimentary tract perforation. Switzerland: Springer International Pu; 2016.

77. Chung KT, Shelat VG. Perforated peptic ulcer - an update. World J Gastrointest Surg 2017;9(1):1.

78. Furukawa A, Sakoda M, Yamasaki M, et al. Gastrointestinal tract perforation: CT diagnosis of presence, site, and cause. Abdom Imaging 2005;30(5):524–34.

79. Hines J, Rosenblat J, Duncan DR, et al. Perforation of the mesenteric small bowel: etiologies and CT findings. Emerg Radiol 2012;20(2):155–61.

80. Lo Re G, Mantia FL, Picone D, et al. Small bowel perforations: what the radiologist needs to know. Seminars Ultrasound, CT MRI 2016;37(1):23–30.
81. Bielecki K, Kamiński P, Klukowski M. Large bowel perforation: morbidity and mortality. Tech Coloproctol 2002;6(3):177–82.
82. Singh JP, Steward MJ, Booth TC, et al. Evolution of imaging for abdominal perforation. Ann R Coll Surg Engl 2010;92(3):182–8.
83. Biondo S, Parés D, Ragué Juan M, et al. Emergency operations for nondiverticular perforation of the left colon. Am J Surg 2002;183(3):256–60.
84. Marshall JC, Maier RV, Jimenez M, et al. Source control in the management of severe sepsis and septic shock: An evidence-based review. Crit Care Med 2004; 32(Supplement).
85. Oldenburg WA, Lau LL, Rodenberg TJ, et al. Acute mesenteric ischemia. Arch Intern Med 2004;164(10):1054.
86. Chang RW. Update in management of mesenteric ischemia. World J Gastroenterol 2006;12(20):3243.
87. Berland T, Oldenburg WA. Acute mesenteric ischemia. Curr Gastroenterol Rep 2008;10(3):341–6.
88. Wyers MC. Acute mesenteric ischemia: diagnostic approach and surgical treatment. Semin Vasc Surg 2010;23(1):9–20.
89. Reginelli A, Iacobellis F, Berritto D, et al. Mesenteric ischemia: the importance of differential diagnosis for the surgeon. BMC Surg 2013;13(Suppl 2). https://doi.org/10.1186/1471-2482-13-s2-s51.
90. Baiu I, Shelton A. Sigmoid volvulus. JAMA 2019;321(24):2478.
91. Rakinic J. Colonic Volvulus. In: Beck DE, Roberts PL, Saclarides TJ, et al, editors. The ASCRS Textbook of Colon and Rectal Surgery. New York, NY: Springer; 2011.
92. Madiba TE, Thomson SR, Church JM. The management of cecal volvulus. Dis Colon Rectum 2002;45(2):264–7.
93. Berger JA, van Leersum M, Plaisier PW. Cecal volvulus: case report and overview of the literature. Eur J Radiol Extra 2005;55(3):101–3.

Resuscitation and Preparation of the Emergency General Surgery Patient

Brett Harden Waibel, MD*, Andrew James Kamien, MD

KEYWORDS

- Emergency general surgery • Resuscitation • Sepsis • Patient preparation
- Perioperative management

KEY POINTS

- The emergency general surgery patient, due to the time-dependent nature of the emergency, may require an altered workflow usually seen in traditional elective surgery patients.
- The initial resuscitation and interventions depend largely on the nature of the emergency (bleeding vs sepsis).
- Understanding common medical comorbidities and their effects on an emergency general surgery patient is often necessary in their treatment.

INTRODUCTION

Traditionally, the workflow surrounding a general surgery patient allows for a period of evaluation and optimization of underlying medical issues to allow for risk modification; however, in the emergency, this optimization period is largely truncated due to its time dependent nature. As the lack of optimization can lead to complications, it behooves the surgeon to be able to identify the emergent patient who cannot undergo a traditional workflow with comorbidity optimization. The extent of medical intervention preceding procedural intervention largely depends on the urgency of the matter, which itself is often based on the physiology of the patient. Additionally, the emergency general surgery patient's medical comorbidities are often poorly controlled due to the stress of the surgical emergency, further causing derangements in the patient's underlying physiology.

Division of Acute Care Surgery, Department of Surgery, University of Nebraska Medical Center, 983280 Nebraska Medical Center, Omaha, NE 68198-3280, USA
* Corresponding author.
E-mail address: brett.waibel@unmc.edu

Surg Clin N Am 103 (2023) 1061–1084
https://doi.org/10.1016/j.suc.2023.05.011
0039-6109/23/© 2023 Elsevier Inc. All rights reserved.

INITIAL EVALUATION

As with any other patient, the initial history and physical examination are key to developing a treatment strategy in the emergency general surgery patient. Following a strategy similar to that in a trauma patient (another time-dependent surgical process), in a patient *in extremis*, this initial evaluation may need to be truncated with a focus on stabilization of the patient's physiology.

The *initial* history in these patients may be best directed via an AMPLE history. [1] In a time-dependent situation, a focused history can allow for quicker initiation of interventions. The areas of focus are allergies, medications, past medical history (medical and surgical), last mealtime, and event(s) leading to presentation. Medications of importance include those of high risk such as insulin, anticoagulants, and cardiovascular medications. Past medical history can both identify potential intraoperative issues (such as multiple prior abdominal surgeries) or perioperative complications (such as pulmonary issues in patients with severe chronic obstructive pulmonary disease [COPD]). Time of last meal can help predict potential aspiration risk with induction at surgery.

The physical examination should focus on identifying the disease process needing surgical intervention and the severity of illness. The first identifies the need for surgery/intervention, whereas the second determines the time period allowed for medical optimization. This second point largely focuses on identifying signs of shock in the patient. Common, though nonspecific, findings of shock may include tachycardia and tachypnea (activation of the sympathetic system and potential compensation of underlying metabolic acidosis). As the shock state worsens, this may include hypotension and altered mental status (organ hypoperfusion causing dysfunction).

Laboratory and imaging studies performed should focus on identifying the primary surgical issue, as well as helping to guide resuscitation. Common labs obtain include basic metabolic panel (BMP), complete blood count, coagulation studies (PTT, PT/INR, fibrinogen levels, thromboelastography), and blood gas analysis. BMP and other electrolytes can identify electrolyte abnormalities common in the severely ill patient. The complete blood count, along with coagulation studies, can help identify the potential for a bleeding diathesis. However, care should be taken in interpreting hematocrit/hemoglobin levels, as they often do not reflect the true absolute red cell mass present, with their decline lagging behind the blood loss until the plasma volume is replaced. Blood gas analysis is helpful with identification of the metabolic disturbances and their etiology, along with lactate levels and base deficit.[2–4] Imaging studies should be chosen with care, so as not to prolong the preoperative time period in the unstable patient with obvious surgical needs, while balancing providing preoperative information needed to guide the intervention.

INITIAL RESUSCITATION

The initial operation for trauma patients in a damage control situation is for bleeding and/or contamination control. In a similar fashion, the emergency general surgery patient's shock state is often driven from one of these issues as well. As such, control of a bleeding source (such as a duodenal peptic ulcer disease with erosion into the gastroduodenal artery) or septic source (such as intra-abdominal abscess, necrotizing soft tissue infection, perforated viscus) is the goal of the procedural intervention. The triad of acidosis, hypothermia, and coagulopathy should be identified and addressed in quick fashion as they can exacerbate the shock state. The underlying etiology of the shock state (bleeding vs septic) dictates the resuscitation. For the purposes of discussion, we are referring to patients with sepsis being those who fulfill the criteria of the Sepsis-3 definition. Sepsis involves "life-threatening organ dysfunction caused by a dysregulated host response to infection."[5] As such, these patients will demonstrate a suspected infectious source with end-organ dysfunction. Additionally, those patients who demonstrate circulatory and/or metabolic abnormalities requiring vasopressor agents with elevated lactate levels despite adequate volume resuscitation with ongoing hypotension represent the subset of septic shock.

Bleeding Etiology

In the actively bleeding patient, the resuscitation is limited to maintaining organ perfusion. Attempts to normalize hemodynamics may worsen blood loss and, therefore, permissive hypotension in a patient that is clinically achieving end organ perfusion is valid and can improve mortality.[6–8] Focus should be on reestablishing organ perfusion with predominant product resuscitation without normalization of hemodynamics until definitive control of the bleeding source is obtained.[9] Time to intervention (surgical, interventional radiology, endovascular) is the driving focus in the resuscitation of these patients.

A balanced product resuscitation with monitoring of coagulation status is forefront in the resuscitation, as the degree of coagulopathy present is inversely proportional to the injury severity and already present on admission.[10] Monitoring can include sequential laboratory values (prothrombin time [PT]/PTT/International normalized ratio [INR], platelet levels, fibrinogen levels, calcium (clotting factor IV), thromboelastography), as well as clinical manifestation of bleeding in the operating room. Regulation of the patient's temperature is also needed, as hypothermia can worsen bleeding through disruption of the coagulation cascade and platelet function. Additionally, acidosis should be monitored and addressed, as it also worsens bleeding issues. Depending on the rate of bleeding, the speed of resuscitation may outstrip the monitoring of laboratory values. In this case, maintaining a balanced transfusion ratio (1:1:1 packed red blood cells [pRBC]:plasma:platelets) until definitive control is obtained may be required. In these scenarios, hypocalcemia can manifest as a result of the patient disease and resuscitation efforts; steps to include proper calcium replacement is imperative as part of the resuscitation effort.[11] After obtaining control, a more focused resuscitation of the patient's deficits can then occur.

One should focus their attention on control of hemorrhage and restoration of bleeding, not performing a definitive operation. Damage control and other operative strategies have been described for over several decades.[12–15] Definitive repair is not necessary and can contribute to patient morbidity and mortality. Vascular shunts have been demonstrated to be effective in maintaining their patency and allowing for limb salvage.[16–23] Endovascular techniques can be used as temporizing or definitive therapy for hemorrhage control.[17,19,23] Although long-term studies are needed, endovascular repair of vascular injuries have been demonstrated to be safe even in unstable patients and may provide improvements in morbidity, iatrogenic injury, and wound complications when compared to open repair.[18–22]

Septic Etiology

In the septic patient, some preoperative resuscitation to improve hemodynamics before anesthesia is usually possible. The Surviving Sepsis guidelines can be used to guide the initial resuscitation and therapy of the septic patient.[24] Some core tenants of the Surviving Sepsis Campaign involve aggressive volume expansion in the hypoperfused patient, restoration of blood pressure, early initiation of antibiotic therapy, and early source control of the septic focus. The recommended volume of expansion in the hypoperfused/septic shock patient is at least 30 mL per kilogram of intravenous crystalloid in the first 3 hours of identifying sepsis. The aggressiveness of this resuscitation has slowly developed over the last 2 decades, starting with River's work in 2001.[25] Although the goal-directed resuscitation studies of the last decade (ProCESS, ARISE, ProMISE) failed to show outcome improvements over a nonprotocolized resuscitation, a more aggressive crystalloid resuscitation had become the standard by that time, with similar infusion volumes between the protocol and standard therapy arms of each study (4–5 L before and up to 6 hours postrandomization across the 3 studies). [26–29] Additionally, failure to achieve this initial resuscitation has been linked with increased mortality, even in the presence of end-stage renal disease and heart failure.[30] In one study looking at bundle compliance, mortality benefits with increased resuscitation fluid volumes were seen in the heart failure and end-stage renal disease patient populations.[31]

Some data do exist giving concerns that over-resuscitation may have negative outcomes with increased mortality rates.[32–34] This prompted the CLASSIC and CLOVERS trials looking at restriction of intravenous fluid after the initial resuscitation (CLASSIC up to 90 days while in the ICU, CLOVERS for the initial 24 hours).[35,36] Both looked at 90 day all-cause mortality, with no difference in mortality in either study. The CLOVERS trial did show an increased use of vasopressor use (initiation and duration) in the restrictive fluid group. Serious adverse event rates were similar in both arms. Currently, the Surviving Sepsis Campaign recommends using dynamic measurements (evaluating changes in cardiac output, stroke volume, pulse pressure, echocardiography vs fluid challenges or passive leg raise challenge) over static measurements of hemodynamics in guiding ongoing resuscitation.[37,38] Given the CLASSIC and CLOVERS trials, a more restrictive fluid resuscitation after the initial volume expansion does appear viable as a treatment strategy; however, care should be taken to ensure that the shock state does resolve.

Balanced crystalloid solutions are recommended over normal saline based on improved mortality and decreased renal dysfunction in multiple studies; though the recent BaSICS and PLUS trials did not support this conclusion, as no mortality difference was noted between fluid types.[39–44] Albumin is not recommended as a first-line resuscitation fluid because of no proven outcomes benefits with higher cost.[45,46] However, the Surviving Sepsis Campaign guidelines did recommend using albumin in large volume crystalloid resuscitation due to demonstrated increased blood pressure, static filling pressures, and decreased net fluid balances; though what defines a large volume resuscitation has not been determined.[46,47]

At present, norepinephrine is the preferred first line vasopressor agent in septic shock with a mean arterial pressure (MAP) goal of 65 mm Hg. This is largely due to studies against other agents showing either no difference or improved mortality with norepinephrine, along with other considerations such as cost and other complications.[48–50] For example, agents with beta-adrenergic activity (dopamine, epinephrine) show increased risk of arrhythmias (β-1 mediated) and increased lactate production from muscle (β-2 mediated).[51–53] Vasopressin is used as an adjunct in patients with ongoing malperfusion despite adequate volume resuscitation and norepinephrine use to reduce the adrenergic burden via a catecholamine sparing effect, along with some data showing reduced mortality compared to norepinephrine alone.[24,50,54,55] Sepsis can induce myocardial dysfunction with associated worsening outcomes in septic shock.[56] Inotropic therapy (dobutamine, epinephrine, milrinone) may be necessary in those patients, though it is associated with an increased mortality when used. [57] At present, the Surviving Sepsis Campaign recommends epinephrine or dobutamine for an inotropic agent when needed for persistent hypoperfusion due to cardiac dysfunction. [24]

Hydrocortisone (200 mg per day in divided doses) is currently recommended for patients with ongoing vasopressor therapy (norepinephrine or epinephrine $\geq$ 0.25 mcg/kg/min) of greater than 4 hours duration to maintain mean arterial pressure.[24] This recommendation was based on 3 randomized controlled trials and a meta-analysis showing quicker resolution of the shock state; though the optimal dose, initiation, and duration has not been determined from studies at present.[50,58–60]

In addition to aggressive resuscitation and reestablishing blood pressure, early administration of antibiotics is recommended in the septic patient.[61–63] Currently, the recommendation is immediate (within 1 hour) initiation of broad-spectrum antibiotics to cover the source for patients with definitive/probable sepsis and those patients with possible sepsis with shock. This recommendation is predominantly based on the observation that patients with septic shock are the most likely to benefit from early antibiotic use.[63–65] In patients with possible sepsis without shock, the recommendation is a rapid assessment for other noninfectious causes with initiation of antibiotics within 3 hours on those patients for whom infection still is a concern. This is due to the studies being less consistent for benefit with immediate antibiotic use, but observational studies suggesting an increased mortality if antibiotics are delayed more than 3 to 5 hours from diagnosis.[64–67] Additionally, antibiotic use is not without potential complications. These include allergic reactions, increased risk of iatrogenic infection (*Clostridioides difficile*), organ dysfunction, and antibiotic resistance.[68–73]

Ultimately, early antibiotic therapy is not a replacement for source control, which often is the deciding factor in the patient's outcome.[67,74,75] Source control can take many different forms, depending on the etiology of the infection, including removal of implanted devices.[76] Although the benefit of source control has been observed, there is limited data on the optimal time which it should be obtained. Although small studies suggest control within 6 to 12 hours, earlier timeframes may be more advantageous.[77–83] At present, the Surviving Sepsis Campaign guidelines recommend source control at the earliest time possible, including recommending not prolonging medical stabilization for severely ill patients.[67,84]

Direct peritoneal resuscitation (DPR) holds promise in helping to improve outcomes in these patient populations with an open abdomen.[85–87] DPR involves infusing a hypertonic glucose-based peritoneal dialysis fluid into the peritoneal cavity after surgery. The fluid is generally removed via a negative pressure abdominal dressing. The effect of the dialysis fluid is to improve the microvascular splanchnic perfusion to reduce tissue injury by increasing visceral blood flow. This helps to decrease the time of ischemia reperfusion injury, the release of inflammatory mediators, and their subsequent effect on the gastrointestinal tract. As such, it is an adjunct to the resuscitation, resulting in decreased time to abdominal closure, increased primary fascial closure rates, and decreased intra-abdominal complications.[87,88] Additionally, evidence exists showing improvement in the underlying physiology of these patients.

ORGAN SYSTEM SPECIFIC ISSUES

Emergency surgeries, in addition to being time restrictive processes, also carry an increased burden from patient comorbidities compared to elective surgical cases. This is directly due to the inability to optimize the patient preoperatively; as well as the shock state associated with the emergency process can often exacerbate these same underlying medical comorbidities. Thus, in addition to managing the emergency, the surgeon may also have to deal with other physiologic/metabolic disorders at the same time. Although not exhaustive, we present several common problems that can complicate the perioperative management of the emergency surgery patient, which need to be addressed at admission.

Neurological

An altered mental status can be a common occurrence in the emergency general surgery patient. This may be due to malperfusion from a shock state and/or acute delirium. Additionally, as the general population is aging, other chronic neurologic processes may be superimposed in the presentation. Family and/or friends may be useful in determining the baseline mental status of the patient.

Substance use disorders are not uncommon in the emergency general surgery population. Chronic opioid use should be identified to provide an adequate baseline opioid level both to prevent opioid withdrawal and achieve adequate pain relief. Attempts to minimize opioid use to prevent masking the physical examination should be avoided. Additionally, a multimodal approach for analgesia should be used, as that has demonstrated a decreased need for opiates.[89]

Alcohol use disorders are also common in this population. Although the prevalence of alcohol use disorder in the general population is approximately 9%, those patients presenting to the emergency department (approximately 40%) or requiring ICU admission (up to 60%) have increased rates of alcohol use disorder.[90,91] In the past, the Clinical Institute Withdrawal Assessment for Alcohol (CIWA) was used to monitor severity of symptoms and initiate interventions.[92] This approach can cause delays in intervention (designed to measure the severity, not the risk of withdrawal) or lead to increased sedation with prophylactic use of sedative hypnotics in patients who do not need intervention. The Brief Alcohol Withdrawal Scale (BAWS), similar to CIWA, also awaits symptom manifestation before starting treatment.[93] Predictive scoring systems, which do not depend on symptom manifestation, include the Alcohol Use Disorders Identification Test (AUDIT) and Prediction of Alcohol Withdrawal Severity Scale (PAWSS).[94,95] AUDIT with the addition of 2 or more abnormal biological markers has a lower positive predictive value (47% vs 93%) for the development of alcohol withdrawal than PAWSS, which will lead to a higher prophylaxis rate among patients who would not benefit from such, but has a higher sensitivity (100% vs 93%).[96,97]

Pulmonary

Tachypnea is a common presenting symptom with metabolic illness in the emergency general surgery patient. This is due to increased sympathetic tone and/or correction of the metabolic acidosis through offloading of carbon dioxide. A significant amount of cardiac output may go to support pulmonary function in the ill patient.[98] This can lead to exhaustion as demonstrated through accessory muscle use and paradoxical breathing effort as exhaustion develops. Although oxygenation can often be measured noninvasively with pulse oximetry, ventilation may require blood gas analysis to better monitor. Oxygenation may also require blood gas analysis in those patients in whom pulse oximetry cannot be obtained due to vasoconstriction.

Care should be taken in intubating these patients, as the loss of sympathetic tone during intubation may result in a code event. Rapid sequence intubation with short-term paralytics and induction agents may be preferable. Etomidate is often used in this situation because of its limited hemodynamic effects; however, it is a known suppressant of the adrenal system after a single dose and for up to 24 hours.[99–102] Its use has previously been critiqued in the septic patient; however, these effects may have been overstated when looking at clinical outcomes compared to other agents.[101–103] After intubation, a lung protective strategy (tidal volume 6 cc/kg based on ideal body weight) may help to mitigate the risk of developing acute respiratory distress syndrome.[104] This may require accepting a lower pH with retention of some carbon dioxide (permissive hypercapnia) in some patients.

Cardiovascular

In the emergent situation, the ability to optimize the cardiovascular status of the patient is limited. This can be seen in the multiple guidelines that do not recommend further testing in this patient population.[105] However, knowledge of underlying cardiovascular disease, such as congestive heart failure and/or valvular disease, may alter subsequent management.[105] Basic perioperative interventions, such as correction of metabolic derangements, supplemental oxygen, continuation of beta-blockade, and adequate volume management, should be employed.

Congestive heart failure patients may have more complex volume management issues. Care must be taken not to induce a volume overload state; however, we often tend to under resuscitate these patients. These patients may benefit from ongoing management with more invasive monitoring techniques intraoperatively and perioperatively, such as a transesophageal echocardiogram; however, there remains no overall mortality benefit for the use of pulmonary artery catheters.[106–109] Inotropic support may be needed with pressors to improve contractility in those with acute or chronic heart failure. Common medications used in the chronic management of these patients include beta-blockade, diuretic therapy, ACE inhibitors, and digoxin. Early initiation of beta-blockers reduces the rate of nonfatal myocardial infarction, but increases the rate of hypotension, bradycardia, stroke, and all-cause mortality.[110] Diuretics should be used depending on the patient's clinical status to maintain euvolemia. ACE inhibitors are avoided given their risk of perioperative hypotension and acute kidney injury (AKI).[111] The use of digoxin should be routinely held due to concern for increased cardiac risk.[112,113]

Dysrhythmias, especially atrial fibrillation, are common in critically ill patients, particularly those in septic shock.[114–116] Although cardiac ischemia is often an underlying concern, usually the sympathetic tone, severe systemic inflammation, and potential atrial distention from volume expansion are the etiologies for the dysrhythmia.[117,118] Judicious volume management, along with correction of electrolyte disturbances, may help mitigate this risk. When present, atrial node blockade with beta-blocker or cardiac (nondihydropyridine) calcium-channel blockers, along with magnesium, may help control the rate and improve conversion to sinus rhythm.[119]

Renal

Acute renal injury is a common complication associated with these critically ill patients.[120] This is often due to relative hypovolemia/malperfusion leading to prerenal azotemia or acute tubular necrosis.[121] This can exacerbate the metabolic acidosis issues common in this patient population as well. Aggressive resuscitation strategies, preferably with buffered crystalloid solutions, may help ameliorate some of the effects.[41,122,123] Avoidance of nephrotoxic drugs (both those that are directly nephrotoxic and those that alter renal hemodynamics) is important, as they may be more injurious in patients with shock.[121] As inflammation and hypoperfusion are the driving forces behind AKI, control of the inflammatory process and restoration of hemodynamics are of utmost importance.[124] Despite these efforts, a significant percentage of the critically ill population will require renal replacement therapy (13.5% in the AKI-EPI study).[125] Additionally, renal replacement therapy does not provide good clearance of elevated lactate levels,[126–128] and early addition of renal replacement therapy may lead to chronic dependence without any benefit on mortality.[129]

Hepatic

Cirrhosis is becoming more prevalent in the population, especially due to the rise in patients with nonalcoholic fatty liver disease, as well as alcohol-related liver disease, with approximately 3% of intensive care unit admissions due to cirrhosis.[130–134] At baseline, the risk of mortality is greatly increased as the severity of the disease worsens. This risk is correlated with the Child-Pugh score and Model End-Stage Liver Disease (MELD) score, though these do not include surgery specific risks.[135–140] More recent scoring systems, including the Mayo Risk score and Veterans Outcomes and Cost Associated with Liver Disease-Penn (VOCAL-Penn) score, include surgery specific risk factors in determining the mortality risk.[141–144] These scoring systems can be useful in discussions concerning the perioperative risk with the patient or their family, with calculators available on the internet showing predicted mortality at several different time points.

Determining the coagulation status of cirrhotic patients, as many have thrombocytopenia and derangements in their hepatically synthesized coagulation factors, is a common problem.[145] Despite these lab abnormalities, a low platelet count may not correlate with actual bleeding risk, as higher levels of von Willebrand factor compensate for the thrombocytopenia, save for instances of severe thrombocytopenia ($<50 \times 10^9$/L).[146–148] Standard therapy relies on replacement of deficient factors; however, there is little data that support this practice. Newer research supports the use of thromboelastography in guiding blood product resuscitation, as this has been demonstrated to reduce the amount of blood products that are transfused with similar rates of re-bleeding related complications, and in some cases, mortality benefit at 6 weeks.[149–151]

Volume status, as well as cardiac function, may be altered in advanced hepatic disease. Functionally, the cirrhotic liver can lead to a high output cardiac failure state, along with maladaptive expansion of the fluid compartments of the body. The actual intravascular component can be difficult to determine on clinical examination alone. Thus, advanced monitoring options, such as arterial lines, pulmonary artery catheters, ultrasonography, and other techniques, are often required in monitoring the patient with goal directed resuscitation.[152,153] The cirrhotic patient additionally has issues with sodium management. Although the hyponatremic cirrhotic patient may require some volume loading with isotonic fluids, care should be taken in both the volume given and the sodium content of the fluids used to prevent excessive volume and/or sodium expansion. Use of albumin is also often recommended in the resuscitation of the hypotensive cirrhotic patient, especially associated with spontaneous bacterial peritonitis, large-volume paracentesis, or hepatorenal syndrome. [154]

Associated syndromes with cirrhosis include hepatorenal, hepatic encephalopathy, and hepatopulmonary syndrome. Hepatorenal syndrome (HRS) is a maladaptive response in sodium and volume management with worsening cirrhosis that results in ascites and renal dysfunction. [155–157] Type 1 HRS (now HRS-AKI) involves an acute change in renal function (AKI) in the presence of cirrhosis with ascites (**Box 1**). [157] This must be differentiated from the traditional AKI phenotypes (prerenal, intrinsic, postrenal). Prerenal AKI, the most common cause, can usually be identified by clinical presentation and response to volume expansion. Additionally, because postrenal failure is rare, in patients who are not responsive to volume expansion, the diagnosis is usually between HRS-AKI and intrinsic renal failure (usually acute tubular necrosis/ATN). Although urine microscopy and fractional excretion of sodium (FENa) or urea (FEU) may be helpful in differentiating these 2 etiologies, there is considerable overlap in

---

Box 1
Diagnostic criteria for hepatorenal syndrome-acute kidney injury

Diagnostic criteria

- Cirrhosis; acute liver failure; acute-on-chronic liver failure

- Increase in serum creatinine $\geq$0.3 mg/dL within 48 h or $\geq$50% from baseline value according to ICA consensus document
  and/or
  Urinary output $\leq$0.5 mL/kg BW $\geq$6 h*

- No full or partial response, according to the ICA consensus document,[205] after at least 2 days of diuretic withdrawal and volume expansion with albumin. The recommended dose of albumin is 1 g/kg of body weight per day to a maximum of 100 g/d

- Absence of shock

- No current or recent treatment with nephrotoxic drugs

- Absence of parenchymal disease as indicated by proteinuria >500 mg/d, microhaematuria (>50 red blood cells per high power field), urinary injury biomarkers (if available) and/or abnormal renal ultrasonography**.

- Suggestion of renal vasoconstriction with FENa of <0.2% (with levels <0.1% being highly predictive).

- The evaluation of this parameter requires a urinary catheter.

- This criterion would not be included in cases of known pre-existing structural chronic kidney disease (eg, diabetic or hypertensive nephropathy). AKI, acute kidney injury; FENa, fractional excretion of sodium; HRS, hepatorenal syndrome; ICA, International Club of Ascites.

From Angeli P, Garcia-Tsao G, Nadim MK, Parikh CR. News in pathophysiology, definition and classification of hepatorenal syndrome: A step beyond the International Club of Ascites (ICA) consensus document. J Hepatol. 2019;71(4):811-822; with permission.

---

presentation.[157–159] Because of the baseline sodium retention issues in cirrhosis, a FENa less than 1% is typical, even in the presence of ATN. It is recommended using a lower cutoff (0.2%) in differentiating between HRS-AKI and intrinsic renal failure.[160] Urinary biomarkers (neutrophil gelatinase-associated lipocalin being the most promising) are currently under investigation to help in this diagnosis, but are not widely available at present.[157,161]

The severity of AKI determines management in the cirrhotic patient. In stage 1A (plasma creatinine < 1.5 mg/dL), discontinuation of diuretics along with albumin volume expansion (1 g/kg/d 20%–25% intravenous albumin for 2 days) will usually improve the AKI. In more advanced cases of AKI, this therapy is less likely to work. EASL (European Association for the Study of the Liver) guidelines recommend the addition of vasopressors with albumin in the treatment of HRS-AKI in stage 1B or higher.[161] Three vasoconstrictor therapies have been validated in the treatment of HRS: midodrine with octreotide, norepinephrine, and terlipressin.[161–163] Terlipressin has only recently been approved for use in the United States, but may have a higher reversal rate for HRS-AKI.

Hepatopulmonary syndrome is a result of intrapulmonary shunts that develop with worsening cirrhosis causing an abnormal arterial oxygenation (partial pressure of oxygen determines severity) with widening of the alveolar-arterial gradient ($\geq$15 mm Hg).[164] Contrast echocardiography and lung perfusion scans can help in the diagnosis.[165–167] Clinically, symptoms will include dyspnea, hypoxia, orthodeoxia, and platypnea. At present, supportive care with supplemental oxygen is the only therapy as no effective treatment except liver transplantation exists.[167]

Hepatic encephalopathy is also common in advance cirrhosis, often resulting from a precipitating event.[168] In addition to addressing the precipitating event, osmotic laxatives are the first-line therapy.[169] Lactulose is often the primary pharmacologic agent used in treating hepatic encephalopathy. An alternative therapy exists with a 4 L polyethylene glycol purge, with one study showing shorter time to improvement.[170] Rifaximin can also be given as an adjunct therapy. The combination of rifaximin and lactulose has demonstrated decreased mortality and hospital length of stay in one study compared to lactulose alone.[171]

Endocrine

Hyperglycemia is another common finding in the acute stress state of the emergency general surgery patient. With the elevated hormonal responses to stress, increased glucose levels occur secondary to elevated levels of cortisol, glucagon, and epinephrine. These hormone elevations can also lead to peripheral insulin resistance that further worsens the hyperglycemia. Although multiple observational studies have shown worse outcomes, it is not known if this is due to the hyperglycemia or just a marker of illness severity.[172–175] Multiple studies were performed in the 2000s looking at tight glycemic control with intensive insulin therapy with conflicting results.[176–182] Overall, although improved glycemic control (goal < 180 mg/dL) over that of the last century appears beneficial, iatrogenic hypoglycemic events associated with intensive glucose control (80–110 mg/dL) can nullify the benefit/worsen outcomes. Thus, the current goal of glycemic control in the critically ill patient is between 140 and 180 mg/dL.

Diabetic patients may be at increased risk for hyperglycemic issues, including hyperglycemic crises (diabetic ketoacidosis [DKA] and hyperosmolar hyperglycemic state [HHS]). This is due to the stress states created by the emergency in the presence of insulin deficiency/resistance along with excess stress hormones resulting in this hyperglycemic crisis through impaired peripheral glucose use, increased gluconeogenesis, and increased glycogenolysis.[183] When insulin production and replacement is absent, a high anion gap metabolic acidosis (DKA) occurs due to the production of ketoacids (beta-hydroxybutyric and acetoacetic acids) and D-lactate.[184] Both states (DKA and HHS) are associated with the development of an increased plasma osmolality, hyponatremia, osmotic diuresis from glucosuria, and potassium deficit (generally 300–600 mEq).[185] Generally, plasma potassium levels are normal to elevated despite the global potassium deficit at diagnosis.

Treatment involves correction of the fluid and electrolyte abnormalities with close monitoring of the potassium levels during resuscitation, along with insulin therapy. With correction of the acidosis (DKA) and intracellular shifting of the potassium with insulin administration, severe hypokalemia can develop while the global deficit is being replaced. Additionally, hyponatremia is a common finding secondary to the hyperglycemia. A corrected sodium level (approximately 2 mEq per 100 mg/dL of excess glucose from normal) needs to be determined to guide the resuscitation until the hyperosmolar state is resolved. Additionally, in patients with DKA and functional kidneys, the acidosis will shift from a high anion gap to normal anion gap acidosis as the ketoacidosis resolves with insulin therapy due to bicarbonate loss (in the form of ketoacid anions in the urine).[186,187]

Hematological

Given the aging population, along with medical comorbidities needing chronic anticoagulation, the use of systemic anticoagulation at baseline has become more common.[188] Reversal of this anticoagulation is often needed for emergent interventions,

Table 1
Reversal agents and their targets

Reversal Agent	Anticoagulant	Mechanism of Action	Dose
Vitamin K	Warfarin	Cofactor for production of factors II, VII, IX, and X	10 mg IV
Protamine	Heparin, enoxaparin	Binds bound and unbound heparin	*Heparin* (based on time from last heparin dose) 0 min: 1–1.5 mg/100 units of heparin 30–60 min: 0.5–0.75 mg/100 units of heparin Up to max of 50 mg Enoxaparin 1 mg/mg of enoxaparin up to max of 50 mg
4-factor PCC	Warfarin	Replenishes inactivated factors II, VII, IX, and X	Warfarin Major bleeding: 25 units/kg Minor bleeding: 12.5 units/kg DOACs 2000 units
Activated PCC	Warfarin	Replenishes activated factor VII, and factors II, IX, and X	25–50 units/kg
Idarucizumab	Dabigatran	Binds free and thrombin-bound dabigatran	5 g IV (two 2.5/50 mL vials given 15 min apart)
Andexanet alfa	Apixaban, rivaroxaban	Binds to the active site of the Xa inhibitors	High dose: 800 mg IV followed by 8 mg/min for 120 min Low dose: 400 mg IV followed by 4 mg/min for 120 min
Ciraparantag	Heparin, enoxaparin, rivaroxaban, apixaban, dabigatran	Binds anticoagulants	Not available yet, still in clinical trials

From Josef AP, Garcia NM. Systemic Anticoagulation and Reversal. Surg Clin North Am. 2022;102(1):53-63; with permission.

either for active bleeding or the potential for bleeding with the intervention.[189] A multitude of agents have been developed over the years that affect the coagulation cascade at different points, necessitating the surgeon to be comfortable with understanding the coagulation cascade, the pharmacologic agents used, and their reversal agents.

Most anticoagulants either work through inhibition of the vitamin K dependent clotting factors (warfarin) or inhibition of thrombin (clotting factor II) and/or the Xa complex action. This later group can either be indirect action through anti-thrombin III (heparin, enoxaparin, fondaparinux) or direct acting inhibitors of the clotting factors. The direct acting inhibitors include older intravenous agents (argatroban, lepirudin, bivalirudin) and the newer direct acting oral anticoagulants (DOACs) such as rivaroxaban, apixaban, edoxaban, and dabigatran.

Obviously, reversal of the anticoagulation depends on the agent used (**Table 1**). Although its use has declined with the creation of novel oral anticoagulants, warfarin is still prescribed in the community.[188,190] Replacement of the vitamin K dependent clotting factors using fresh-frozen plasma (FFP) or prothrombin complex concentrates (PCC) is needed for reversing warfarin. Plasma can require a significant volume of infusion to achieve its results, a potential problem in patients who cannot tolerate this, such as heart failure. PCCs may confer some advantages in being approximately 25 times more concentrated and thus requiring less volume.[191,192] Prothrombin complex concentrates come in 4 and 3 factor forms. The 4 factor forms include factors II, VII, IX, and X, whereas the 3 factor form lacks factor VII. Kcentra, a 4 factor PCC includes proteins C and S, along with anti-thrombin III and heparin.[193] FEIBA (factor VIII inhibitor bypassing activity) is another 4 factor PCC that has demonstrated activity in reducing life-threatening bleeds from warfarin.[193,194] Profilnine-SD and Bebulin, 3 factor PCCs used for hemophilia B patient factor IX replacement, are not currently recommended in warfarin reversal due to lack of factor VII.[193,195] Vitamin K is an adjunct to FFP and PCC in the reversal of warfarin.[196,197]

Some of the systemic anticoagulants have specific reversal agents. Protamine can reverse the heparinoid inhibition of factor II and partially reverse the inhibition of factor Xa.[198] Additionally, it can scavenge and bind heparin.[199] This allows for good reversal of heparin, and partial reversal of low molecular weight heparin. Care should be taken, because higher doses (>50 mg) can lead to factor V inhibition, leading to anticoagulation.[198] Fondaparinux, additionally, is not reversed by protamine. [200]

The DOACs now have some reversal agents available. Dabigatran can be reversed using idarucizumab, a monoclonal antibody fragment that binds dabigatran with higher affinity than factor II.[201,202] Andexanet alfa is a factor Xa decoy protein that binds Xa inhibitors, preventing their action on the Xa complex.[203] Both these agents work through binding of the drug to reduce its effects. Additional experimental agents are in development (Ciraparantag, universal heparin reversal agent).[204]

SUMMARY

In an emergency, the focus shifts from the traditional process of comorbidity optimization before surgery to resuscitation with rapid progression to intervention. As such, complications associated with medical comorbidities are more common. Additionally, these comorbidities can exacerbate the situation and alter the perioperative management and resuscitation of the patient. Understanding the management of bleeding and septic patients and their medical comorbidities is critical in having a successful outcome.

CLINICS CARE POINTS

- Identification of the etiology of the emergency is important, as it determines the resuscitation, interventions, and timing of them.

- Bleeding patients usually require quicker time to intervention while monitoring coagulopathy and undergoing a balanced product resuscitation. A goal-directed product resuscitation usually follows control of the bleeding source.

- Septic patients often have more time for resuscitation prior to intervention. At present, we recommend an initial volume expansion with balanced crystalloid solutions. Additionally, focus should be on restoration of hemodynamics, early initiation of antibiotics, and source control.

- Other resuscitative adjuncts are common in the septic patient. These include pressors (norepinephrine primarily), vasopressin, and steroids.

- DPR may help facilitate abdominal wall closure in patients with open abdomens.

- Substance use disorders are common in the emergency general surgery population. Predictive scoring systems may help in identifying patients in whom prophylactic intervention can help.

- Common medical comorbidities (cardiac, renal, hepatic, diabetes) can be exacerbated in the emergency situation. These states need to be identified and addressed with admission, as they can alter the resuscitation and perioperative management of the patient.

- Systemic anticoagulation has become more common in the past few decades. Knowledge of common anticoagulants and their reversal agents is needed.

DISCLOSURE

The authors have nothing to disclose.

REFERENCES

1. American College of Surgeons. Advanced trauma life support: student course manual. 10th edition. Chicago, IL: American College of Surgeons; 2018.
2. Chang MC, Rutherford EJ, Morris JA Jr. Base deficit as a guide to injury severity and volume resuscitation. J Tenn Med Assoc 1993;86(2):59–61.
3. Rutherford EJ, Morris JA Jr, Reed GW, et al. Base deficit stratifies mortality and determines therapy. J Trauma Inj Infect Crit Care 1992;33(3):417–23.
4. Juern J, Khatri V, Weigelt J. Base excess: a review. J Trauma Acute Care Surg 2012;73(1):27–32.
5. Singer M, Deutschman CS, Seymour CW, et al. The Third International Consensus Definitions for Sepsis and Septic Shock (Sepsis-3). JAMA 2016; 315(8):801–10.
6. Bickell WH, Wall MJ Jr, Pepe PE, et al. Immediate versus delayed fluid resuscitation for hypotensive patients with penetrating torso injuries. N Engl J Med 1994;331(17):1105–9.
7. Dutton RP, Mackenzie CF, Scalea TM. Hypotensive resuscitation during active hemorrhage: impact on in-hospital mortality. J Trauma Inj Infect Crit Care 2002;52(6):1141–6.
8. Schreiber MA, Meier EN, Tisherman SA, et al. A controlled resuscitation strategy is feasible and safe in hypotensive trauma patients: results of a prospective randomized pilot trial. J Trauma Acute Care Surg 2015;78(4):687–95 [discussion: 695-7].

9. Borgman MA, Spinella PC, Perkins JG, et al. The ratio of blood products transfused affects mortality in patients receiving massive transfusions at a combat support hospital. J Trauma Inj Infect Crit Care 2007;63(4):805–13.

10. Brohi K, Singh J, Heron M, et al. Acute traumatic coagulopathy. J Trauma Inj Infect Crit Care 2003;54(6):1127–30.

11. Giancarelli A, Birrer KL, Alban RF, et al. Hypocalcemia in trauma patients receiving massive transfusion. J Surg Res 2016;202(1):182–7.

12. Waibel BH, Rotondo MM. Damage control surgery: it's evolution over the last 20 years. Rev Col Bras Cir 2012;39(4):314–21.

13. Waibel BH, Rotondo MF. Damage control for intra-abdominal sepsis. Surg Clin 2012;92(2):243–57, viii.

14. Rotondo MF, Schwab CW, McGonigal MD, et al. Damage control: an approach for improved survival in exsanguinating penetrating abdominal injury. J Trauma Inj Infect Crit Care 1993;35(3):375–82 [discussion: 382-3].

15. Feliciano DV, Mattox KL, Jordan GL Jr. Intra-abdominal packing for control of hepatic hemorrhage: a reappraisal. J Trauma Inj Infect Crit Care 1981;21(4):285–90.

16. Subramanian A, Vercruysse G, Dente C, et al. A decade's experience with temporary intravascular shunts at a civilian level I trauma center. J Trauma Inj Infect Crit Care 2008;65(2):316–24 [discussion: 324-6].

17. White R, Krajcer Z, Johnson M, et al. Results of a multicenter trial for the treatment of traumatic vascular injury with a covered stent. J Trauma Inj Infect Crit Care 2006;60(6):1189–95 [discussion: 1195-6].

18. Stewart DK, Brown PM, Tinsley EA Jr, et al. Use of stent grafts in lower extremity trauma. Ann Vasc Surg 2011;25(2):264, e9-13.

19. Scott AR, Gilani R, Tapia NM, et al. Endovascular management of traumatic peripheral arterial injuries. J Surg Res 2015;199(2):557–63.

20. MC OD, Shah J, Martin JG, et al. Emergent Endovascular Treatment of Penetrating Trauma: Solid Organ and Extremity. Tech Vasc Intervent Radiol 2017;20(4):243–7.

21. Maynar M, Baro M, Qian Z, et al. Endovascular repair of brachial artery transection associated with trauma. J Trauma Inj Infect Crit Care 2004;56(6):1336–41 [discussion: 1341].

22. Gilani R, Tsai PI, Wall MJ Jr, et al. Overcoming challenges of endovascular treatment of complex subclavian and axillary artery injuries in hypotensive patients. J Trauma Acute Care Surg 2012;73(3):771–3.

23. Desai SS, DuBose JJ, Parham CS, et al. Outcomes after endovascular repair of arterial trauma. J Vasc Surg 2014;60(5):1309–14.

24. Evans L, Rhodes A, Alhazzani W, et al. Surviving Sepsis Campaign: International Guidelines for Management of Sepsis and Septic Shock 2021. Crit Care Med 2021;49(11):e1063-143.

25. Rivers E, Nguyen B, Havstad S, et al. Early goal-directed therapy in the treatment of severe sepsis and septic shock. N Engl J Med 2001;345(19):1368–77.

26. Pro CI, Yealy DM, Kellum JA, et al. A randomized trial of protocol-based care for early septic shock. N Engl J Med 2014;370(18):1683–93.

27. Investigators A, Group ACT, Peake SL, et al. Goal-directed resuscitation for patients with early septic shock. N Engl J Med 2014;371(16):1496–506.

28. Henning DJ, Shapiro NI. Goal-Directed Resuscitation in Septic Shock: A Critical Analysis. Clin Chest Med 2016;37(2):231–9.

29. Mouncey PR, Osborn TM, Power GS, et al. Trial of early, goal-directed resuscitation for septic shock. N Engl J Med 2015;372(14):1301–11.

30. Kuttab HI, Lykins JD, Hughes MD, et al. Evaluation and Predictors of Fluid Resuscitation in Patients With Severe Sepsis and Septic Shock. Crit Care Med 2019;47(11):1582–90.

31. Liu VX, Morehouse JW, Marelich GP, et al. Multicenter Implementation of a Treatment Bundle for Patients with Sepsis and Intermediate Lactate Values. Am J Respir Crit Care Med 2016;193(11):1264–70.

32. Boyd JH, Forbes J, Nakada TA, et al. Fluid resuscitation in septic shock: a positive fluid balance and elevated central venous pressure are associated with increased mortality. Crit Care Med 2011;39(2):259–65.

33. Micek ST, McEvoy C, McKenzie M, et al. Fluid balance and cardiac function in septic shock as predictors of hospital mortality. Crit Care 2013;17(5):R246.

34. Sadaka F, Juarez M, Naydenov S, et al. Fluid resuscitation in septic shock: the effect of increasing fluid balance on mortality. J Intensive Care Med 2014;29(4): 213–7.

35. Meyhoff TS, Hjortrup PB, Wetterslev J, et al. Restriction of Intravenous Fluid in ICU Patients with Septic Shock. N Engl J Med 2022;386(26):2459–70.

36. The National Heart L, and Blood Institute Prevention and Early Treatment of Acute Lung Injury Clinical Trials Network. Early Restrictive or Liberal Fluid Management for Sepsis-Induced Hypotension. N Engl J Med 2023;388(6):499–510.

37. Fleischmann-Struzek C, Mellhammar L, Rose N, et al. Incidence and mortality of hospital- and ICU-treated sepsis: results from an updated and expanded systematic review and meta-analysis. Intensive Care Med 2020;46(8):1552–62.

38. Cherpanath TG, Hirsch A, Geerts BF, et al. Predicting Fluid Responsiveness by Passive Leg Raising: A Systematic Review and Meta-Analysis of 23 Clinical Trials. Crit Care Med 2016;44(5):981–91.

39. Rochwerg B, Alhazzani W, Sindi A, et al. Fluid resuscitation in sepsis: a systematic review and network meta-analysis. Ann Intern Med 2014;161(5):347–55.

40. Semler MW, Wanderer JP, Ehrenfeld JM, et al. Balanced Crystalloids versus Saline in the Intensive Care Unit. The SALT Randomized Trial. Am J Respir Crit Care Med 2017;195(10):1362–72.

41. Brown RM, Wang L, Coston TD, et al. Balanced Crystalloids versus Saline in Sepsis. A Secondary Analysis of the SMART Clinical Trial. Am J Respir Crit Care Med 2019;200(12):1487–95.

42. Zampieri FG, Machado FR, Biondi RS, et al. Effect of Intravenous Fluid Treatment With a Balanced Solution vs 0.9% Saline Solution on Mortality in Critically Ill Patients: The BaSICS Randomized Clinical Trial. JAMA, J Am Med Assoc 2021;326(9):818–29.

43. Finfer S, Micallef S, Hammond N, et al. Balanced Multielectrolyte Solution versus Saline in Critically Ill Adults. N Engl J Med 2022;386(9):815–26.

44. Semler MW, Self WH, Wanderer JP, et al. Balanced Crystalloids versus Saline in Critically Ill Adults. N Engl J Med 2018;378(9):829–39.

45. Lewis SR, Pritchard MW, Evans DJ, et al. Colloids versus crystalloids for fluid resuscitation in critically ill people. Cochrane Database Syst Rev 2018;8: CD000567.

46. Martin GS, Bassett P. Crystalloids vs. colloids for fluid resuscitation in the Intensive Care Unit: A systematic review and meta-analysis. J Crit Care 2019;50: 144–54.

47. Caironi P, Tognoni G, Masson S, et al. Albumin Replacement in Patients with Severe Sepsis or Septic Shock. N Engl J Med 2014;370(15):1412–21.

48. Avni T, Lador A, Lev S, et al. Vasopressors for the Treatment of Septic Shock: Systematic Review and Meta-Analysis. PLoS ONE [Electronic Resource] 2015; 10(8):e0129305.

49. Myburgh JA, Higgins A, Jovanovska A, et al. A comparison of epinephrine and norepinephrine in critically ill patients. Intensive Care Med 2008;34(12): 2226–34.

50. Gordon AC, Mason AJ, Thirunavukkarasu N, et al. Effect of Early Vasopressin vs Norepinephrine on Kidney Failure in Patients With Septic Shock: The VANISH Randomized Clinical Trial. JAMA 2016;316(5):509–18.

51. De Backer D, Creteur J, Silva E, et al. Effects of dopamine, norepinephrine, and epinephrine on the splanchnic circulation in septic shock: which is best? Crit Care Med 2003;31(6):1659–67.

52. Regnier B, Safran D, Carlet J, et al. Comparative haemodynamic effects of dopamine and dobutamine in septic shock. Intensive Care Med 1979;5(3): 115–20.

53. Cui J, Wei X, Lv H, et al. The clinical efficacy of intravenous IgM-enriched immu-noglobulin (pentaglobin) in sepsis or septic shock: a meta-analysis with trial sequential analysis. Ann Intensive Care 2019;9(1):27.

54. Russell JA, Walley KR, Singer J, et al. Vasopressin versus norepinephrine infu-sion in patients with septic shock. N Engl J Med 2008;358(9):877–87.

55. Ukor IF, Walley KR. Vasopressin in Vasodilatory Shock. Crit Care Clin 2019; 35(2):247–61.

56. Walley KR. Sepsis-induced myocardial dysfunction. Curr Opin Crit Care 2018; 24(4):292–9.

57. Wilkman E, Kaukonen KM, Pettila V, et al. Association between inotrope treat-ment and 90-day mortality in patients with septic shock. Acta Anaesthesiol Scand 2013;57(4):431–42.

58. Annane D, Renault A, Brun-Buisson C, et al. Hydrocortisone plus Fludrocorti-sone for Adults with Septic Shock. N Engl J Med 2018;378(9):809–18.

59. Venkatesh B, Finfer S, Cohen J, et al. Adjunctive Glucocorticoid Therapy in Pa-tients with Septic Shock. N Engl J Med 2018;378(9):797–808.

60. Rygard SL, Butler E, Granholm A, et al. Low-dose corticosteroids for adult pa-tients with septic shock: a systematic review with meta-analysis and trial sequential analysis. Intensive Care Med 2018;44(7):1003–16.

61. Ferrer R, Artigas A, Suarez D, et al. Effectiveness of treatments for severe sepsis: a prospective, multicenter, observational study. Am J Respir Crit Care Med 2009;180(9):861–6.

62. Kalil AC, Johnson DW, Lisco SJ, et al. Early Goal-Directed Therapy for Sepsis: A Novel Solution for Discordant Survival Outcomes in Clinical Trials. Crit Care Med 2017;45(4):607–14.

63. Seymour CW, Gesten F, Prescott HC, et al. Time to Treatment and Mortality dur-ing Mandated Emergency Care for Sepsis. N Engl J Med 2017;376(23): 2235–44.

64. Liu VX, Fielding-Singh V, Greene JD, et al. The Timing of Early Antibiotics and Hospital Mortality in Sepsis. Am J Respir Crit Care Med 2017;196(7):856–63.

65. Door-to-Antibiotic Time and Long-term Mortality in Sepsis. In: Peltan ID, Brown SM, Bledsoe JR, et al, editors. Chest 2019;155(5):938–46.

66. Alam N, Oskam E, Stassen PM, et al. Prehospital antibiotics in the ambulance for sepsis: a multicentre, open label, randomised trial. Lancet Respir Med 2018;6(1):40–50.

67. Bloos F, Ruddel H, Thomas-Ruddel D, et al. Effect of a multifaceted educational intervention for anti-infectious measures on sepsis mortality: a cluster randomized trial. Intensive Care Med 2017;43(11):1602–12.
68. Baggs J, Jernigan JA, Halpin AL, et al. Risk of Subsequent Sepsis Within 90 Days After a Hospital Stay by Type of Antibiotic Exposure. Clin Infect Dis 2018;66(7):1004–12.
69. Branch-Elliman W, O'Brien W, Strymish J, et al. Association of Duration and Type of Surgical Prophylaxis With Antimicrobial-Associated Adverse Events. JAMA Surgery 2019;154(7):590–8.
70. Hranjec T, Rosenberger LH, Swenson B, et al. Aggressive versus conservative initiation of antimicrobial treatment in critically ill surgical patients with suspected intensive-care-unit-acquired infection: a quasi-experimental, before and after observational cohort study. Lancet Infect Dis 2012;12(10):774–80.
71. Ong DSY, Frencken JF, Klein Klouwenberg PMC, et al. Short-Course Adjunctive Gentamicin as Empirical Therapy in Patients With Severe Sepsis and Septic Shock: A Prospective Observational Cohort Study. Clin Infect Dis 2017;64(12): 1731–6.
72. Tamma PD, Avdic E, Li DX, et al. Association of Adverse Events With Antibiotic Use in Hospitalized Patients. JAMA Intern Med 2017;177(9):1308–15.
73. Teshome BF, Vouri SM, Hampton N, et al. Duration of Exposure to Antipseudomonal beta-Lactam Antibiotics in the Critically Ill and Development of New Resistance. Pharmacotherapy 2019;39(3):261–70.
74. Kim H, Chung SP, Choi SH, et al. Impact of timing to source control in patients with septic shock: A prospective multi-center observational study. J Crit Care 2019;53:176–82.
75. Martinez ML, Ferrer R, Torrents E, et al. Impact of Source Control in Patients With Severe Sepsis and Septic Shock. Crit Care Med 2017;45(1):11–9.
76. Jimenez MF, Marshall JC. Source control in the management of sepsis. Intensive Care Med 2001;27(Suppl 1):S49–62.
77. Azuhata T, Kinoshita K, Kawano D, et al. Time from admission to initiation of surgery for source control is a critical determinant of survival in patients with gastrointestinal perforation with associated septic shock. Crit Care 2014;18(3):R87.
78. Bloos F, Thomas-Ruddel D, Ruddel H, et al. Impact of compliance with infection management guidelines on outcome in patients with severe sepsis: a prospective observational multi-center study. Crit Care 2014;18(2):R42.
79. Chao WN, Tsai CF, Chang HR, et al. Impact of timing of surgery on outcome of Vibrio vulnificus-related necrotizing fasciitis. Am J Surg 2013;206(1):32–9.
80. Karvellas CJ, Abraldes JG, Zepeda-Gomez S, et al. The impact of delayed biliary decompression and anti-microbial therapy in 260 patients with cholangitis-associated septic shock. Aliment Pharmacol Therapeut 2016; 44(7):755–66.
81. Moss RL, Musemeche CA, Kosloske AM. Necrotizing fasciitis in children: prompt recognition and aggressive therapy improve survival. J Pediatr Surg 1996;31(8):1142–6.
82. Wong CH, Chang HC, Pasupathy S, et al. Necrotizing fasciitis: clinical presentation, microbiology, and determinants of mortality. J Bone Joint Surg Am 2003; 85(8):1454–60.
83. Buck DL, Vester-Andersen M, Moller MH. Surgical delay is a critical determinant of survival in perforated peptic ulcer. Br J Surg 2013;100(8):1045–9.
84. Solomkin JS, Mazuski JE, Bradley JS, et al. Diagnosis and management of complicated intra-abdominal infection in adults and children: guidelines by

the Surgical Infection Society and the Infectious Diseases Society of America. Clin Infect Dis 2010;50(2):133–64.

85. Pera SJ, Schucht J, Smith JW. Direct Peritoneal Resuscitation for Trauma. Adv Surg 2022;56(1):229–45.

86. Ribeiro-Junior MAF, Costa CTK, de Souza Augusto S, et al. The role of direct peritoneal resuscitation in the treatment of hemorrhagic shock after trauma and in emergency acute care surgery: a systematic review. Eur J Trauma Emerg Surg 2022;48(2):791–7.

87. Smith JW, Neal Garrison R, Matheson PJ, et al. Adjunctive treatment of abdominal catastrophes and sepsis with direct peritoneal resuscitation: indications for use in acute care surgery. J Trauma Acute Care Surg 2014;77(3):393–8 [discussion 398-9].

88. Smith JW, Garrison RN, Matheson PJ, et al. Direct peritoneal resuscitation accelerates primary abdominal wall closure after damage control surgery. J Am Coll Surg 2010;210(5):658–64.

89. Chou R, Gordon DB, de Leon-Casasola OA, et al. Management of Postoperative Pain: A Clinical Practice Guideline From the American Pain Society, the American Society of Regional Anesthesia and Pain Medicine, and the American Society of Anesthesiologists' Committee on Regional Anesthesia, Executive Committee, and Administrative Council. J Pain 2016;17(2):131–57.

90. Grant BF, Stinson FS, Dawson DA, et al. Prevalence and co-occurrence of substance use disorders and independent mood and anxiety disorders: results from the National Epidemiologic Survey on Alcohol and Related Conditions. Arch Gen Psychiatr 2004;61(8):807–16.

91. Holt S, Stewart IC, Dixon JM, et al. Alcohol and the emergency service patient. Br Med J 1980;281(6241):638–40.

92. Sullivan JT, Sykora K, Schneiderman J, et al. Assessment of alcohol withdrawal: the revised clinical institute withdrawal assessment for alcohol scale (CIWA-Ar). Br J Addict 1989;84(11):1353–7.

93. Rastegar DA, Applewhite D, Alvanzo AAH, et al. Development and implementation of an alcohol withdrawal protocol using a 5-item scale, the Brief Alcohol Withdrawal Scale (BAWS). Subst Abuse 2017;38(4):394–400.

94. World Health O, Babor TF, Higgins-Biddle JC, et al. AUDIT: the alcohol use disorders identification test : guidelines for use in primary health care. 2nd edition. Geneva: World Health Organization; 2001.

95. Maldonado JR, Sher Y, Ashouri JF, et al. The "Prediction of Alcohol Withdrawal Severity Scale" (PAWSS): systematic literature review and pilot study of a new scale for the prediction of complicated alcohol withdrawal syndrome. Alcohol 2014;48(4):375–90.

96. Dolman JM, Hawkes ND. Combining the audit questionnaire and biochemical markers to assess alcohol use and risk of alcohol withdrawal in medical inpatients. Alcohol Alcohol 2005;40(6):515–9.

97. Maldonado JR, Sher Y, Das S, et al. Prospective Validation Study of the Prediction of Alcohol Withdrawal Severity Scale (PAWSS) in Medically Ill Inpatients: A New Scale for the Prediction of Complicated Alcohol Withdrawal Syndrome. Alcohol Alcohol 2015;50(5):509–18.

98. Coast JR, Krause KM. Relationship of oxygen consumption and cardiac output to work of breathing. Med Sci Sports Exerc 1993;25(3):335–40.

99. Malerba G, Romano-Girard F, Cravoisy A, et al. Risk factors of relative adrenocortical deficiency in intensive care patients needing mechanical ventilation. Intensive Care Med 2005;31(3):388–92.

100. den Brinker M, Hokken-Koelega AC, Hazelzet JA, et al. One single dose of eto-midate negatively influences adrenocortical performance for at least 24h in children with meningococcal sepsis. Intensive Care Med 2008;34(1):163–8.

101. Albert SG, Sitaula S. Etomidate, Adrenal Insufficiency and Mortality Associated With Severity of Illness: A Meta-Analysis. J Intensive Care Med 2021;36(10):1124–9.

102. Du Y, Chen YJ, He B, et al. The Effects of Single-Dose Etomidate Versus Propofol on Cortisol Levels in Pediatric Patients Undergoing Urologic Surgery: A Randomized Controlled Trial. Anesth Analg 2015;121(6):1580–5.

103. Lipiner-Friedman D, Sprung CL, Laterre PF, et al. Adrenal function in sepsis: the retrospective Corticus cohort study. Crit Care Med 2007;35(4):1012–8.

104. Umbrello M, Marino A, Chiumello D. Tidal volume in acute respiratory distress syndrome: how best to select it. Ann Transl Med 2017;5(14):287.

105. Fleisher LA, Fleischmann KE, Auerbach AD, et al. ACC/AHA guideline on perioperative cardiovascular evaluation and management of patients undergoing noncardiac surgery: executive summary: a report of the American College of Cardiology/American Heart Association Task Force on practice guidelines. Developed in collaboration with the American College of Surgeons, American Society of Anesthesiologists, American Society of Echocardiography, American Society of Nuclear Cardiology, Heart Rhythm Society, Society for Cardiovascular Angiography and Interventions, Society of Cardiovascular Anesthesiologists, and Society of Vascular Medicine Endorsed by the Society of Hospital Medicine. J Nucl Cardiol 2015;22(1):162–215.

106. Burns JM, Sing RF, Mostafa G, et al. The role of transesophageal echocardiography in optimizing resuscitation in acutely injured patients. J Trauma Inj Infect Crit Care 2005;59(1):36–40 [discussion 40-2].

107. Griffee MJ, Singleton A, Zimmerman JM, et al. The Effect of Perioperative Rescue Transesophageal Echocardiography on the Management of Trauma Patients. A A Case Rep 2016;6(12):387–90.

108. Binanay C, Califf RM, Hasselblad V, et al. Evaluation study of congestive heart failure and pulmonary artery catheterization effectiveness: the ESCAPE trial. JAMA, J Am Med Assoc 2005;294(13):1625–33.

109. Radaideh Q, Abusnina W, Ponamgi S, et al. Meta-Analysis of Use of Pulmonary Artery Catheter and Mortality in Patients With Cardiogenic Shock on Mechanical Circulatory Support. Am J Cardiol 2022;180:165–6.

110. Wijeysundera DN, Duncan D, Nkonde-Price C, et al. Perioperative beta blockade in noncardiac surgery: a systematic review for the 2014 ACC/AHA guideline on perioperative cardiovascular evaluation and management of patients undergoing noncardiac surgery: a report of the American College of Cardiology/American Heart Association Task Force on practice guidelines. J Am Coll Cardiol 2014;64(22):2406–25.

111. Prowle JR, Forni LG, Bell M, et al. Postoperative acute kidney injury in adult noncardiac surgery: joint consensus report of the Acute Disease Quality Initiative and PeriOperative Quality Initiative. Nat Rev Nephrol 2021;17(9):605–18.

112. Freeman JV, Reynolds K, Fang M, et al. Digoxin and risk of death in adults with atrial fibrillation: the ATRIA-CVRN study. Circ 2015;8(1):49–58.

113. Vamos M, Erath JW, Hohnloser SH. Digoxin-associated mortality: a systematic review and meta-analysis of the literature. Eur Heart J 2015;36(28):1831–8.

114. Meierhenrich R, Steinhilber E, Eggermann C, et al. Incidence and prognostic impact of new-onset atrial fibrillation in patients with septic shock: a prospective observational study. Crit Care 2010;14(3):R108.

115. Salman S, Bajwa A, Gajic O, et al. Paroxysmal atrial fibrillation in critically ill patients with sepsis. J Intensive Care Med 2008;23(3):178–83.

116. Kanji S, Williamson DR, Yaghchi BM, et al. Epidemiology and management of atrial fibrillation in medical and noncardiac surgical adult intensive care unit patients. J Crit Care 2012;27(3):326.e1–8.

117. Sibley S, Muscedere J. New-onset atrial fibrillation in critically ill patients. Can Respir J 2015;22(3):179–82.

118. Seguin P, Launey Y. Atrial fibrillation is not just an artefact in the ICU. Crit Care 2010;1(4):182.

119. Joshi KK, Tiru M, Chin T, et al. Postoperative atrial fibrillation in patients undergoing non-cardiac non-thoracic surgery: A practical approach for the hospitalist. Hosp Pract 2015;43(4):235–44.

120. Hoste EA, Clermont G, Kersten A, et al. RIFLE criteria for acute kidney injury are associated with hospital mortality in critically ill patients: a cohort analysis. Crit Care 2006;10(3):R73.

121. Pickkers P, Darmon M, Hoste E, et al. Acute kidney injury in the critically ill: an updated review on pathophysiology and management. Intensive Care Med 2021;47(8):835–50.

122. Brienza N, Giglio MT, Marucci M, et al. Does perioperative hemodynamic optimization protect renal function in surgical patients? A meta-analytic study. Crit Care Med 2009;37(6):2079–90.

123. Grocott MP, Dushianthan A, Hamilton MA, et al. Perioperative increase in global blood flow to explicit defined goals and outcomes after surgery: a Cochrane Systematic Review. British journal of anaesthesia 2013;111(4):535–48.

124. Zarbock A, Koyner JL, Hoste EAJ, et al. Update on Perioperative Acute Kidney Injury. Anesth Analg 2018;127(5):1236–45.

125. Hoste EA, Bagshaw SM, Bellomo R, et al. Epidemiology of acute kidney injury in critically ill patients: the multinational AKI-EPI study. Intensive Care Med 2015; 41(8):1411–23.

126. Bellomo R. Bench-to-bedside review: Lactate and the kidney. Crit Care 2002; 6(4):322.

127. Levraut J, Ciebiera JP, Jambou P, et al. Effect of continuous venovenous hemofiltration with dialysis on lactate clearance in critically ill patients. Crit Care Med 1997;25(1):58–62.

128. Luft FC. Lactic acidosis update for critical care clinicians. J Am Soc Nephrol 2001;12(Suppl 17):S15–9.

129. Investigators S-A. Canadian Critical Care Trials G, Australian, et al. Timing of Initiation of Renal-Replacement Therapy in Acute Kidney Injury. N Engl J Med 2020;383(3):240–51.

130. Gallegos-Orozco JF. The Growing Challenge of Advanced Liver Disease Due to Alcohol Use in the United States. Am J Gastroenterol 2019;114(11):1712–3.

131. Dang K, Hirode G, Singal AK, et al. Alcoholic Liver Disease Epidemiology in the United States: A Retrospective Analysis of 3 US Databases. Am J Gastroenterol 2020;115(1):96–104.

132. Christiansen CF, Christensen S, Johansen MB, et al. The impact of pre-admission morbidity level on 3-year mortality after intensive care: a Danish cohort study. Acta Anaesthesiol Scand 2011;55(8):962–70.

133. O'Brien AJ, Welch CA, Singer M, et al. Prevalence and outcome of cirrhosis patients admitted to UK intensive care: a comparison against dialysis-dependent chronic renal failure patients. Intensive Care Med 2012;38(6):991–1000.

134. Chandna S, Zarate ER, Gallegos-Orozco JF. Management of Decompensated Cirrhosis and Associated Syndromes. Surg Clin 2022;102(1):117–37.
135. Pugh RN, Murray-Lyon IM, Dawson JL, et al. Transection of the oesophagus for bleeding oesophageal varices. Br J Surg 1973;60(8):646–9.
136. Child CG III, Turcotte JG. Surgery and Portal Hypertension. The liver and portal hypertension. Philadelphia, PA: Saunders; 1964.
137. Hoteit MA, Ghazale AH, Bain AJ, et al. Model for end-stage liver disease score versus Child score in predicting the outcome of surgical procedures in patients with cirrhosis. World J Gastroenterol 2008;14(11):1774–80.
138. Northup PG, Friedman LS, Kamath PS. AGA Clinical Practice Update on Surgical Risk Assessment and Perioperative Management in Cirrhosis: Expert Review. Clin Gastroenterol Hepatol 2019;17(4):595–606.
139. Child CG, Turcotte JG. Surgery and portal hypertension. Major Probl Clin Surg 1964;1:1–85.
140. Kamath PS, Wiesner RH, Malinchoc M, et al. A model to predict survival in patients with end-stage liver disease. Hepatology 2001;33(2):464–70.
141. Mahmud N, Fricker Z, Hubbard RA, et al. Risk Prediction Models for Post-Operative Mortality in Patients With Cirrhosis. Hepatology 2021;73(1):204–18.
142. Mahmud N, Fricker Z, Lewis JD, et al. Risk Prediction Models for Postoperative Decompensation and Infection in Patients With Cirrhosis: A Veterans Affairs Cohort Study. Clin Gastroenterol Hepatol 2022;20(5):e1121–34.
143. Mahmud N, Fricker Z, Panchal S, et al. External Validation of the VOCAL-Penn Cirrhosis Surgical Risk Score in 2 Large, Independent Health Systems. Liver Transplant 2021;27(7):961–70.
144. Teh SH, Nagorney DM, Stevens SR, et al. Risk factors for mortality after surgery in patients with cirrhosis. Gastroenterology 2007;1(4):1261–9.
145. Giannini E, Botta F, Borro P, et al. Platelet count/spleen diameter ratio: proposal and validation of a non-invasive parameter to predict the presence of oesophageal varices in patients with liver cirrhosis. Gut 2003;52(8):1200–5.
146. Ferro D, Quintarelli C, Lattuada A, et al. High plasma levels of von Willebrand factor as a marker of endothelial perturbation in cirrhosis: relationship to endotoxemia. Hepatology 1996;23(6):1377–83.
147. La Mura V, Reverter JC, Flores-Arroyo A, et al. Von Willebrand factor levels predict clinical outcome in patients with cirrhosis and portal hypertension. Gut 2011;60(8):1133–8.
148. Northup PG, Caldwell SH. Coagulation in liver disease: a guide for the clinician. Clin Gastroenterol Hepatol 2013;11(9):1064–74.
149. Kumar M, Ahmad J, Maiwall R, et al. Thromboelastography-Guided Blood Component Use in Patients With Cirrhosis With Nonvariceal Bleeding: A Randomized Controlled Trial. Hepatology 2020;71(1):235–46.
150. Rout G, Shalimar GD, Mahapatra SJ, et al. Thromboelastography-guided Blood Product Transfusion in Cirrhosis Patients With Variceal Bleeding: A Randomized Controlled Trial. J Clin Gastroenterol 2020;54(3):255–62.
151. De Pietri L, Bianchini M, Montalti R, et al. Thrombelastography-guided blood product use before invasive procedures in cirrhosis with severe coagulopathy: A randomized, controlled trial. Hepatology 2016;63(2):566–73.
152. Bleszynski MS, Bressan AK, Joos E, et al. Acute care and emergency general surgery in patients with chronic liver disease: how can we optimize perioperative care? A review of the literature. World J Emerg Surg 2018;13:32.
153. Davenport A, Ahmad J, Al-Khafaji A, et al. Medical management of hepatorenal syndrome. Nephrol Dial Transplant 2012;27(1):34–41.

154. Paugam-Burtz C, Levesque E, Louvet A, et al. Management of liver failure in general intensive care unit. Anaesth Crit Care Pain Med 2020;39(1):143–61.
155. Angeli P, Gines P, Wong F, et al. Diagnosis and management of acute kidney injury in patients with cirrhosis: revised consensus recommendations of the International Club of Ascites. J Hepatol 2015;62(4):968–74.
156. Piano S, Rosi S, Maresio G, et al. Evaluation of the Acute Kidney Injury Network criteria in hospitalized patients with cirrhosis and ascites. J Hepatol 2013;59(3): 482–9.
157. Angeli P, Garcia-Tsao G, Nadim MK, et al. News in pathophysiology, definition and classification of hepatorenal syndrome: A step beyond the International Club of Ascites (ICA) consensus document. J Hepatol 2019;71(4):811–22.
158. Patidar KR, Kang L, Bajaj JS, et al. Fractional excretion of urea: A simple tool for the differential diagnosis of acute kidney injury in cirrhosis. Hepatology 2018; 68(1):224–33.
159. Belcher JM, Sanyal AJ, Peixoto AJ, et al. Kidney biomarkers and differential diagnosis of patients with cirrhosis and acute kidney injury. Hepatology 2014; 60(2):622–32.
160. Diamond JR, Yoburn DC. Nonoliguric acute renal failure associated with a low fractional excretion of sodium. Ann Intern Med 1982;96(5):597–600.
161. EAftSot Liver. EASL Clinical Practice Guidelines for the management of patients with decompensated cirrhosis. J Hepatol 2018;69(2):406–60.
162. Facciorusso A, Chandar AK, Murad MH, et al. Comparative efficacy of pharmacological strategies for management of type 1 hepatorenal syndrome: a systematic review and network meta-analysis. Lancet Gastroenterol Hepatol 2017;2(2): 94–102.
163. Israelsen M, Krag A, Allegretti AS, et al. Terlipressin versus other vasoactive drugs for hepatorenal syndrome. Cochrane Database Syst Rev 2017;9: CD011532.
164. Rodriguez-Roisin R, Krowka MJ. Hepatopulmonary syndrome—a liver-induced lung vascular disorder. N Engl J Med 2008;358(22):2378–87.
165. Krowka MJ, Tajik AJ, Dickson ER, et al. Intrapulmonary vascular dilatations (IPVD) in liver transplant candidates. Screening by two-dimensional contrast-enhanced echocardiography. Chest 1990;97(5):1165–70.
166. Abrams GA, Jaffe CC, Hoffer PB, et al. Diagnostic utility of contrast echocardiography and lung perfusion scan in patients with hepatopulmonary syndrome. Gastroenterology 1995;109(4):1283–8.
167. Krowka MJ, Fallon MB, Kawut SM, et al. International Liver Transplant Society Practice Guidelines: Diagnosis and Management of Hepatopulmonary Syndrome and Portopulmonary Hypertension. Transplantation 2016;100(7): 1440–52.
168. Cordoba J, Ventura-Cots M, Simon-Talero M, et al. Characteristics, risk factors, and mortality of cirrhotic patients hospitalized for hepatic encephalopathy with and without acute-on-chronic liver failure (ACLF). J Hepatol 2014;60(2):275–81.
169. Rose CF, Amodio P, Bajaj JS, et al. Hepatic encephalopathy: Novel insights into classification, pathophysiology and therapy. J Hepatol 2020;73(6):1526–47.
170. Rahimi RS, Singal AG, Cuthbert JA, et al. Lactulose vs polyethylene glycol 3350–electrolyte solution for treatment of overt hepatic encephalopathy: the HELP randomized clinical trial. JAMA Intern Med 2014;174(11):1727–33.
171. Sharma BC, Sharma P, Lunia MK, et al. A randomized, double-blind, controlled trial comparing rifaximin plus lactulose with lactulose alone in treatment of overt hepatic encephalopathy. Am J Gastroenterol 2013;108(9):1458–63.

172. Becker CD, Sabang RL, Nogueira Cordeiro MF, et al. Hyperglycemia in Medically Critically Ill Patients: Risk Factors and Clinical Outcomes. Am J Med 2020;133(10):e568–74.
173. Falciglia M, Freyberg RW, Almenoff PL, et al. Hyperglycemia-related mortality in critically ill patients varies with admission diagnosis. Crit Care Med 2009;37(12): 3001–9.
174. Krinsley JS. Association between hyperglycemia and increased hospital mortality in a heterogeneous population of critically ill patients. Mayo Clin Proc 2003; 78(12):1471–8.
175. Vedantam D, Poman DS, Motwani L, et al. Stress-Induced Hyperglycemia: Consequences and Management. Cureus 2022;14(7):e26714.
176. Investigators N-SS, Finfer S, Chittock DR, et al. Intensive versus conventional glucose control in critically ill patients. N Engl J Med 2009;360(13):1283–97.
177. Malmberg K, Ryden L, Wedel H, et al. Intense metabolic control by means of insulin in patients with diabetes mellitus and acute myocardial infarction (DIGAMI 2): effects on mortality and morbidity. Eur Heart J 2005;26(7):650–61.
178. Patel A, MacMahon S, Chalmers J, et al. Intensive blood glucose control and vascular outcomes in patients with type 2 diabetes. N Engl J Med 2008; 358(24):2560–72.
179. Action to Control Cardiovascular Risk in Diabetes Study G, Gerstein HC, Miller ME, *et al.* Effects of intensive glucose lowering in type 2 diabetes. N Engl J Med 2008;358(24):2545–59.
180. van den Berghe G, Wouters P, Weekers F, et al. Intensive insulin therapy in critically ill patients. N Engl J Med 2001;345(19):1359–67.
181. Van den Berghe G, Wilmer A, Hermans G, et al. Intensive insulin therapy in the medical ICU. N Engl J Med 2006;354(5):449–61.
182. Annane D, Cariou A, Maxime V, et al. Corticosteroid treatment and intensive insulin therapy for septic shock in adults: a randomized controlled trial. JAMA 2010;303(4):341–8.
183. Kitabchi AE, Umpierrez GE, Miles JM, et al. Hyperglycemic crises in adult patients with diabetes. Diabetes Care 2009;32(7):1335–43.
184. Lu J, Zello GA, Randell E, et al. Closing the anion gap: contribution of D-lactate to diabetic ketoacidosis. Clin Chim Acta 2011;412(3–4):286–91.
185. Kreisberg RA. Diabetic ketoacidosis: new concepts and trends in pathogenesis and treatment. Ann Intern Med 1978;88(5):681–95.
186. Oh MS, Carroll HJ, Goldstein DA, et al. Hyperchloremic acidosis during the recovery phase of diabetic ketosis. Ann Intern Med 1978;89(6):925–7.
187. Oh MS, Carroll HJ, Uribarri J. Mechanism of normochloremic and hyperchloremic acidosis in diabetic ketoacidosis. Nephron 1990;54(1):1–6.
188. Navar AM, Kolkailah AA, Overton R, et al. Trends in Oral Anticoagulant Use Among 436 864 Patients With Atrial Fibrillation in Community Practice, 2011 to 2020. J Am Heart Assoc 2022;11(22):e026723.
189. Josef AP, Garcia NM. Systemic Anticoagulation and Reversal. Surg Clin 2022; 102(1):53–63.
190. Ko D, Lin KJ, Bessette LG, et al. Trends in Use of Oral Anticoagulants in Older Adults With Newly Diagnosed Atrial Fibrillation, 2010-2020. JAMA netw 2022; 5(11):e2242964.
191. Chai-Adisaksopha C, Hillis C, Siegal DM, et al. Prothrombin complex concentrates versus fresh frozen plasma for warfarin reversal. A systematic review and meta-analysis. Thromb Haemostasis 2016;116(5):879–90.

192. Chaudhary R, Singh A, Chaudhary R, et al. Evaluation of Direct Oral Anticoagulant Reversal Agents in Intracranial Hemorrhage: A Systematic Review and Meta-analysis. JAMA netw 2022;5(11):e2240145.

193. Simon EM, Streitz MJ, Sessions DJ, et al. Anticoagulation Reversal. Emerg Med Clin 2018;36(3):585–601.

194. Wójcik C, Schymik ML, Cure EG. Activated prothrombin complex concentrate factor VIII inhibitor bypassing activity (FEIBA) for the reversal of warfarin-induced coagulopathy. Int J Emerg Med 2009;2(4):217–25.

195. Holland L, Warkentin TE, Refaai M, et al. Suboptimal effect of a three-factor prothrombin complex concentrate (Profilnine-SD) in correcting supratherapeutic international normalized ratio due to warfarin overdose. Transfusion 2009;49(6): 1171–7.

196. Nee R, Doppenschmidt D, Donovan DJ, et al. Intravenous versus subcutaneous vitamin K1 in reversing excessive oral anticoagulation. Am J Cardiol 1999;83(2): 286–8. A6-7.

197. Mottice BL, Soric MM, Legros E. Effect of Intravenous Versus Subcutaneous Phytonadione on Length of Stay for Patients in Need of Urgent Warfarin Reversal. Am J Therapeut 2016;23(2):e345–9.

198. Yee J, Kaide CG. Emergency Reversal of Anticoagulation. West J Emerg Med 2019;20(5):770–83.

199. Bower MM, Sweidan AJ, Shafie M, et al. Contemporary Reversal of Oral Anticoagulation in Intracerebral Hemorrhage. Stroke 2019;50(2):529–36.

200. Giangrande PL. Fondaparinux (Arixtra): a new anticoagulant. Int J Clin Pract 2002;56(8):615–7.

201. Pollack CV Jr, Reilly PA, van Ryn J, et al. Idarucizumab for Dabigatran Reversal - Full Cohort Analysis. N Engl J Med 2017;377(5):431–41.

202. Pollack CV Jr, Reilly PA, Eikelboom J, et al. Idarucizumab for Dabigatran Reversal. N Engl J Med 2015;373(6):511–20.

203. Connolly SJ, Crowther M, Eikelboom JW, et al. Full Study Report of Andexanet Alfa for Bleeding Associated with Factor Xa Inhibitors. N Engl J Med 2019; 380(14):1326–35.

204. Smetana KS, Counts J, Sodhi A, et al. Review of Target-Specific Anticoagulation Reversal Agents. Crit Care Nurs Q 2022;45(2):180–8.

205. Angeli P, Merkel C. Pathogenesis and management of hepatorenal syndrome in patients with cirrhosis. J Hepatol 2008;48(Suppl 1):S93–100.

Thoracic Emergencies for the General Surgeon

Jane Zhao, MD, MS, Desmond M. D'Souza, MD*

KEYWORDS

- Thoracic surgery emergencies • Acute care surgery • Chest trauma
- Penetrating trauma • Blunt trauma • Rib fractures
- Strangulated paraesophageal hernia • Esophageal perforation

KEY POINTS

- Depending on the type of thoracic emergency, treatment may range from multimodal analgesia, thoracotomy in the emergency room bay, or transfer to higher level of care to a system equipped to handle such emergencies. It is important for the non-thoracic trained surgeon to be able to recognize which scenarios call for which intervention.
- The thorax encompasses the region between the base of the neck to the abdomen. Knowledge of anatomy is critical for the purposes of operative planning.
- Critical thoracic injuries can be identified quickly and efficiently using ATLS protocol providing attention to airway, breathing and circulation.

INTRODUCTION AND NATURE OF THE PROBLEM

Thoracic disease affects a significant portion of the population and encompasses the entire thorax, which spans the chest and foregut. Thoracic scenarios are well within the scope of the general surgeon, even in the context of medicine's increasing subspecialization. This article serves to review common and uncommon general surgery thoracic emergencies, provide work up and management guidance, and lay out the algorithm for appropriate escalation of patient care when the severity of the thoracic disease indicates subspecialist involvement.

This review will be divided into basic anatomy, common diagnostic tests, ways to gain access into the thoracic cavity, trauma scenarios and other thoracic emergencies, common procedures, when to call the thoracic surgeon, and a summary of key points.

ANATOMY

The thorax encompasses the region between the base of the neck to the abdomen. The diaphragm divides the thorax into the chest superiorly and the abdomen inferiorly.

Division of Thoracic Surgery, Department of Surgery, The Ohio State Wexner Medical Center, 410 West 10th Avenue, N835 Doan Hall, Columbus, OH 43210, USA
* Corresponding author.
E-mail address: Desmond.D'Souza@osumc.edu

Surg Clin N Am 103 (2023) 1085–1095
https://doi.org/10.1016/j.suc.2023.07.005
0039-6109/23/Published by Elsevier Inc.
surgical.theclinics.com

Chest Wall

The chest wall is composed of ribs, vertebrae, cartilage, sternum, and muscle. Of the 12 ribs, the first 7 are considered true ribs, as they articulate with the sternum anteriorly. False ribs 8 through 10 have cartilaginous extensions that communicate with the sternum, and floating ribs 11 and 12 do not communicate with the sternum at all. Intercostal neurovascular bundles run underneath the ribs. Chest wall muscles include the intercostal, latissimus dorsi, serratus anterior, and pectoralis major and minor muscles. Rectus abdominus muscles form the core of the anterior abdominal wall.

Mediastinum and Pleural Cavities

The chest can be divided into the mediastinum and the right and left pleural cavities. The pleural cavities contain the lungs and the visceral and parietal pleura. Within the mediastinum sits the heart, which has four chambers, consisting of the right atrium, right ventricle, left atrium, and left ventricle. The right-sided chambers are lower pressured and thinner walled. The right ventricle is often the most susceptible to injury, given its anterior location posterior to the sternum. The thymus, which is responsible for some remnant immunologic functions in infancy, sits superiorly and anteriorly to the heart and ascending aorta.

Airway

The trachea is composed of 16 to 20 C-shaped hyaline cartilaginous rings before it bifurcates into the right and left main bronchi at the carina. The left main bronchus angles to the left at a nearly horizontal orientation relative to the carina and passes underneath the aortic arch. The right main bronchus continues at a near-vertical orientation relative to the carina. Blood is supplied to the carina by the pulmonary and bronchial arteries.

Esophagus

The esophagus is typically 40 cm long when measured from incisors to gastroesophageal junction. Food is bolused from the mouth to the stomach via the esophagus by peristalsis. The upper esophageal sphincter and lower esophageal sphincter prevent retrograde reflux of esophageal or gastric contents. The esophagus is composed of the following layers: mucosa, submucosa, muscularis propria, and adventitia. Unlike elsewhere in the gastrointestinal tract, the esophagus does not have a distinct serosa.

Thoracic Duct

The thoracic duct is typically 5 to 7 mm wide and transports up to 4 L of lymphatic fluid daily. It arises out of the abdomen into the chest through the diaphragmatic hiatus at the T12 vertebral level and crosses over into the left side of the chest, where it empties into the systemic circulation at the junction of the left subclavian and left internal jugular veins.

Diagnostic Tests

Chest Radiography, Computed Tomography, and Fluoroscopy

Conventional radiography is one of the most widely used tests for diagnosing thoracic disease.[1] Chest x-rays can be performed upright, supine, or in lateral decubitus, with posteroanterior and lateral or portable anteroposterior views. Plain films can reveal consolidation consistent with pneumonia, a pneumothorax, a hemothorax, rib fractures, mucus plugging, pneumoperitoneum, hiatal hernia, among many other classic thoracic diagnoses.

Chest computed tomography (CT) is useful when a 3 dimensional approach is necessary. Typically a non-contrasted CT is sufficient for the evaluation of a pneumonia or empyema. If pulmonary embolism or vascular injury is part of the differential diagnosis, then intravenous (IV) contrast is necessary. If there is a concern for esophageal perforation, then a CT esophagram or an esophagram under fluoroscopy can provide information about the presence or absence of a contained or uncontained perforation.

Ultrasonography, Including Echocardiography

Ultrasound is useful in that it is fast and can provide real-time information. It can be used as an adjunct for thoracentesis, evaluation for pericardial or peritoneal fluid, and increasingly, as part of the extended focused assessment with sonography in trauma (E-FAST) examination to evaluate for presence of a pneumothorax.

Angiography

Angiography is helpful to localize bleeding. When performed by interventional radiology or vascular surgery, it can also be used for therapeutic and diagnostic intent.

Endoscopy

Esophagogastroduodenoscopy (EGD) is a diagnostic and therapeutic modality that can be used for the evaluation and temporization or treatment of perforations, gastrointestinal bleeding, ingested foreign bodies, and incarcerated paraesophageal hernias. Bronchoscopy can be used to treat mucus plugging, diagnose bronchopleural fistulas, and extract inhaled foreign bodies.

ACCESS CONSIDERATIONS
Anterolateral Thoracotomy

The left anterolateral thoracotomy is a versatile and expeditious approach, particularly in trauma surgery, as most cardiac injuries and aortic injuries can be addressed via this incision.[2] Superficial landmarks include the breast and pectoralis major and serratus anterior muscles. A bump to elevate the ipsilateral chest optimizes exposure. An incision is made in the inframammary crease and the pectoralis major muscle is divided to gain access into the fourth interspace. The breast can be partially elevated to avoid inadvertent cutting through breast tissue. The lateral limit is the long thoracic nerve found in the midaxillary line. A right-sided thoracotomy is useful for right-sided pulmonary parenchymal and tracheal injuries. Thoracotomies should be closed in a layered manner, with re-approximation of the ribs to represent the first layer. Large sutures are placed around the ribs and secured once all the sutures are placed. Compression of the intercostal nerves may result in post-thoracotomy pain. Each divided muscle group should be repaired anatomically.

Median Sternotomy

This is the most used incision for isolated cardiac and certain central vascular injuries.[2] This incision provides exposure to the thymus, innominate vein, superior vena cava, aorta and arch vessels, pulmonary artery, heart, middle and distal trachea, and left mainstem bronchus. The posterior mediastinum is difficult if not impossible to expose via a median sternotomy, so this approach is not indicated for descending aortic injuries. The sternum is most narrow below the angle of Louis, where the second rib inserts, so identifying midline is critical in this location. The sternum can be divided starting inferiorly or superiorly. Ventilation is usually held to reduce the chance of pleural injury. Sternal closure is greatly facilitated by a midline split of the manubrium and sternal body. The xiphoid process can often be misleading, so it is helpful to palpate the sternal edges at a minimum of 3 points superiorly and inferiorly along the sternum to maintain an even split of the bone. If the sternum is to be divided with the saw starting superiorly, the infraclavicular ligament will need to be divided to facilitate the jaw of the saw gaining good purchase of the sternal notch. Stainless steel wires (approximately 6 gauge) are used. Manubrial wires are brought through the bone, and wires are generally placed around the lateral sternal edges of the sternal body below the angle of Louis.

Standard Posterolateral Thoracotomy

This is the most common approach for pulmonary resection, descending aortic abnormalities, and for exposure of the thoracic esophagus. It should not be used for hemodynamically unstable patients.[2] It provides the best exposure for parenchymal injuries. The patient is positioned as for a lateral approach, but the sterile field is extended to include the spine and high back. Landmarks include the spine, scapular tip, and axilla. A curvilinear incision is made approximately one fingerbreadth below the tip of the scapula and extended anteriorly to the midaxillary line and posteriorly to a midpoint between the scapula and spine. The latissimus dorsi muscle is divided and the serratus anterior muscle is spared by anterior mobilization. When additional rib distraction is required, the posterior aspect of a given rib can be shingled, meaning the periosteum and intercostal pedicle are elevated off the rib posteriorly, close to the paraspinous muscles, and then rib shears are used to resect approximately half an inch to an inch of the rib, permitting much wider distraction.

Chamberlain Procedure

Also known as an anterior mediastinotomy, this small left anterior thoracotomy via the second interspace is useful for gaining access to the internal mammary pedicle or the left subclavian artery. In cases where more exposure is required to gain hemostatic control, the incision can be extended and supplemented with a median sternotomy to create what is known as an "open book" thoracotomy.

Upper Midline Abdominal Incision

Indications include subxiphoid pericardial window, gastroesophageal access, and omental flap harvest. For subxiphoid exploration, hemostasis is critical to avoid any question as to the nature of the pericardial fluid once the window is made. A 2 inch vertical incision is typically required for a window. The patient is positioned supine with a roll placed underneath the lumbar spine. A small midline incision is made beginning at the xiphoid tip and carried through the linea alba but not the peritoneum. The preperitoneal fat and peritoneum are bluntly dissected off the diaphragm. Resection of the xiphoid may be necessary to improve exposure. A small incision is made through the pericardium (which may be bulging with a large pericardial effusion), and the effusion is drained. The window can be enlarged by resecting a portion of the pericardium under direct vision. Take care to not injure the right ventricle or posterior descending artery, especially if the pericardium is adherent to the heart.

Thoracosternotomy

Also known as a clamshell incision, this approach is preferred when one or both hemithoraces, in addition to anterior and middle mediastinal spaces, need exposure. Outside of lung transplantation, its biggest application is in the trauma scenario. The full clamshell begins with the patient in the supine position. Depending on body habitus, the arms can either be tucked laterally or flexed at the elbows and suspended over the head. The latter approach tends to favor more petite patients, such as female patients with a thin habitus and a long torso. The skin incision is made via the infra-mammary crease, and bilateral anterior thoracotomies are typically made through the fourth interspace. The sternum is divided transversely to connect the 2 thoracotomy incisions. The internal mammary pedicles must be securely controlled superiorly and inferiorly on either side of the sternum.

TRAUMA
Penetrating Chest Trauma

Pulmonary injuries

Typically parenchymal injuries will self-resolve with chest tube drainage, lung expansion, and time. Occasionally, ongoing issues related to bleeding or large air leaks, including bronchopleural fistulas will require operative evaluation and treatment, which can consist of suture repair, stapled wedge resection, or even a pedicled muscle flap. A hemothorax after trauma may benefit from a thoracoscopic evaluation and washout. Life-threatening hemorrhage may necessitate an emergent lobectomy or pneumonectomy. A damage control strategy to gain control of pulmonary hilar bleeding consists of taking down the inferior pulmonary ligament and twisting the entire lung 180° around the hilum (the direction of the twist matters less than the actual 180° twist itself). However, this can obscure operative exposure, so another approach that does not require division of the inferior pulmonary ligament would be applying a clamp from superiorly to inferiorly.

Diaphragm injuries

These injuries can be the result of both penetrating and blunt trauma. One must have a high index of suspicion based on mechanism of injury and the patient's history because physical examination and imaging may not always be revealing. Generally, the surgeon should start with a diagnostic laparoscopy and be prepared to convert to an open incision if unable to proceed with a laparoscopic repair. Primary repairs of the diaphragm injury are best performed using permanent suture. Felt pledgets are helpful when tissue quality is poor.

Cardiac injuries

Typically cardiac injuries in a penetrating trauma scenario involve a laceration to the right ventricle. The patient should be lined up with large bore IV catheters for resuscitation and an arterial line for continuous blood pressure monitoring. Massive transfusion is typically warranted. Median sternotomy or a left-sided anterolateral thoracotomy is used to gain quick access into the mediastinum. A horizontal mattress suture using pledgeted prolene is typically sufficient to gain control of the bleeding. If this does not fix it, point pressure over the area of injury to prevent ongoing exsanguination is recommended, while allowing time for the blood bank to send up more product, and anesthesia to catch up with resuscitation. It would also be prudent to consider calling the perfusionist and cardiac surgeon for consideration of repair on cardiopulmonary bypass if the challenging injury is isolated to the heart.

Great vessel injuries

Injuries to the aorta, innominate vein, vena cava, and head vessels are some of the most terrifying scenarios encountered in thoracic trauma. These are situations where the bleeding is audible and the patient can quickly bleed out if unable to get control of the bleeding quickly enough. In these scenarios, once access into the chest is gained, the following thoughts should be running through the general surgeon's head: whether proximal and distal control are feasible, controlling the bleeding with strategic packing until anesthesia is ready with blood products, having cell-saver readily available, and calling for the perfusionist and cardiothoracic surgeon for the possibility of cardiopulmonary bypass.

Esophageal perforation

The patient's clinical presentation can be very telling in situations related to esophageal perforation. For example, if the perforation is iatrogenic after an intervention such as a balloon dilation, and the perforation is contained on imaging and the patient is nontoxic appearing with a benign examination, the patient can typically tolerate conservative measures, including being made *nil per os*, resuscitation with IV fluids, being placed on broad spectrum antibiotics and antifungal coverage, and being transferred to a center with a thoracic surgeon on staff. On the other hand, if the patient is starting to demonstrate early symptoms and signs of sepsis and has imaging concerning for an uncontained perforation, then an intervention should be entertained. Unless the surgeon on staff is someone who is trained to perform esophageal stenting or endo-vac therapy, the most appropriate solution in these situations is surgery. Access into the chest is best through a posterolateral thoracotomy.[3] If the injury is in the upper two-thirds of the chest, the injury would be best approached via the right chest, and if the injury is in the lower one-third of the chest toward the esophagogastric junction, then the more optimal approach would be via the left chest. If the injury is acute and the tissue quality is good, the devitalized tissue can be debrided and primary repair in 2 layers can be entertained, taking care to leave the area widely drained. Otherwise, the appropriate approach is esophageal diversion with creation of a left cervical esophagostomy. If unable to perform or not within the skillset of the general surgeon on call, the injured area of esophagus can be resected and left in discontinuity, and a nasoesophageal tube can be guided into the esophagus to sit in the blind pouch above the staple line for drainage, as a form of damage control surgery, until the patient is able to be transferred to a center with a thoracic surgeon. Regardless of whether diversion is successfully performed, the chest should be widely drained with chest tubes, and consideration should be given for a gastrostomy for drainage (taking care to stay away from the right gastro-epiploic arcade to avoid compromise to the gastric conduit for future reconstruction) and a feeding jejunostomy when the patient is stabilized.

BLUNT CHEST TRAUMA
Rib Fractures

Isolated rib fractures typically can be managed nonoperatively. However, care must be paid to provide adequate analgesia and low threshold for close monitoring particularly in older and frailer patients, as the pain is typically not terrible on day of presentation but rather peaks by 72 hours. Patients with rib fractures are at risk for splinting and developing pneumonia. Patients with multiple rib fractures or a flail chest may be better suited to undergo early rib plating to stabilize the chest wall. Rib plating can be performed either open or via thoracoscopy. Patients with rib fractures will almost always have an underlying pulmonary contusion. Aggressive pulmonary toileting and multimodal analgesia are a must in these individuals given the elevated risk for pneumonia.

Sternal Fractures

Typically sternal fractures can be monitored nonoperatively with recommendations for sternal precautions for 4 to 6 weeks. If the sternum is significantly displaced then sternal plating can be offered as a solution. Anyone with a sternal injury should be evaluated for blunt cardiac injury. At baseline, troponins and an electrocardiogram should be checked. Any suspicion for troponin leak or new heart block should trigger additional workup with an echocardiogram.

Hemothorax

Patients who present with a effusion on chest Xray (CXR) after blunt trauma have a hemothorax until proven otherwise and should undergo chest tube drainage. If the output is greater than 1000 to 1500 mL of blood immediately or greater than 200 mL/hour for 2 consecutive hours, then they should be taken for surgical exploration.[4] Often, the source of the bleeding is an intercostal artery that can be cauterized under direct vision but a pulmonary laceration or a hilar injury can also be the culprit until proven otherwise. If the patient is stable, it is not unreasonable to start with thoracoscopy, but there should be no hesitation to start with or convert to a thoracotomy if doing so will facilitate the exposure and save the patient's life.

Anyone who has residual hemothorax on follow-up imaging despite chest tube drainage should be taken for thoracoscopic washout, as retained blood in the chest places patients at undue risk for empyema or fibrothorax.

OTHER THORACIC EMERGENCIES
Inhaled Foreign Body

Patients—typically children—will present with a story of something going down the wrong way, followed by coughing, salivating, or dyspnea. If the history is unclear and the object is radiopaque, a PA and a lateral CXR can be helpful to confirm the diagnosis. Treatment is with rigid bronchoscopy.

Massive Hemoptysis

These patients are typically self-explanatory, as they present with large volume hemoptysis. The number one priority for these patients is to make sure they are stabilized, with a protected airway and IV access for large volume resuscitation. If intubation is required, try to advance the endotracheal tube into the non-affected side, to isolate it off from ongoing bleeding from the opposite airway. The patient will also benefit from being positioned in a lateral decubitus position, with the affected lung in the dependent position. A bronchoscopy is useful for diagnosis and treatment in these scenarios. Interventional radiology may be beneficial as well. Recurrent episodes of hemoptysis without a discrete source may necessitate a lobectomy for hemostatic control.

Tension Pneumothorax

Tension pneumothorax should be a clinical diagnosis based on physical examination alone, with distended jugular veins, absent ipsilateral breath sounds, tachycardia, and hypotension. If a CXR was to be obtained, the side of lung collapse will appear hyperlucent, and the mediastinum will be shifted toward the contralateral lung. If the patient is hemodynamically unstable, the patient can be temporarily stabilized with a needle thoracostomy in the second intercostal space at the midclavicular line or with a finger thoracostomy at the fourth or fifth intercostal space at the anterior axillary line. This will allow the trapped air to escape and temporize the situation until a formal chest tube can be placed.

Caution should always be used for patients who appeared have a hyperlucent lung field on CXR but seem to be hemodynamically stable. In these patients, particularly those with a history of COPD and emphysema, large bullae may masquerade as a pneumothorax. In stable patients, additional CT imaging may be prudent to avoid the inadvertent placement of a chest tube into a large bullae.

Incarcerated or Strangulated Paraesophageal Hernia

When patients present with their stomach and/or other intraabdominal organs in their chest and have complaints consistent with obstruction, the inability to pass a nasogastric tube is pathopneumonic for gastric volvulus. EGD is helpful in these situations to (1) evaluate for any evidence of esophageal or gastric mucosal ischemia or necrosis and (2) pass a nasogastric tube under direct visualization if the mucosa appears viable.[5,6] Successful passage of a nasogastric tube for decompression converts a surgical emergency into a situation that can be temporized. If, on the other hand, the patient has symptoms and signs consistent with septic shock due to strangulation, then the patient must proceed to the operating room for an upper midline exploratory laparotomy and damage control surgery in much the same way as one would for a distal esophageal perforation.

Acute Respiratory Distress Syndrome

General surgeons are typically not involved in the process of cannulating or managing patients for extracorporeal life support but may encounter patients who have reached the limits of support that can be provided by mechanical ventilation, prone positioning, and paralysis and should be able to recognize which patients deserve to be provided the opportunity for transfer for the option of extracorporeal life support. Each institution will have its own set of inclusion and exclusion criteria but typically patients should have evidence of no other end-organ failure, have suffered a treatable acute pulmonary insult (eg, pulmonary embolism, fat embolism, viral pneumonia), and not have other significant life-limiting comorbid diseases.

Tracheoinnominate Fistula

Tracheoinnominate fistulas are fortunately rare occurrences. When they do occur, it is usually in a fairly debilitated person who has a prolonged tracheostomy in place and can present initially with a sentinel bleed or with hemoptysis. Thus no bleeding following a tracheostomy should be discounted. When a tracheoinnominate fistula does present itself, it is important to try and remain calm and recruit help. First and foremost, it is important to get control of the bleeding to prevent the patient from hemorrhaging to death. The easiest way to do this is to hyperinflate the cuff of the tracheostomy to tamponade the bleeding. However if this does not work, then the tracheostomy should be removed, a gloved finger should be placed in the tracheostomy tract to achieve hemostasis with digital pressure, and the patient should be intubated from above for airway protection.

Traditionally the treatment for tracheoinnominate fistula has been in the operating room with median sternotomy and direct repair of the fistula; however, in modern practice, given that the patients who typically develop this rare complication are typically so debilitated and sick at baseline, many have taken to attempting endovascular stenting or embolization as a temporizing measure, with surgery only being offered if the patient's condition improves to a point where he or she becomes strong enough to not only tolerate but also recover from surgical repair.

PROCEDURES
Tube Thoracostomy

Chest tubes are indicated for pneumothorax or hemothorax and are usually placed in the fifth intercostal space, midaxillary line (though an alternate site for a pure pneumothorax is the second intercostal space in the midclavicular line). Make a transverse incision approximately 1 to 1.5 inches long. Tunnel superiorly to enter the pleural space along the superior border of the fifth rib. Digitally explore the wound to ensure the entrance is into the chest and not the abdominal cavity and to ensure the lack of dense adhesions. Make sure the proximal hole is within the chest. Order a chest x-ray to evaluate for reinflation of the lung. Antibiotics prophylactically are controversial. One dose of a first-generation cephalosporin at the time of placement before incision should be sufficient.

Tractotomy

Tractotomy is useful in scenarios of pulmonary bleeding after penetrating injury.[4] Insert one jaw of a GIA stapler into the tract made by the bullet or blade and the other jaw over healthy lung. Use the stapler to transect the healthy lung to expose the inside of the tract caused by the penetrating injury. Once the injury is exposed, take absorbable suture to gain hemostatic control.

Rib Plating

Rib plating is recommended when there are 3 or more ribs are fractured resulting in flail chest or if the fractures are severely displaced and there are pulmonary derangements and/or failure to wean off the ventilator.[2] Rib plating is absolutely contraindicated in the setting of a contaminated field. CT imaging with 3 dimensional reconstruction is helpful to plan the incision once a patient has been identified. Multiple devices exist for plating with no singular study suggesting the superiority of one device to another. Most common ribs repaired are fourth through tenth as these are the most mobile and tend to be the greatest source of pain. If the fractures are lateral or posterior then a lateral decubitus position is preferable, but if the fractures are anterior then having the patient remain supine is acceptable. The incision should be strategically placed in the middle of the segment to be repaired. A skin flap should be raised, muscle should be spared, and the periosteum of the rib should remain in place and not excessively dissected. When plates are used, there should be enough space to reduce the rib fracture and provide a landing zone for the screws.

Often the pleura will already have been violated by the initial trauma. If not, it is generally recommended to enter the pleura to ensure full reduction of the ribs, protect the underlying lung, and evacuate any remaining hemothorax. Some advocate for video-assisted thoracoscopy during the same operation to optimally inspect the lungs and diaphragm.

Video-assisted Thoracoscopic Surgery

Video-assisted thoracoscopic surgery (VATS) is helpful for diagnostic and therapeutic purposes. For the general surgeon, VATS will most often be used to evacuate retained hemothorax, diagnose ongoing bleeding within the chest cavity, or perform a decortication for an empyema. The chest should be positioned with the injured side facing up. The hip should be overlying the break in the operating table to allow for optimal expansion of the ribs with the bed flexed. All pressure points should be padded. Coordination with anesthesia is important to coordinate single lung ventilation with either a dual lumen endotracheal tube or a bronchial blocker. Access into the chest can be obtained with the ipsilateral lung isolated at the lateral most aspect of the chest wall, taking care to avoid injury to the underlying lung parenchyma and staying superior to the rib to avoid injury to the intercostal bundle. Once access into the chest is gained, the chest should be thoroughly inspected and additional ports can be placed in a triangulated manner as needed to facilitate the operation at hand. If there is any possibility of conversion to open thoracotomy, some surgeons find it helpful to place the initial port where it may be incorporated into the thoracotomy incision.

Endoscopy

The ability to use EGD and flexible and rigid bronchoscopy for diagnostic and therapeutic purposes is an important skillset that shares overlap between general and thoracic surgery. In the acute setting, endoscopy can be used for retrieving a swallowed foreign body, clearing out a mucus plug, and diagnosing the extent of an esophageal injury, among other uses.

More complex endoscopic interventions such as esophageal or airway stenting, or endovac therapy, are not necessary tools in the general surgeon's armamentarium but the general surgeon should be aware that such interventions exist so that appropriate referrals to the thoracic can be made if the occasion arise.

Cervical Esophagostomy

In the unlikely event that a general surgeon will have to perform a cervical esophagostomy, the following encapsulate the key steps for the general surgeon to remember. Once the proximal esophagus has been mobilized as much as possible via thoracotomy, the chest incision should be closed and the patient should be positioned supine with the neck hyperextended and the face turned slightly to the right. The incision should be made along the anterior border of the sternocleidomastoid muscle. The middle and inferior thyroid arteries are divided, as is the omohyoid muscle. A plane is created between the esophagus and the spine down to the thoracic inlet, taking care to avoid the recurrent laryngeal nerve. Most of the dissection will be blunt. Surgeons use different strategies to facilitate identification of the esophagus during this portion of the operation, whether that is a penrose drain looped to the esophagus during the thoracotomy or leaving a tube within the lumen of the esophagus. Once an adequate length of the esophagus has been mobilized, it is tunneled within the subcutaneous tissue over the clavicle, with the stoma sited inferior to the clavicle for optimal cosmesis.

WHEN TO CALL THE THORACIC SURGEON

There is never too early a time to call the thoracic surgeon if there is a concern, including before the patient arrives. Generally, if the patient is hemodynamically unstable, the first thought should be to stabilize the patient before escalation of care or consideration of transfer. Straightforward pneumothorax or hemothorax situations can typically be managed by the general surgeon without involvement by the thoracic surgeon. However, more complicated scenarios that involve the lung not being able to fully expand or lend the possibility of a bronchopleural fistula should lead to the thoracic surgeon being involved sooner rather than later.

Almost all esophageal scenarios should involve a phone call to the thoracic surgeon. Bleeding scenarios can usually be handled as a trauma scenario, but if cardiopulmonary bypass is deemed necessary, then the thoracic surgeon should be made aware of the situation as quickly as possible. Depending on the institution, management of extracorporeal life support may or may not involve thoracic surgery. If there is any possibility of the patient requiring lung transplantation, then the process should be started right away to facilitate the transfer of the patient to an appropriate lung transplant center with an accepting thoracic surgeon.

SUMMARY

Thoracic surgery encompasses a broad array of disease processes with varying levels of acuity. Common scenarios fall well within the scope of a general surgeon, particularly in the acute or global setting when a specialty trained thoracic surgeon may not be readily available. The objective of this article was to review common and uncommon general surgery thoracic emergencies, provide guidance for the appropriate workup and management for these situations, review different approaches into the chest cavity depending on the target anatomy, and how to recognize when further escalation of care is indicated. We hope that this review helps the general surgeon out in a bind for the management of patients who present with thoracic emergencies and time permitting, point the general surgeon in the direction of further focused reading as needed.

CLINICS CARE POINTS

- Air and blood in the chest resulting in lung collapse require drainage. If the lung does not expand on follow up chest x-ray, additional drainage, bronchoscopy, or a VATS may be indicated. If additional procedures are necessary, call the thoracic surgeon.

- Different imaging modalities exist to help for operative planning. Noncontrasted studies are useful when evaluating the lung. CT studies with IV contrast are important when evaluating for bleeding. Upper gastrointestinal series under fluoroscopy are helpful for evaluating the esophagus in real time.

- Consider the target anatomy when deciding patient position and type of incisional access. If starting with a minimally invasive approach, consider the possibility of having to convert to open.

- Rib fractures can often be dealt with nonoperatively but be generous with multimodal analgesia as pain tends to peak around 72 hours following the injury and splinting as a result of undertreated pain predisposes patients to the development of pneumonia.

- Thoracic emergencies often require systems equipped to care for patients, so once the patient is stabilized by the general surgeon, a low threshold should be in place to transfer the patient to a center with thoracic surgical capabilities.

DISCLOSURE

No relevant disclosures.

REFERENCES

1. Crawford T, Kemp C, Yang S. Thoracic Trauma. Surgery of the Chest 2016;100–30.
2. Murthy S and DeCamp M. Chapter 48: Thoracic Incisions (Web Only Chapter). Mastery of Surgery. Fiftzh Edition. 2006.
3. Beck A. Chapter 21: thoracic trauma. Third Edition. Parkland Trauma Handbook; 2009. p. 165–79.
4. Galante J and Coimbra R. Thoracic Surgery for the Acute Care Surgeon. Hot Topics in Acute Care Surgery and Trauma 2021.
5. de Moya M, Nirula R, Biffl W. Rib fixation: Who, What, When? Trauma Surgery & Acute Care Open 2017;2:e000059.
6. Raymond D, Watson T. Esophageal Diversion. Operat Tech Thorac Cardiovasc Surg 2008;13(2):138–46.

Gastric, Duodenal, and Small Bowel Emergencies

Brianna S. Williams, MD[a], Teresa A. Huynh, MD[a],
Ahmed Mahmoud, MD, FRCS[b],*

KEYWORDS

- Paraesophageal hernia (PEH) • Gastric volvulus/incarceration
- Perforated peptic ulcers • Bleeding peptic ulcers • Small bowel obstruction
- Acute mesenteric ischemia • Small bowel hemorrhage • Meckel's diverticulum

KEY POINTS

- Paraesophageal hernias presenting with gastric volvulus, incarceration or strangulation require emergent decompression and may require immediate exploration if necrosis is visualized on endoscopy.
- While most bleeding ulcers can be treated with endoscopy/embolization, hemodynamically unstable patients, patients who have failed endoscopic treatment, and patients who have ongoing transfusion may require surgical intervention.
- Patients with small bowel obstruction without clinical or radiographic signs of ischemia may undergo a trial of nonoperative management at the discretion of the surgeon.
- Oral or nasogastric contrast studies can be used as a tool to predict failure of conservative management and further select for those patients who are in need of an operation.
- High clinical suspicion of acute mesenteric ischemia and prompt diagnosis, preferably by computed tomography (CT) angiogram, is needed to expedite patient care, as mortality rates remain high.

GASTRIC EMERGENCIES
Gastric Volvulus

Introduction

Most of the paraesophageal hernias (PEHs) are asymptomatic, found incidentally on imaging studies. Symptoms typically manifest as gastroesophageal reflux and most commonly occur in sliding PEHs. PEHs, however, can also present acutely especially when associated with gastric volvulus, which can lead to acute incarceration or strangulation of viscera.

a Riverside Community Hospital, 4445 Magnolia Avenue, Riverside, CA 92501, USA; b University of California Riverside, Riverside Community Hospital, , 4445 Magnolia Avenue, Riverside, CA 92501, USA
* Corresponding author. 4510 Brockton Avenue, Riverside, CA 92501.
E-mail addresses: ahmed.mahmoud@hcahealthcare.com; Mahmoud@medsch.ucr.edu

Surg Clin N Am 103 (2023) 1097–1112
https://doi.org/10.1016/j.suc.2023.05.012
0039-6109/23/© 2023 Elsevier Inc. All rights reserved.

surgical.theclinics.com

Gastric volvulus is defined as an abnormal rotation of the stomach more than 180° and can occur along an organoaxial (59%) or mesoaxial axis (29%) (**Fig. 1**). A combined type is described in 2% of cases and 10% remain of unclassified type.[1] The more common organoaxial torsion has a diaphragmatic defect and more than 180 torsion. Borchardt's triad was first coined more than a century ago to define gastric volvulus comprises of three classic symptoms: severe upper abdominal pain, retching with little vomitus, and inability to pass a nasogastric tube.[1] Imaging studies, for example, CT abdomen or chest and contrast studies such as upper GI, which would demonstrate the hernia and its twisting, can aid in diagnosing gastric volvulus. Delay in

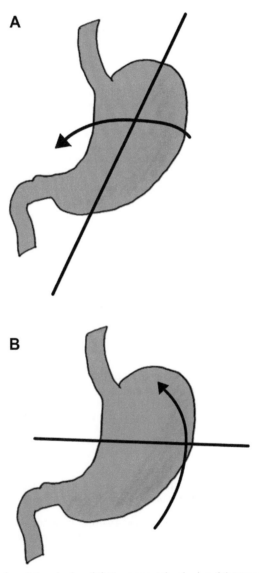

Fig. 1. Two types of gastric volvulus. (*A*) Organoaxial volvulus. (*B*) Mesoaxial volvulus.

patient presentation, diagnosis, or intervention are the most common causes of mortality, with rates as high as 20%.[2,3]

Management

Once gastric volvulus is diagnosed (or even suspected), rapid decompression of the stomach followed by detorsion is critical to avoid gastric necrosis. In most cases, nasogastric tube is efficacious, although some cases may require image or endoscopic guidance. Repeated attempts at placement of nasogastric tube (NG or NGT) tubes are not recommend as multiple blind attempts can lead to gastric perforation typically at the gastroesophageal (GE) junction.

The following steps should be taken to ensure rescue of gastric volvulus patients.

1. NGT placement can be attempted under fluoroscopic guidance.
2. If unsuccessful, immediate esophagogastroduodenoscopy (EGD) with gastric decompression and assessment of gastric mucosa for ischemia or necrosis should be performed. Ischemic mucosa indicates emergency operation, whether laparoscopic or open.
3. If EGD is successful in decompression of the stomach and the mucosa is not ischemic, patient is admitted for volume resuscitation and optimization for urgent or semi-elective repair which is typically performed laparoscopically or robotically.

The timing of semi-elective surgery after successful detorsion of the stomach and nonischemic gastric mucosa has been discussed in several retrospective studies. Delay for resuscitation and optimization is likely safe, but significant delay should be avoided because of high risk of recurrence (30% in 1 month in one study), if possible, surgical repair should be performed during the index hospitalization.[4]

Surgical intervention

Surgical repair when performed after successful gastric decompression can be performed open, laparoscopic, or robotic, though minimally invasive is more common in present days. Technical steps entail reduction of stomach to the abdomen, restoration of intrabdominal esophagus (3 cm length), excision of hernia sac in mediastinum, and approximation of the diaphragmatic crura without excessive pressure on the esophagus. The addition of partial fundoplication is recommended to decrease recurrence but should be judged based on vascular appearance of the fundus at the end of reduction.[5] In some cases, fundus congestion is worrisome after gastric reduction, and fundus necrosis may develop if it is used for wrapping. The use of gastropexy or gastrostomy to decrease recurrence is controversial.[6] Mesh closure of the hiatus is occasionally needed in elective cases but is discouraged in emergency or urgent cases of gastric volvulus surgery due to infection risk.

Occasionally, a transthoracic approach may be required as in cases of perforated stomach in chest. The typical site for perforation is the left lower chest, necessitating a left lower thoracotomy, in addition to transabdominal access.

Peptic Ulcer Disease

Introduction

Elective peptic ulcer surgery has declined dramatically over last 50 years, with the introduction of H2 receptor antagonists in 1977 and utilization of proton-pump inhibitors (PPIs) in the 1980s.[2] The discovery and understanding of *Helicobacter Pylori* (*H pylori*) in pathogenesis of peptic ulcer disease (PUD) has also dramatically progressed effective medical treatment.[7]

It is estimated that *H pylori* is present in 85% of patients with PUD (90% of duodenal ulcer and 75% of gastric ulcer). Several mechanisms have been postulated to explain

H pylori effects on gastroduodenal mucosa; the inflammation and local alkalization that accompany *H pylori* decrease antral somatostatin secretion (antral D cells) and disrupt the inhibitory control of gastrin release (antral G cells). The result is a hypergastrinemia state promoting parietal cell hypertrophy and hypersecretion of gastric acid.[8]

Despite advancements in medical treatment, PUD remains a problem. Approximately 20% of PUD are associated with NSAID use, and complications from PUD are more common in patients taking non-steroidal anti-inflammatory drug (NSAID).[9] Inhibition of prostaglandin production by NSAID exposes the gastric mucosa to hydrogen chloride (HCl) effects. Cigarette smoking doubles the risk of developing PUD.

Critically ill patients especially in respiratory failure with ventilation support or coagulopathy are at increased risk developing stress-related gastritis.

Other less common risk factors are trauma, sepsis, burns, head injury, and Zollinger–Ellison syndrome. The complications of PUD that require emergency surgical consultation and possible intervention include perforation, bleeding, and less frequently gastric outlet obstruction.

Perforated peptic ulcer disease

It is estimated that 10% to 20% of patients with peptic ulcer disease will experience a complication and 2% to 14% will perforate.[10] Despite occurring with approximately one-sixth the frequency of bleeding, perforation is the most common cause for emergency surgical intervention in PUD patients.

Clinical presentation of perforated peptic ulcer disease is described as a three-stage process. Initially, within 2 hours of perforation, patients have abrupt upper abdominal pain. Between 2 and 12 hours of perforation, abdominal pain worsens and can be experienced in right lower quadrant secondary to succus migrating along mesenteric root. Twelve hours after perforation, patient may have fever, abdominal distention, and signs of hypovolemia.

Abdominal examination will typically reveal peritoneal signs of board such as rigidity, rebound tenderness, and distention. Some patients may present early on the onset of abrupt abdominal pain and before peritoneal signs develop. A history of previously diagnosed PUD is present only in 20% of patients presenting with perforation.

The presence of free air on upright chest x-ray or CT scan is diagnostic. However, in up to 20% of cases, no free air is identified on CT scan.[11] If clinical suspicion remains high, an upper gastrointestinal (GI) study or CT scan with oral contrast may be helpful to identify the area of perforation. Abdominal exploration based on peritoneal signs in the absence of pneumoperitoneum is justified. Laboratory tests of leukocytosis with slight elevation of amylase are characteristic of perforation.[12]

On confirming the diagnosis, emergent surgical exploration by open technique or laparoscopically should be undertaken. Volume resuscitation and antibiotics may be required in few cases with severe hypovolemia or sepsis but should not delay surgery. Emergency surgery for perforated ulcers has a 6% to 30% mortality risk.[13]

The first part of duodenum and pyloric channel are the most common sites of perforation and are grouped together as duodenal perforation. The duodenal bulb is the perforation site in 62% of cases and 20% of perforation are in the pylorus channel. The gastric body is site of perforation in 18%.[14] Most of these perforations occur on anterior wall of the duodenum and can be clearly identified in laparotomy or laparoscopy. Graham patch (free omentum) or omentopexy using an omental pedicle (Cellan-Jones) is the most commonly used technique to close these perforations. In this technique, the ulcer is not closed but rather a vascularized pedicle of omentum is sutured over the perforation with interrupted sutures. In case of paucity of omentum, the falciform ligament has been used instead by some surgeons. Leak tests of repair are not routine.[15]

The simple technique using the omental patch is highly successful in the classic perforations 1 cm or less in size and at typical anterior duodenal location. Management of larger perforations and posteriorly located perforation with surrounding inflammation is challenging. The failure of omental patch and postoperative leak occur in up to 12% of perforations exceeding 2 cm in size.[16] Multiple procedures have been tried to help dealing with these situations ranging from adding internal tube duodenostomy, jejunal serosal patch, and pyloric exclusion with gastrojejunostomy and up to antrectomy with Billroth II construction. In some situations, the "difficult duodenal stump" is commonly used to describe larger perforations in tenuous locations, with management requiring complex methods for closure such as the Nissen or Bancroft closure[17] (**Fig. 2**).

Gastric perforation has twice the mortality of duodenal perforation and patients are usually elder. Malignancy is reported in 10% to 16%.[18] Local resection followed by patch repair is feasible. For gastric ulcers at greater curvature, antrum, or body of stomach, simple wedge resection is possible and achieves closure as well as tissue biopsy. In the lesser curvature, the left gastric pedicle and GE junction make resection more challenging. Distal gastric ulcers can be treated by distal gastrectomy with Billroth II construction in hemodynamically stable patients. For high lesser curvature ulcer, distal gastrectomy with tongue-shaped excision of lesser curvature and Roux-en-Y esophagogastrojejunostomy is appropriate in stable patients (Csendes procedure).

The need for definitive ulcer operation during surgical treatment of perforation has almost been eliminated because of our better understanding the role of *H pylori* and the effective medical treatment. In rare circumstances, patients may have negative *H pylori* and perforation or life time need to use NSAID. In these patients, a definitive ulcer operation can be undertaken during emergency surgery as long as patient is stable to tolerate a longer surgical procedure.

Recently, endoscopic closure of perforated ulcers has been used with increasing success.

Bleeding peptic ulcer

Bleeding occurs in 15% to 20% of PUD patients, and only 40% of patients with bleeding from PUD have previous documented history of PUD. PUD makes up to 90% non-variceal upper GI bleeding.[10,13] Most (80%) of PUD bleeding will cease with medical management without therapeutic endoscopy or surgical intervention. Risk factors for bleeding from PUD include NSAID use (dose-dependent), *H pylori* infection, use of anticoagulation, smoking, and critical illness. Prolonged ventilation (more than 48 hours) is a high-risk factor in developing bleeding stress ulcer in intensive care unit patients.

Bleeding PUD typically presents as hematemesis and/or melena. Hematochezia may develop in patients with severe bleeding where blood may pass quickly down the GI tract without being digested.

Nasogastric tube will reveal bleeding from upper GI and the presence of clear bile excludes upper GI bleeding.

Rapid resuscitation by volume replacement and air way protection are the key initial steps in management.

Several scoring systems to predict the course of bleeding and mortality risks have been developed (Blatchford score and Rockall score)[19] (**Table 1**).

Upper endoscopy is an essential step which must be performed as soon as patient resuscitation is initiated. Delay in endoscopy has the direct effect on mortality and

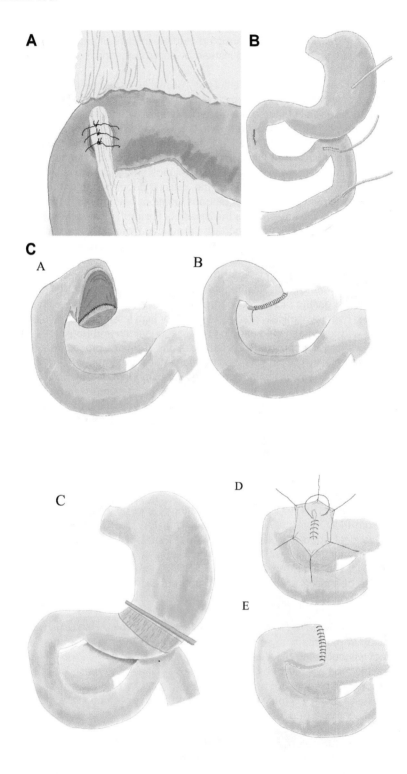

Table 1 Rockall scoring system*		
Variables	**Score**	
Age	<60	0
	60–79	1
	>80	2
Comorbidities	No comorbidities	0
	Congestive heart failure, ischemic heart disease	2
	Renal failure, liver disease, metastasis	4
Shock	No shock (systolic blood pressure [SBP] > 100, HR < 100)	0
	Tachycardia (heart rate [HR] > 100)	1
	Hypotension (SBP < 100 mmHg)	2
Source of bleeding	None or Mallory–Weiss	0
	All other diagnoses, for example, esophagitis	1
	Malignancy	2
Stigma	None	0
	Adherent clot, visible vessel	2

* Score of <3 is minor, 3-8 is moderate, >8 is major. Mortality rate is approximately 10% for score of 3, 40% for score of 5, and 50% for score of 7.

overall outcome. With more refined endoscopic techniques, successful control of bleeding is seen in 80% of cases. Even when endoscopy fails to control the bleeding, exclusion of varices and proper localization of bleeding site are of vital importance to surgeons.

Treatment of bleeding PUD
Immediate acid suppression with intravenous bolus followed by continuous infusion of PPI should be initiated. This treatment has been shown to reduce the risk of recurrent bleeding and subsequent need for surgery.

Traditional teaching indicates that the transfusion of more than 6 units of packed red blood cells (PRBC) in 24 is an indication for surgery. Current practices, however, are more inclined toward mitigation of coagulopathy and early endoscopic intervention.

Endoscopy within 24 hours or less of upper GI bleeding onset has become a quality metric for management of upper GI bleeding. Most of upper GI bleeding will be controlled by medical management and upper endoscopy saving the patients from surgical or radiological intervention, in recurrent bleeding, endoscopic measures should be attempted once more.[20]

Therapeutic endoscopic options include injection of epinephrine, thermal coagulation, vasoactive medications, and clipping of visible vessels. Injection therapy should be used in conjunction with clipping and not alone because it has a high bleeding recurrence rate when used in isolation. The recurrence of bleeding is seen in

Fig. 2. Methods for surgical management of gastroduodenal perforation and management of the difficult duodenal stump. (A) Modified graham patch repair. (B) Proximal and distal drainage with feeding jejunostomy tube placement. (C) a. Nissen closure, the duodenum is transected and the duodenal stump is anastamosed to the pancreatic capsule b. Bancroft closure. The stomach is transected proximal to they pylorus, the gastric mucosa in the duodenal stump is dissected away from the submucosal layer, and secured with pursestring suture. The seromuscular layer is closed over the stump.

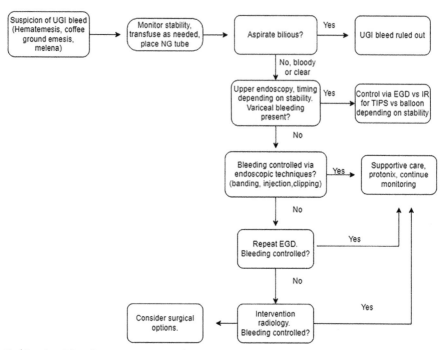

Fig. 3. Algorithm for management of upper gastrointestinal series (UGI) bleed.

approximately 13% of patients and re-endoscopy should be attempted with interventional radiology and/or surgery is in close stand by (**Fig. 3**).

Forrest classification of endoscopic description of bleeding ulcer is helpful in anticipating the need for further intervention and overall mortality.[21]

Celiac angiogram can reveal a blush within the lumen and embolization or coiling of the vessel can control bleeding. The most common vessels involved in descending order are the gastroduodenal artery, left gastric artery, right gastric artery, and splenic artery. Active extravasation is seen only in 50% of patients sent to interventional radiology (IR), but empiric successful embolization is reported in 90% of patients. Approximately 30% of patients will have recurrent bleeding.[4]

Surgical intervention
Patients who fail endoscopic and radiologic interventions will require surgery, commonly undertaken during active bleeding. The main goal in these patients is to stop the bleeding by ligation of the bleeding vessel. The gastroduodenal artery is the most common vessel which typically erodes in the posterior wall of the duodenum within 2 cm distal to the pylorus. The bleeding can be exposed by a 3 cm anterior duodenotomy extending just proximal to the pylorus. The bleeding once localized can be controlled by the well-described three-point ligation (**Fig. 4**). The anterior pyloroduodenotomy can then be closed transversally creating a pyloroplasty. Patients who remain stable after control of bleeding as such should be highly considered for adding truncal vagotomy if surgeon is comfortable with the procedure. It has been shown that ligation of bleeding only has higher mortality compared with truncal vagotomy pyloroplasty. Rarely, antrectomy may be required if bleeding could not be controlled through anterior pyloroduodenotomy.[22]

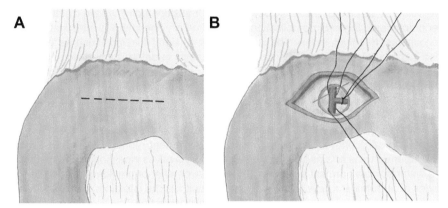

Fig. 4. Control of bleeding ulcer. (*A*) Transverse incision over the pylorus. (*B*) 3-point ligation of the gastroduodenal artery, superior, inferior and medial

Small Bowel Emergencies

Introduction: nature of the problem

Small bowel obstruction (SBO) remains a nuanced problem to emergency abdominal surgery. This problem accounts for 300,000 to 350,000 hospital admissions and can amount to 960,000 admission days to the hospital. There is also accrual of significant financial burden, especially in the United States, to the tune of 2 to 3 billion each year.[23,24] SBO is defined as mechanical or functional impediment of intraluminal contents. This leads to upstream accumulation of gas and fluids; the stasis of which can nourish bacterial growth and translocation. Subsequent bowel wall edema occurs, and eventually, venous return becomes impaired. Variations in obstruction range from partial to complete. Strangulation indicates compromise of the intestinal blood flow leading to necrosis. Closed-loop obstruction denotes obstruction at two separate points of the bowel (which may include a competent ileocecal valve) predisposing that segment to volvulus and ischemia. A myriad of causes of mechanical SBO exist. The most common in the developed world is adhesive disease (75%), hernia, malignancy, previous radiation exposure, inflammatory bowel disease, intussusception, Meckel's diverticulum (MD), foreign bodies, and internal hernia.[24]

Evaluation and treatment

Classically, patients present with symptoms of nausea, vomiting, abdominal distension, and constipation that may lead to obstipation. Initial evaluation, after history and physical examination, includes laboratory studies (complete blood count [CBC], comprehensive metabolic panel [CMP], amylase, lactic acid) and radiographic studies. The patient should be kept nil per os, vital signs and urinary output should be observed in a monitored setting for acute changes. The correction of electrolytes and acidosis noted on routine laboratory studies is also crucial. Broad spectrum antibiotics should be administered given the potential for perforation and exposure to intestinal bacteria. Plain abdominal x-ray is widely available and able to quickly evaluate small bowel and gastric dilation. SBO is characterized by dilation of small bowel to over 3 cm, presence of air fluid levels, and absence of distal or colonic gas. Computed tomography of the abdomen and pelvis with intravenous contrast is the most sensitive and specific. It has also become more widely available in the emergency setting. Although scar tissue may not be discernible on imaging, distinctive features of intestinal obstruction on CT are noted by dilation of the small bowel and a "transition point" where distal bowel is decompressed. Signs of complication include free air, pneumatosis intestinalis, portal venous gas, free fluid, mesenteric edema, or "swirl sign." Findings such as these can also guide surgical planning. CT can be more useful in determining etiology of bowel obstruction and elucidating worrisome features in patients who may be sicker than they seem (ie, immunocompromised, incapacitated).[24,25]

Most SBOs which are due to adhesive disease can be managed nonoperatively. The mainstay of initial management has been nasogastric decompression followed by a contrast study in stable patients. In fact, there are many studies focused on the use of Gastrografin contrast as an evaluation and treatment modality. A contrast study (also referred to as a "small bowel follow through") involves ingestion of a hyperosmolar, water soluble contrast solution such as Gastrografin, or omnipaque, and taking a series of abdominal x-rays following contrast as it fills the intestines. Failure to reach the colon by 4 hours is considered at least partial obstruction. Failure of the contrast to reach the colon at 24 hours has been used as a threshold for surgical exploration. The hyperosmolar quality of the fluid ingested is theorized to shift edema into the lumen of the bowel and relieve obstruction, lessening the need for surgery.[26] A caveat to this method is that it should not be used in patients whom the clinician suspects has a perforation of the bowel, as the leakage of this fluid can worsen peritonitis.

Knowing when to operate as an acute care surgeon is nuanced. There is little debate as to aggressive operative management for cases of perforation, closed-loop obstruction, or strangulated hernia, as these will not resolve without intervention. The timing of operative intervention is diverse among abdominal surgeons. Surgery has typically been reserved for patients with suspected complication, peritonitis, failure to progress with conservative management, or failure of contrast to reach the colon on contrast study. Early recognition by the surgeon facilitates prompt treatment. Extended delay may resort in higher morbidity such as extensive bowel resection. Predicting patients who will fail nonoperative measures has been a fraught subject. Observation periods of up to 3 to 5 days have been used as a typical trial for nonoperative management. Unsuccessful contrast studies have also been used as a signifier for operating. In a study by Behman and colleagues published a retrospective cohort study out of Canada analyzing recurrence and readmission rates of patients with SBO treated operatively versus nonoperatively. In a matched cohort of nearly 28,000 patients over a 10-year period (2005–2014), those with adhesive SBO who underwent operative intervention at the index admission had a lower risk of recurrence at 5 years when compared with those undergoing nonoperative management (11.2% vs 19.2%; $P < .001$). In addition, the more episodes of SBO that occurred, the more likely subsequent episodes would occur. Thus, some would argue that if a patient is fit for operation, earlier surgical intervention may benefit the patient. The method in which this is undertaken has shifted attitudes over the past decade. Laparoscopy as an initial strategy for exploration has been demonstrated as a safe approach with no major difference in morbidity and may decrease the length of stay.[27] Minimally invasive techniques have been theorized to create fewer adhesions, which might lower the burden of future need for additional exploration. Barriers to performing successful treatment with laparoscopy include the lack of training in advanced laparoscopy, excessive bowel distention, and dense matted adhesions. Exploratory laparotomy has been the gold standard for surgery due to SBO. Through a midline incision, using any previous laparotomy scar, the abdominal cavity is entered. Ideally, this is through a virgin plane extending beyond any previous scar. Adhesions to the abdominal wall and between small bowel loops should be lysed, typically with sharp dissection to avoid iatrogenic enterotomy. The bowel and its mesentery should be examined in an organized fashion between the ligament of Treitz and the ileocecal valve. Any twisting of the mesentery should be corrected, and any defect should be closed. Nonviable bowel should be resected; these include areas of necrosis, perforation, and appearance of venous thrombosis within the distal mesentery. Areas that are pink or erythematous are less likely to be nonviable, whereas areas that are violaceous are borderline and should be kept warm and then reexamined at a later point in the operation. Other techniques used to determine viability include intravenous use of fluorescent dyes and direct visualization of blood flow under a Woods lamp or specialized camera. Sterile Doppler can be placed on the antimesenteric border of the bowel to assess the most distal area of perfusion to that segment. Primary anastomosis can usually take place at the index operation provided the patient is hemodynamically stable. In the face of multiple pressor use or other circumstances prohibiting a longer operation, a second look operation may be planned after stabilization to restore continuity.

Summary
SBO remains one of the most common reasons for surgical admission to the hospital. The etiology for obstruction can determine the decision for immediate surgery versus conservative management with observation. Ancillary testing with a per os (PO) contrast study may govern which patients are likely to need surgical intervention.

Acute Mesenteric Ischemia

Introduction
Acute mesenteric ischemia (AMI) requires special attention as a surgical emergency given its high mortality rate (50%–80%), though incidence is quite low.[28] Vascular supply of the small bowel is primarily through the superior mesenteric artery with collateral flow contributed by the celiac axis via the pancreaticoduodenal arteries and inferior mesenteric artery. The narrow takeoff angle from the aorta itself makes the SMA particularly vulnerable to emboli, though the typical course of an acute embolus lands in a distal portion of the artery. Hence, the key ischemic pattern is noted as sparing the proximal jejunum and colon. The source of the embolus is most commonly from the left atrium, with emboli formed from atrial fibrillation or poor ventricular function. Less common is the source from an atherosclerotic plaque or thrombus in the aorta. Thrombosis of the superior mesenteric artery (SMA) accounts for approximately 25% of the incidence of mesenteric ischemia and occurs in patients with underlying atherosclerotic disease. Thus, there may be an acute on chronic picture during presentation, though vasculitis and mycotic aneurysm are also sources. Special consideration should be made to patients who are positive for SARS Coronavirus-19 as this novel virus has not just affected the respiratory tract but is also associated with multiorgan involvement, including thromboembolic complications.[29] Nonocclusive mesenteric ischemia (NOMI) pathophysiology is due to a vasoconstrictive or hypovolemic state to the splanchnic blood flow (20%). There is a global effect on the gut; therefore, all of the small bowel and ileocolic territories are threatened by this low-flow state. Mesenteric venous thrombosis is the least common (10%) etiology of mesenteric ischemia, in which thrombophilic states cause impaired venous return of the splanchnic vascularity to the portal vein.

Evaluation
Early diagnosis is the key to avoiding irreversible ischemia and the morbidity of extensive bowel resection or death. Diffuse abdominal pain is acute and unrelenting. "Pain out of proportion to exam" is a finding that should raise clinical suspicion, especially in an elderly patient accompanied by fever and bloody stools. One must be mindful that

only a third of patients will have all these signs. Septic shock may be a late sign of extensive bowel ischemia. Surgeons should tease out the underlying pathophysiology through gathering a detailed history. Often there is a history of diffuse post-prandial abdominal pain or extensive weight loss due to "food fear," history of cardiac disease, or thromboembolic event. In already hospitalized, critically ill patients, there may be an extended period of vasopressor use. The patient should be kept nil per os with naso-gastric tube to avoid metabolic stress on the bowel. No laboratory tests can specif-ically rule out mesenteric ischemia, though lactic acid and D-dimer have been used as adjuncts in diagnosis but must be supported by the overall clinical picture.[28] The trend of lactic acidosis may guide resuscitation efforts. Multiphase computed tomog-raphy angiography of the abdomen and pelvis should be obtained STAT to confirm the diagnosis as its positive and negative predictive values reach nearly 100%[28] (**Fig. 5**). Along with arterial and venous anatomy, imaging may demonstrate other signs of complications from ischemia, including bowel wall thickening, pneumatosis intestina-lis, portal venous gas, or free air from perforated viscus.

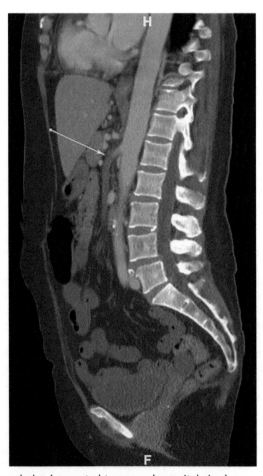

Fig. 5. Acute SMA embolus (computed tomography sagital view).

Treatment
Once the diagnosis is made, prompt resuscitation should be initiated in the form of volume infusion with crystalloid, being careful to avoid excessive fluid overload. Suggested vasopressor agents such as dobutamine, dopamine, and milrinone should help to optimize cardiac performance while minimizing the effect on mesenteric blood flow. Unless contraindicated, systemic anticoagulation should be started in the form of heparin to stabilize any clot that has formed, and broad-spectrum antibiotics should also be administered as the intestinal mucosal barrier is assumed to be compromised. Laparotomy is the method of choice in critically ill patients with the principle first step being to reestablish blood supply to the mesenteric territory threatened. The SMA is identified by tracing the middle colic artery down to the mesentery which can be palpated for a pulse. Sterile Doppler or angiography using a hybrid operating room can be done in cases of uncertainty. Exposure of the artery and thromboembolectomy with Fogarty balloon catheter is performed, then closure of the arteriotomy either primarily or patch angioplasty. Extensive atherosclerotic disease or thrombosis at the origin of the SMA requires a bypass procedure, usually retrograde from the iliac artery. The use of a synthetic graft is a difficult choice that the surgeon must make especially in the face of a contaminated field. Autologous vein grafts using the femoral or saphenous vein are a consideration, though they may be prone to kinking. In the presence of mesenteric venous thrombosis or NOMI, this vascular manipulation is unnecessary and systemic anticoagulation should suffice without necessarily needing an operation. Abdominal exploration after restoration of blood flow should then aim to resect any necrotic or perforated bowel and, if stable, restore continuity. Damage control laparotomy with planned reexplanation is perfectly acceptable given the need to correct any physiologic derangements such as coagulopathy, temperature, and acidosis. Endovascular approaches have gained traction as a more attractive treatment option especially in cases of partial occlusion or chronic mesenteric ischemia. The caveat being there should be no evidence of perforation or advanced bowel ischemia, and the patient cannot have a contraindication to thrombolytic therapy. If endovascular treatment is not successful or not technically achievable patients would still need to be referred for open revascularization which remains the standard at this time. Therefore, endovascular techniques are typically reserved for chronic mesenteric ischemia, which is not the focus of this summary.

Summary
Quality of life depends on prompt recognition of AMI and its underlying pathology leading to expedient treatment. Failure to recognize this condition can result in bowel ischemia requiring extensive bowel resection leading to short gut syndrome or complete small bowel necrosis which is incompatible with life.

Consideration of Other Miscellaneous Small Bowel Conditions

Meckel's diverticulum
Gastrointestinal bleeding from the small intestine is a diagnostic dilemma and typically considered after other origins of upper and lower GI bleeding have been investigated, and the patient continues to have bleeding episodes, typically per rectum. MD is a congenital anomaly of the omphalomesenteric duct (2:1 male-to-female predominance) which infrequently causes problems in the adult population. Although the incidence of Meckel's may be somewhere on the scale of 2% in cadaver studies, complications from it are more of a burden in the pediatric population and decrease exponentially with age. The most common ectopic tissue found in the MD is gastric and pancreatic tissue.

Gastrointestinal stromal tumors

Although gastrointestinal stromal tumors (GISTs) are rare mesenchymal tumors that account for less than 2% of all GI malignancies,[30] they are the most common form of sarcoma of the GI tract. They derive from the interstitial cells of Cajal and are associated with activating mutations in *c-KIT* and platelet derived growth factor receptor alpha (PDGFRA). They most commonly arise in the stomach (60%), with the small intestine (30%) being the second most prevalent area of origin.[31]

Evaluation and treatment

The cornerstone of treatment involves maintaining physiologic stability with fluid and blood product. All gastrointestinal bleeding should be evaluated systematically; typically excluding an upper GI source with upper endoscopy or gastric lavage. CT angiography is also typically performed. Direct visualization of the bowel by endoscopy, followed by capsule endoscopy, may be able to localize bleeding or anomalies with more specificity. At specialized centers with a capable endoscopist, double-balloon enteroscopy may also be attempted. The use of a Meckel's scan with radionucleotide tracer (Technetium-99) may be less sensitive in adults compared with pediatrics.[32]

There has been some investigation of the benefit of tranexamic acid (TXA) in ameliorating death from gastrointestinal bleeding, as TXA has been demonstrated to have benefit in bleeding due to trauma and postpartum; however, in a large-scale international randomized control trial, there seemed to be no benefit in reduction of mortality and subsequently observed higher rates of venous thromboembolic events.[33]

Once a diagnosis has been established, surgical resection should be undertaken to remove the affected bowel. Laparoscopy may be the surgical method of choice; however, laparotomy is still an accepted standard approach. In the case of a bleeding MD, segmental bowel resection is typically done given the pathologic tissue and possibly adjacent ulcerated mucosa. Controversy around whether to resect incidentally found MD should be undertaken; the general consensus is that resection is acceptable for pediatric patients, but not in the adult population; however, if a patient is presenting with acute bleeding, obstruction, or perforation, the MD is presumed to be pathologic and should be addressed.

Follow-up

GIST encountered on final pathology should take into consideration the resection margin, size, and mitotic index; typically, at least 1 to 2 cm is considered adequate. Notation of rupture during the operation is also taken into consideration, which is especially relevant in situations where the tumor is resected under emergent circumstances, as this can increase the risk of local recurrence. Lymph node involvement is rare and not considered in oncologic resection unless clinical suspicion is high at the time of surgery. Oncology specialist review and multidisciplinary committee can determine need for adjuvant therapy with a tyrosine kinase inhibitor, such as imatinib, and the patient can be followed for long-term surveillance.[31,34]

CLINICS CARE POINTS

- Although the presence of pneumoperitoneum is seen in most perforated peptic ulcers, up to 20% are not evident on CT imaging. High suspicion needs to be obtained and further imaging is recommended with contrast studies.

- Most bleeding ulcers can be managed nonoperatively. In relatively stable patients who respond to resuscitation, endoscopy should be attempted twice, and radiologic intervention should attempted before consideration of operative exploration.

- Depending on the skill set and comfort of the individual surgeon, minimally invasive techniques can be used as an operative modality during exploration for small bowel obstruction.
- Laparotomy for acute mesenteric ischemia remains the standard for restoring vascularity to the bowel circulation, though there has been a growing interest in endovascular methods.
- When encountering neoplastic tumors during emergency surgery, care should be taken to prevent rupture and obtain a grossly disease-free margin when possible.

DISCLOSURE

The authors have nothing to disclose. This research was supported (in whole or in part) by HCA Healthcare and/or an HCA Healthcare affiliated entity. The views expressed in this publication represent those of the author(s) and do not necessarily represent the official views of HCA Healthcare, United States or any of its affiliated entities.

REFERENCES

1. Johnson JA 3rd, Thompson AR. Gastric volvulus and the upside-down stomach. J Miss State Med Assoc 1994;35(1):1–4.
2. Fuccio L, Minardi ME, Zagari RM, et al. Meta-analysis: duration of first-line proton-pump inhibitor based triple therapy for Helicobacter pylori eradication. Ann Intern Med 2007;147(8):553–62.
3. Stylopoulos N, Rattner DW, et al. Paraesophageal hernias: operation or observation? Ann Surg 2002;236(4):492–500, discussion 500-1.
4. Akhtar A, Siddiqui FS, Sheikh AA, et al. Gastric Volvulus: A Rare Entity Case Report and Literature Review. Cureus 2018;10(3):e2312.
5. Coleman C, et al. Incarcerated paraesophageal hernia and gastric volvulus: Management options for the acute care surgeon, an Eastern Association for the Surgery of Trauma master class video presentation. J Trauma Acute Care Surg 2020; 88(6):e146–8.
6. Dhamija A, Hayanga JA, Abbas KA, Abbas G. Common Tenets in Repair of Primary Paraesophageal Hernias: Reducing Tension and Maximizing Length. Thorac Surg Clin 2019;29(4):421–5.
7. Sonnenberg A. Review article: historic changes of Helicobacter pylori-associated diseases. Aliment Pharmacol Ther 2013;38(4):329–42.
8. Olbe L. Mechanisms involved inHelicobacter pyloriinduced duodenal ulcer disease: an overview. World J Gastroenterol 2000;6(5):619.
9. Lanza FL, Chan FK, Quigley EM, et al. Guidelines for prevention of NSAID-related ulcer complications. Am J Gastroenterol 2009;104(3):728–38.
10. Tarasconi A, Coccolini F, Biffl WL, et al. Perforated and bleeding peptic ulcer: WSES guidelines. World J Emerg Surg 2020;15:3.
11. Grassi R, Romano S, Pinto A, Romano L. Gastro-duodenal perforations: conventional plain film, US and CT findings in 166 consecutive patients. Eur J Radiol 2004;50(1):30–6.
12. Chung KT, Shelat VG. Perforated peptic ulcer - an update. World J Gastrointest Surg 2017;9(1):1.
13. Lee CW, Sarosi GA. Emergency ulcer surgery. Surg Clin 2011;91(5):1001–13.
14. Bertleff MJ, Lange JF. Laparoscopic correction of perforated peptic ulcer: first choice? A review of literature. Surg Endosc 2010;24(6):1231–9.

15. Gupta S, Kaushik R, Sharma R, Attri A. The management of large perforations of duodenal ulcers. BMC Surg 2005;5:15.
16. Jani K, Saxena AK, Vaghasia R. Omental plugging for large-sized duodenal peptic perforations: A prospective randomized study of 100 patients. South Med J 2006;99(5):467–71.
17. Burch JM, Cox CL, Feliciano DV, et al. Management of the difficult duodenal stump. Am J Surg 1991;162(6):522–6.
18. Ergul E, Gozetlik EO. Emergency spontaneous gastric perforations: ulcus versus cancer. Langenbeck's Arch Surg 2009;394(4):643–6.
19. Rockall TA, Logan RF, Devlin HB, et al. Risk assessment after acute upper gastro-intestinal haemorrhage. Gut 1996;38(3):316–21.
20. Kovacs TOG, Jensen DM. Endoscopic Therapy for Severe Ulcer Bleeding. Gastrointestinal Endoscopy Clinics of North America 2011;21(4):681–96.
21. Forrest JA, Finlayson ND, Shearman DJ. Endoscopy in gastrointestinal bleeding. Lancet 1974;2(7877):394–7.
22. Laine L, Jensen DM. Management of Patients With Ulcer Bleeding. American College of Gastroenterology | ACG 2012;107(3):345–60.
23. Behman R, Nathens AB, Mason S, et al. Association of Surgical Intervention for Adhesive Small-Bowel Obstruction With the Risk of Recurrence. JAMA Surg 2019;154(5):413–20.
24. Rami Reddy SR, Cappell MS. A Systematic Review of the Clinical Presentation, Diagnosis, and Treatment of Small Bowel Obstruction. Curr Gastroenterol Rep 2017;19(6):28.
25. Ten Broek RPG, Krielen P, Di Saverio S, et al. Bologna guidelines for diagnosis and management of adhesive small bowel obstruction (ASBO): 2017 update of the evidence-based guidelines from the world society of emergency surgery ASBO working group. World J Emerg Surg 2018;13:24.
26. Kuehn F, Weinrich M, Ehmann S, et al. Defining the Need for Surgery in Small-Bowel Obstruction. J Gastrointest Surg 2017;21(7):1136–41.
27. Darbyshire AR, Kostakis I, Pucher PH, et al. The impact of laparoscopy on emergency surgery for adhesional small bowel obstruction: prospective single centre cohort study. Ann R Coll Surg Engl 2021;103(4):255–62.
28. Bala M, Kashuk J, Moore EE, et al. Acute mesenteric ischemia: guidelines of the World Society of Emergency Surgery. World J Emerg Surg 2017;12:38.
29. Ojha V, Mani A, Mukherjee A, et al. Mesenteric ischemia in patients with COVID-19: an updated systematic review of abdominal CT findings in 75 patients. Abdom Radiol (NY) 2022;47(5):1565–602.
30. Şerban C, Constantin GB, Firescu D, et al. Perforated Ileal GIST Associated with Meckel Diverticulum - A Rare Pathological Entity of Surgical Acute Abdomen. Chirurgia (Bucur) 2020;115(3):404–9.
31. von Mehren M, Kane JM, Riedel RF, et al. NCCN Guidelines® Insights: Gastrointestinal Stromal Tumors, Version 2.2022. J Natl Compr Canc Netw 2022;20(11):1204–14.
32. Pattni V, Wright K, Marden P, Terlevich A. Meckel's diverticulum in an adult: an obscure presentation of gastrointestinal bleeding. BMJ Case Rep 2016;2016: bcr2015213852.
33. HALT-IT Trial Collaborators. Effects of a high-dose 24-h infusion of tranexamic acid on death and thromboembolic events in patients with acute gastrointestinal bleeding (HALT-IT): an international randomised, double-blind, placebo-controlled trial. Lancet. 2020;395(10241):1927-1936.
34. Rutkowski P, Skoczylas J, Wisniewski P. Is the Surgical Margin in Gastrointestinal Stromal Tumors Different. Visc Med 2018;34(5):347–52.

Bariatric Surgery Emergencies in Acute Care Surgery

Kalyana C. Nandipati, MBBS, MD[a],*, Kristin C. Bremer, MD[b]

KEYWORDS

- Roux-en-Y gastric bypass • Sleeve gastrectomy • Gastric band • Duodenal switch
- Internal hernia • Marginal ulcer • Enteric leak • Gastric band prolapse

KEY POINTS

- Discuss the anatomic alterations seen in common bariatric procedures.
- Discuss the differential diagnosis and workup of abdominal pain following bariatric surgery.
- Discuss the presentation, workup, and management of surgical emergencies and complications following bariatric surgery.

INTRODUCTION AND BARIATRIC SURGERY ANATOMY

Patients who have undergone bariatric surgery present unique challenges in the acute care surgery setting. Bariatric surgery is a specialized surgical procedure designed to treat obesity and its associated medical conditions. Because the obesity epidemic continues to grow, the demand for bariatric surgery has increased significantly.[1] Acute care surgeons, who specialize in the management of complex surgical emergencies, play a critical role in the management of postoperative complications for patients who have undergone bariatric surgery.

It is essential to have a basic understanding of bariatric surgery anatomy, which will help to manage complications. Although historically, there have been many bariatric surgery procedures that have gone in and out of vogue, most patients have anatomy resembling one of the following 4 most common bariatric surgeries. Bariatric surgeries are either restrictive or malabsorptive.

[a] Division of Clinical Research, Department of Surgery, Creighton University School of Medicine, Minimally Invasive Surgery, Creighton University Education Building, 7710 Mercy Road, Suite 501, Omaha, NE 68124-2368, USA; [b] Department of Surgery, Creighton University School of Medicine, Creighton University Education Building, 7710 Mercy Road, Suite 501, Omaha, NE 68124-2368, USA
* Corresponding author.
E-mail address: KalyanaNandipati@creighton.edu

Surg Clin N Am 103 (2023) 1113–1131
https://doi.org/10.1016/j.suc.2023.05.013
0039-6109/23/© 2023 Elsevier Inc. All rights reserved.
surgical.theclinics.com

Laparoscopic adjustable gastric band (LAGB) is considered as restrictive procedure. It involves dissecting the pars flaccida and creating a tunnel posterior to the superior aspect of the stomach, through which an adjustable gastric band is placed.[2]

Sleeve gastrectomy (SG) is the most common procedure currently performed and is also restrictive. SG is characterized by a vertical gastric pouch, which is created by resecting the greater curvature of the stomach, preserving the antrum and pylorus.[3]

The Roux-en-Y gastric bypass (RYGB), which is restrictive and malabsorptive, is characterized by a small gastric pouch, typically about 50 mL, which is anastomosed to the roux-limb, which can vary in length but is typically between 100 and 150 cm.[4] The majority of surgeons currently do an "antecolic" anastomosis to the stomach, creating Petersen space. This is defined as the defect between the Roux limb mesentery and the transverse mesocolon. This is typically, but not always, closed at the primary operation, although this closure can sometimes be limited by the patient's body habitus. The other approach is "retrocolic," in which the Roux limb crosses through the mesentery and runs behind the transverse colon before anastomosing to the gastric pouch posteriorly (retrogastric).[5]

The duodenal switch (DS) procedure is also restrictive and malabsorptive. It includes an SG, as detailed above. The duodenum is then divided a few centimeters past the pylorus and an intestinal bypass to the ileum is created.[6] A variation of this procedure involves bringing up a loop of ileum to anastomose to the duodenum, a "single anastomosis duodeno-ileal bypass."[7] Anastomotic procedures such as RYGB and DS pose similar challenges when dealing with emergencies in terms of internal hernias and bowel obstructions.

Knowing the anatomy of the procedure will help in management and operative planning while managing complications in bariatric patients. However, keep in mind that there may be minor surgeon-specific variations in the above procedures. Reviewing the individual patients' previous operative notes may be helpful.

ABDOMINAL PAIN FOLLOWING BARIATRIC SURGERY

Abdominal pain is a common postoperative complaint after bariatric surgery, with a reported incidence ranging from 3% to 61%.[8] The cause of abdominal pain after bariatric surgery is diverse and may include both surgical and nonsurgical causes. Therefore, a thorough diagnostic evaluation is necessary to determine the underlying cause of abdominal pain and provide appropriate management.

a. Differential diagnosis
   i. Common bariatric surgical complications that can cause abdominal pain after bariatric surgery include anastomotic leaks, internal hernias, and bowel obstruction. Gastrointestinal (GI) symptoms, such as gastroesophageal reflux disease (GERD), peptic ulcer disease, and gallbladder disease, can cause abdominal pain after bariatric surgery. Other medical conditions such as pancreatitis, appendicitis, and abdominal wall hernias should also be considered in the differential diagnosis.
b. Workup
   i. History and Physical Examination: The initial workup includes a thorough history and physical examination, with attention to the patient's vital signs. To narrow the differential, it will be particularly important to inquire about the type of bariatric surgery, duration from surgery, and any revisions or other surgical procedures. Consultation with a bariatric surgeon, preferably the surgeon who operated on the patient, should be obtained early in the course of evaluation if possible.

ii. Laboratory: Basic laboratory tests should be obtained. One could consider adding magnesium and phosphorus if dehydration or per oral intolerance is suspected, a lipase if there is any concern for pancreatitis, and a lactate if there is concern for bowel ischemia.

iii. Imaging: Ultrasonography is commonly used to diagnose gallstone disease. A computed tomography (CT) scan of the abdomen and pelvis with contrast is most helpful in identifying the most-emergent causes of abdominal pain. An upper GI series may be helpful if a leak is suspected or if a band-related complication such as prolapse is suspected. As with other causes of acute abdomen, if the patient is peritonitic on examination, then no imaging is necessary before proceeding to the operating room.

INTERNAL HERNIA

Small bowel obstruction (SBO), if not diagnosed early, can lead to significant morbidity and possible mortality in the bariatric population. SBO may be caused by internal hernias, adhesions, intussusception, postoperative edema, technical factors, bezoars, or gastric band-related complications. Internal hernia is a protrusion of small bowel or other viscus through a mesenteric defect or other artificial intra-abdominal space. This can lead to obstruction, incarceration, or strangulation of the herniated contents. Internal hernias are of particular concern in patients who have had Roux-en-Y or DS, due to the intermesenteric spaces created during the operation. The incidence of internal hernias following laparoscopic RYGB is estimated to be between 1% and 3%.[9,10] These potential spaces include Petersen's space, the mesomesenteric space and the mesocolic space[11] (**Fig. 1**).

Internal hernias are more common in patients who have retrocolic Roux limb reconstruction[9,10,12] and in patients whose mesenteric defects were not closed at the index operation.[9] Studies have investigated the role of closure of the Petersen's space in preventing internal hernias after bariatric surgery. A systematic review found that the closure of the Petersen's space significantly reduced the incidence of internal hernias compared with nonclosure.[13] Risk factors have been identified for the

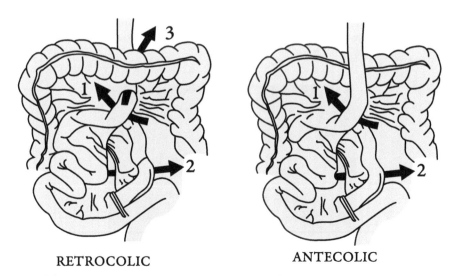

RETROCOLIC   ANTECOLIC

Fig. 1. (1) Petersen's space, (2) mesenteric space, and (3) mesocolic space.

development of internal hernias after bariatric surgery including greater weight loss after surgery[14] and counterclockwise rotation of the small bowel during initial surgery.[15]

a. Presentation

    i. Many patients with symptomatic internal hernias present with nonspecific complaints of abdominal pain, nausea, and vomiting. The most common symptom is acute onset of epigastric and left upper quadrant discomfort, often crampy or colicky in nature.[14] SBO due to internal hernia is often preceded by symptoms of intermittent obstruction, or so called "herald symptoms," such as intermittent abdominal pain associated with bloating and nausea.[16]

b. Workup

    i. CT scan is the preferred imaging modality for the diagnosis of internal hernias. Upper GI series may also show findings consistent with internal hernia, such as clustering of dilated small bowel loops in the left upper quadrant or middle abdomen but this imaging modality is less sensitive and specific than CT scan.[17] In addition to the typical findings of SBO, namely dilated small bowel loops with a transition point, numerous characteristic CT findings have been described in the literature[18,19] (**Fig. 2**):

        1. Mesenteric swirling
        2. Clustering of small bowel loops
        3. Mushroom sign": A mushroom shape of the herniated mesenteric loop due to crowding or stretching of the vessels of the mesenteric root as they travel through the hernia.
        4. Hurricane eye": a tubular or rounded shape of the distal mesenteric fat, surrounded by bowel loops.
        5. Small bowel other than duodenum behind the superior mesenteric artery.
        6. Displaced jejunojejunostomy superiorly or on the right because this anastomosis is routinely made on the left side of the abdomen.
        7. Distended gastric remnant
        8. Altered course of the superior mesenteric artery or superior mesenteric vein
        9. Widening of the jejunojejunostomy
       10. Engorgement of mesenteric lymph nodes
       11. Mesenteric edema
       12. For mesocolic internal hernias: Clustered loops of small intestine cephalad to the transverse colon in the left upper quadrant and a high position of the jejunojejunostomy.

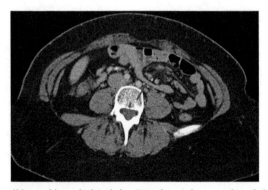

Fig. 2. Note the small bowel loop behind the SMA (*straight arrow*) and the mesenteric swirl (*curved arrow*), which is more apparent on full CT.

ii. Although CT scan can be very useful, it is important to emphasize that approximately 20% of patients with internal hernias have no evidence of internal hernia on CT.[19,20] Thus, normal radiologic studies do not exclude the presence of an internal hernia and a high clinical suspicion, even without radiographic evidence, is enough to warrant surgical exploration.

iii. MRI can be also be used to aid in the diagnosis of internal hernias and bowel obstruction. MRI has been reported to have higher sensitivity and specificity for the diagnosis of bowel obstruction after gastric bypass.[21,22] Thus, MRI may be a useful alternative to CT scan in the diagnosis of bowel obstruction after bariatric surgery.

c. Management

i. Management of internal hernias always requires surgical exploration. A delay in diagnosis and operative intervention can have devastating consequences, most notably the loss of significant lengths of small bowel leading to short gut syndrome.[23] Operative intervention typically consists of diagnostic laparoscopy with the reduction of the internal hernia and closure of all defects. During exploration, running the small bowel in retrograde fashion from the terminal ileum is helpful because the distal small bowel will be decompressed, easier to manipulate, and typically in normal anatomic position. The surgeon must take care not to damage the herniated bowel or the mesentery during the reduction process. Gentle traction of the small bowel will typically reduce the hernia. Hernia reduction can be difficult at times secondary to small bowel necrosis or other factors. An open approach should be considered in technically difficult cases or if the procedure cannot be completed safely with a laparoscopic approach. All potential internal hernia spaces, even those that are incidentally found, need to be examined and closed with a nonabsorbable suture in a running or purse-string fashion. Similarly, any incidentally found mesenteric defects discovered at the time of another surgical procedure should be closed.

OTHER CAUSES OF SMALL BOWEL OBSTRUCTION

In addition to internal hernias, there are other causes of SBO including adhesive disease, obstruction at the jejunojejunostomy, intussusception, intraluminal blood clot, and bezoars. The most common cause of early SBO within the first 30 days following RYGB is obstruction at the jejunojejunostomy, which occurs in approximately 0.4% to 1.2% of patients.[24,25] This can be caused by anastomotic edema, intraluminal clot, angulation of the Roux limb, or technical factors that may increase risk such as stapled closure of the common enterotomy.[24–26] Late SBO often results from internal hernias, ventral hernias, adhesive disease, and intussusception.[24,25,27] Intussusception is rare, with a reported incidence of less than 0.6%.[25,27] It is typically located at the jejunojejunostomy and usually occurs after significant weight loss.[27] Proposed possible lead points include staple lines, sutures, and adhesions.[27] One theory is that separation of the distal jejunum from the duodenal pacemaker causes motility disturbances from ectopic pacemakers.[28] Hemobezoars and phytobezoars, although in the differential diagnosis, are exceedingly rare.[29,30]

a. Presentation

i. Roux limb obstruction typically presents as nausea, bloating, and epigastric pain, which is temporarily relieved by emesis.[25] Biliopancreatic limb obstruction, which leads to gastric remnant distension, typically presents with nausea, bloating, hiccups, shoulder pain, and tachycardia but no vomiting.[25] Common channel obstruction presents with a combination of the above symptoms. Bilious vomiting indicates either a common channel obstruction or biliopancreatic limb obstruction with a gastro-gastric fistula.[25] Given the size of the gastric pouch, obstructed patients do not typically present with large volume emesis unless a gastro-gastric fistula is present.[25]

b. Workup

   i. CT with oral and IV contrast is the study of choice to evaluate for SBO following RYGB because abdominal X-rays are not sufficiently sensitive in this population. However, as described in the internal hernia section, providers should have a low threshold for diagnostic laparoscopy in this population even in the setting of negative imaging given that CT scans may also be nondiagnostic approximately 20% of the time.[19,20] Findings of a transition point at the jejunojejunostomy would suggest jejunojejunal(JJ) obstruction. Findings of a target sign would suggest intussusception.

c. Management

   i. Adhesive disease:
      1. Persistent obstruction requires prompt exploration as the gastric remnant cannot be decompressed with a nasogastric tube and acute gastric distension can result in staple line rupture or gastric wall perforation. Surgical management in patients with adhesive disease consists of lysis of adhesions to relieve the obstruction in addition to placement of a gastrostomy tube for decompression of the gastric remnant.[31]

   ii. Obstruction at jejunojejunostomy:
      1. Given that JJ obstruction is often caused by postoperative edema, a trial of conservative management is reasonable in the stable patient in the early postoperative period.[32] Nasogastric (NG) tubes are typically not recommended and are typically ineffective for decompression regardless given the small size of the gastric pouch. If the patient fails conservative management, operative intervention is warranted, and typically involves creation of a new side-to-side anastomosis proximal to the obstruction site.[31]

   iii. Intussusception:
      1. Intussusception with SBO following RYGB with obstruction requires immediate surgery to rule out bowel ischemia. Thus, there should be a very low threshold to proceed to the operating room if intussusception is suspected.[31] Options for repair include reduction alone, reduction with enteropexy, or resection with reconstruction of the JJ anastomosis. En bloc resection of the affected segment and reconstruction of the jejuno-jejunal anastomosis is recommended for recurrent intussusception.

   iv. Hemobezoar and phytobezoars:
      1. Hemobezoars typically occur shortly after surgery due to blood clots formed from intraluminal bleeding in the postoperative period. Emergent surgical management is warranted, with enterostomy to evacuate the blood clot. Anastomotic revision may also be necessary. Endoscopic management is an option but may be difficult given the distance to reach the JJ anastomosis and the insufflation required could risk perforation. Phytobezoars due to undigested fiber may be amenable to chemical dissolution (eg, with cellulase), endoscopic management, or surgical evacuation.[31]

   v. Obstruction following other bariatric procedures:
      1. For obstruction following DS, the overall principles are similar to what is discussed for RYGB. SBO in gastric sleeve patients should be treated similar to nonbariatric patients. The only caveat is we would recommend against blind

placement of an NG tube in the acute postoperative period following any bariatric procedure to avoid disruption of the healing staple lines, although this is a theoretical risk, which has not been well studied.

LEAK AFTER SLEEVE GASTRECTOMY

The incidence of leaks after SG varies widely in the literature, with reported rates ranging from 0.3% to 4.4%.[33,34] The variation in reported rates may be due to differences in patient populations, surgical techniques, and diagnostic criteria. Leaks after SG are rare but can be difficult to manage. Most leaks occur proximally, near the gastroesophageal junction.[35] Leak rate has been shown to be higher with use of a smaller bougie, less than 40Fr.[33] The benefit of using buttressing materials in the staple line is controversial concerning leak rate[36–38] but has been shown to decrease bleeding along the staple line.[39]

a. Presentation
   i. Leaks typically present within the first 18 days after surgery $\pm$ 14[40] but can occur as late as postop day 120.[41] Patients may present in a stable condition with only mild abdominal pain or may present with sepsis and multiorgan failure. In particular, abdominal pain, tachycardia, fever, and leukocytosis should raise suspicion for a leak.[40]
b. Workup
   i. The imaging study of choice is abdominal CT scan with oral and IV contrast. A positive study may show an intra-abdominal collection, contrast extravasation, pleural effusion, or free air. An upper GI study may also be diagnostic but is less sensitive.[40]
c. Management
   i. Management consists of nutritional support and source control. Patients with signs of sepsis or peritonitis should undergo immediate surgical intervention with washout, laparoscopic drainage, and optional placement of a jejunostomy tube for feeding. Stable patients may be treated nonoperatively with Total Parenteral Nutrition (TPN), antibiotics, and percutaneous drainage.[42] Consultation with an advanced endoscopic should also be strongly considered if such services are available.[43] Endoscopic options used include stenting, clips, glue injection, and vacuum therapy/negative pressure therapy. Endoscopic stenting involves placing a self-expanding metallic stent across the leak site to seal the defect and allow for tissue healing. Stenting has been associated with variable success with some studies reporting success up to 100%.[44] Endoscopic clips and glue have also been shown to promote healing in small retrospective studies.[45] Finally, endoscopic vacuum therapy/negative pressure therapy is a technique, which involves placing a sponge at the leak site and applying negative pressure to promote drainage and tissue healing.[46,47] In conclusion, endoscopic management has become a valuable approach for treating leaks following SG. However, the choice of technique should be individualized based on the patient's clinical condition and the surgeon's experience.
   ii. The above interventions are generally effective but further surgery may be required for refractory leaks. Definitive operative management typically consists of resection of the leaking area with a Roux-en-Y reconstruction versus placing a Roux limb to the site of the fistula.[48,49] Primary repair should only be attempted in the first 48 hours following SG. It is typically advised to wait at least 12 weeks before definitive surgical management, if possible, to avoid dense adhesions.[42] Laparoscopic SG revision involves converting the SG to another bariatric procedure, such as a RYGB[50] or biliopancreatic diversion.

LEAKS AFTER ROUX-EN-Y GASTRIC BYPASS

The incidence of leaks following laparoscopic RYGB has been decreasing with recent literature with a reported incidence of less than 1%.[51] The gastrojejunostomy (GJ) is the most common site of leak but leaks may also occur at the gastric pouch, gastric remnant, or jejunojejunostomy.[52] Risk factors for anastomotic leak after RYGB include increased body mass index (BMI), medical comorbidities, earlier abdominal surgery, longer operative time, and technical factors.[51,53,54] Patients with a BMI of more than 50 are at higher risk for leak compared with patients with a BMI of less than 50.[53] Certain medical conditions such as diabetes, hypertension, and sleep apnea have been associated with an increased risk as well.[55] Patients with earlier abdominal surgery has been identified to be at higher risk compared with the patient with no earlier abdominal surgery.[53] Prolonged surgery time has been identified as a risk factor for leak.[51] Circular staplers may also be associated with higher risk of leak compared with linear staplers.[54] Operative considerations to reduce tension include dividing the greater omentum, scoring the mesentery, or retro colic positioning were also reported impact leaks.[56] An intraoperative leak test is often helpful in identifying intraoperative leaks, allowing many to be repaired during the primary surgery if present but a negative intraoperative leak test does not eliminate the risk of a postoperative leak.[57]

a. Presentation
   i. Enteric leaks following RYGB often present with symptoms of sepsis or peritonitis. The most common symptoms are abdominal pain, tachycardia, fever, and leukocytosis.[52,56]
b. Workup
   i. CT scan with oral contrast (**Fig. 3**) has a high sensitivity and specificity for detecting a leak following gastric bypass. Although less sensitive and specific, an upper GI study (**Fig. 4**) could be considered as a first test given its lower cost but the surgeon should maintain a high index of suspicion in the setting of a negative upper GI study.[56] Of note, the false-negative rate is particularly high for upper GI studies in the setting of a jejunojejunostomy leak, which may lead to an increased morbidity and mortality for these patients due to delayed diagnosis.[58]
c. Management
   i. Principles of management for leak after RYGB are similar to sleeve including hydration and broad-spectrum antibiotics therapy with adequate drainage.

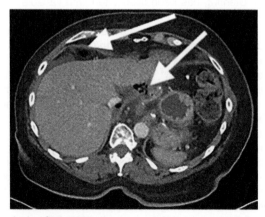

Fig. 3. CT showing leak after RYGB. Arrows pointing toward air outside of the lumen including air under diaphragm.

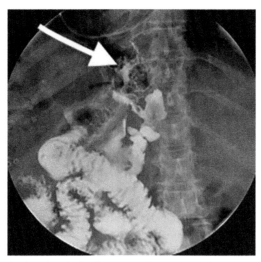

Fig. 4. Upper GI study showing leak after RYGB (*arrow* pointing toward free extravasation of contrast).

Adequate source control typically requires surgical intervention but conservative management can be considered for a well-contained perforation in a stable patient if imaging-guided drainage is possible.[59] Early reoperation within 24 hours of symptom onset is associated with better outcomes.[60] Operative management for GJ leak typically includes abdominal washout with wide drainage and suturing of the perforation with omental pedicle flap reinforcement, versus just wide drainage if not possible. If the defect is severe, anastomotic revision may be necessary, which should be avoided as revision carries at risk. Jejunojejunostomy leaks are typically amenable to repair, rarely requiring anastomotic revision. Placement of a gastrostomy tube in the gastric remnant is also recommended in order to avoid gastric dilation given the likelihood of ileus from contamination and can later be used for nutritional support in the setting of a GJ anastomotic leak or gastric pouch leak. Before resuming oral intake, follow-up imaging should be done to confirm resolution of the leak.[56] Chronic leaks that persist more than 30 days are difficult to treat. Endoscopic management of GJ leaks has been increasingly used. Endoscopic stents, glue, clips, and vacuum therapy have been used with variable success.[61,62] Endoscopic stents have been more commonly reported in retrospective studies with success ranging up to more than 80%.[63] Stent placement has been plagued with migration, which could be a significant issue.[56] These more complex chronic cases are best managed under the guidance of an experienced bariatric surgeon.

MARGINAL ULCER

RYGB has been performed since late 1960s. Since then, marginal ulcers (MUs) have been associated with significant morbidity. A marginal ulcer is an ulceration at or near the GJ of a RYGB patient. The incidence has been quoted as between 0.6% and 25%,[64] and they may occur in the early or late postoperative period.[65] These ulcers typically occur at the anastomosis (50%) or jejunum (40%).[66] The jejunal aspect of the anastomosis is more prone to ulceration because it is not typically exposed to acid in its native location. Risk factors include nonsteroidal anti-inflamatory drug

(NSAID) use, *Helicobacter pylori* infection, obstructive sleep apnea, female sex, smoking, and alcohol dependence.[67] Technical factors such as tension on the anastomosis and having too large of a gastric pouch containing too many parietal cells might also contribute.[68]

Cause of MUs has been widely debated for decades. Several factors have been implicated in the development of marginal ulcer includes pouch size, technique of anastomosis (staple vs hand sewn), suture material (absorbable vs nonabsorbable), Roux limb configuration (antecolic vs retrocolic) and *H pylori*. Smoking and NSAIDs are important factors shown to be associated with the development of MUs.[67] Marginal ulcer may also be secondary to chronic comorbid conditions that induce chronic mucosal damage either secondary to vasculopathy or inflammation. Studies have found smoking to be a strong predictor of MU formation with a greater risk of nonhealing of MUs.[65,66] This is attributed to nicotine-induced vasoconstriction as a key factor in the development on marginal ulceration or recurrence. Just as NSAIDs are also reported to be a major factor in peptic ulcer disease, they are associated with the development of MUs.[64,67] Inhibition of cyclo-oxygenase causes decreased prostaglandin E2 levels, thus interfering with the stomach's natural defense barrier. The role of *H pylori* on MU formation has been under debate for the past decade. *H pylori* screening and eradication before surgery remains controversial but still continues to be a common practice following marginal ulcer diagnosis.

a. Presentation
   i. The most common presenting symptoms for MUs are pain, dysphagia, nausea, and vomiting.[65] The positive predictive value of individual symptoms is as low as 40%.[69] Complications that may occur as the marginal ulcer progresses include bleeding, obstruction, or perforation.

b. Workup
   i. The gold standard of marginal ulcer diagnosis is endoscopy. On endoscopy, the ulcer will be visible at the GJ anastomosis (**Fig. 5**), typically on the jejunal aspect. There may be suture material present, which should be removed endoscopically if possible. If there is acute bleeding from the ulceration, this may also be controlled endoscopically. Imaging studies may also aid in diagnosis. A marginal ulcer may

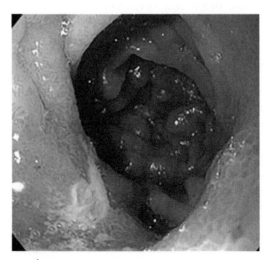

Fig. 5. MU visible on endoscopy.

appear in an Upper GI study as a small collection of contrast within the ulcer near the GJ anastomosis that remains as luminal contrast continues to move distally. A CT with oral contrast may show similar findings to the Upper GI study. Testing for *H pylori* is recommended to complete the workup and assist in the treatment.

c. Management

    ii. Unless the patient is presenting with signs of acute bleeding or perforation, management is typically medical. Medical management is typically with a proton -pump inhibitor (PPI) ± sucralfate. Typical regimens include a PPI bid and sucralfate 1 g qid with repeat endoscopy every few months until the ulcer has healed. Opening the PPI capsules is suggested to have better bioavailability and promote ulcer healing.[70] Management also includes eliminating risk factors such as stopping NSAID use, smoking cessation, and *H pylori* eradiation if applicable.

    iii. GJ revision is needed for more emergent presentations and for complications such as anemia, gastrogastric fistulas, or ulcers that are refractory to conservative management. In order to revise the GJ, the gastric pouch is stapled proximal to the anastomosis and the Roux limb is divided distal to the anastomosis. Endoscopy can be helpful to ensure the entirety of the ulcer is being resected. If necessary, the gastric pouch should be reduced in size to the goal of 20 to 30 mL in volume to reduce the number of acid-producing parietal cells in the pouch. The gastrojejunal anastomosis is then recreated using the method of choice. Truncal vagotomy via either abdominal approach or thoracic approach is another option used with mixed results. If medical management and GJ revision have failed, Roux-en-Y reversal may be considered but this should be performed by a surgeon with experience in complex bariatric surgery revisions. Recently, endoscopic suturing has been used with variable success for complications of MUs such as bleeding ulcers, nonhealing ulcers, and gastrogastric fistulas.[71]

    iv. Perforated MUs are a surgical emergency in the majority of circumstances. Laparoscopic repair of MUs with omental patch reinforcement is associated with low morbidity. Ulcer recurrence is approximately 5%, indicating that these patients need long-term follow-up.[72] Resection and revision has also been done with low recurrence rates in appropriate situations.[73] However, a contained perforation with no evidence of peritonitis can be further evaluated with a contrast study and may be managed with conservative management. Please see the section on enteric leak after RYGB for more details.

    v. Bleeding MUs may be managed similarly to bleeding peptic ulcers. Endoscopic management with conservative treatment is successful in the majority of cases. Failed endoscopic or interventional radiology options require surgical exploration with oversewing the ulcer or resection of the anastomosis with reanastomosis.[74]

GASTRIC BAND PROLAPSE/SLIPPED BAND

LAGB used to be one of the most common weight loss procedures but fewer and fewer gastric bands are placed every year. However, emergencies associated with LAGB are still encountered with relative frequency. Common emergencies associated with LAGB include band slippage, band erosion, and port-related problems. Band prolapse, also known as a slipped band, is defined as herniation of the gastric wall proximally through the adjustable gastric band, with caudal migration of the band.[75] This prolapse can be of the anterior or posterior fundus. This complication is more common when a band is placed using a perigastric approach rather than the pars flaccida technique (16% vs 4%).[76,77] Most bariatric surgeons also plicate the gastric fundus and cardia from under the band to the gastric pouch above the band as another measure to help prevent prolapse, although there has been mixed data on if this helps decrease the rate of prolapse.[78]

a. Presentation
    i. Gastric band prolapse may present with signs of outflow obstruction including nausea, vomiting, food intolerance, dysphagia, or worsening GERD.[75] Acute presentation with abdominal pain, signs of peritonitis, or laboratory abnormalities that do not resolve with fluid resuscitation should raise suspicion for gastric ischemia, volvulus, or perforation, all of which are rare.[79,80]
b. Workup
    i. Workup for band prolapse typically consists of an x-ray or upper GI study. When the band is in the correct position, it lies in an 8 o'clock to 2 o'clock orientation on x-ray. The phi angle, which is the angle between the spine and the bottom of the gastric band, should be less than 58°.[81] These findings would typically indicate an anterior prolapse, given that the band rotates to a horizontal position. Posterior prolapse typically presents with an "O sign," given that the band rotates vertically.[82] An upper GI study would typically show a dilated pouch with abnormal emptying. Endoscopy can also be used but is typically not necessary.
c. Management
    i. When a patient presents with band prolapse, the first thing that should be done is band decompression. This is done by removing all of the fluid from the port in the abdominal wall using a needle and syringe. If symptoms resolve with band decompression, the patient can be discharged on a liquid diet and slow reinflation can be performed under fluoroscopic guidance.[75] If the patient's obstructive symptoms fail to resolve, then emergency surgery is indicated. Laparoscopic removal of the LAGB should be performed to avoid gastric necrosis.
    ii. Surgery typically consists off lysing the adhesions over the band until visualization of the buckle, unbuckling it versus cutting the band, and removal of the band, port, and tubing. Some surgeons will also dismantle the wrap and/or disrupt the band capsule but this is not necessary in the acute setting because it may be done later when the patient returns for revision. Patients should be warned that they will most likely regain the weight they had lost with the band following removal. They could be considered for revisional surgery in the future but this is not typically offered at the time of band removal in the acute setting given that the stomach is typically edematous and friable.[75]

BAND EROSION

Band erosion is a complication of LAGB surgery where the band erodes into the stomach lining. LAGB erosion is a relatively uncommon complication of weight loss surgery. In a systematic review, the incidence of band erosion is around 1.46%.[83] Factors that increase the risk of LAGB erosion include band migration, port infection, band overtightening, and a history of abdominal surgery.

a. Presentation
    i. Patients present with symptoms include abdominal pain, which may be sharp or dull, and may be associated with nausea and vomiting. The patient may have difficulty tolerating oral intake due to the band obstructing the passage of food through the stomach. Infection or bleeding may develop at the site of erosion.
b. Workup
    i. LAGB erosion may be suspected based on imaging studies such as x-rays or CT scans. However, endoscopy is the ideal diagnostic modality because it may be

used to visualize the eroded band, determine the extent of the erosion, and may aid in management.

c. Management

    i. The management of band erosion typically involves band removal with or without revisional surgery. If there is a significant portion of band eroded into the stomach, it can be removed via an endoscopic approach and other components of the tubing and port can be removed with a laparoscopic approach. Before undergoing any revisional surgery, the patient may need to receive antibiotics to treat any infection and stabilize their condition.

POSTOPERATIVE HEMORRHAGE

Postoperative hemorrhage is correlated with increased hospital stay, morbidity, and mortality in bariatric patients.[84,85] In general, the algorithm is the same as in nonbariatric patients but there are a few considerations in this population, which we will discuss in this section.

a. Presentation

    i. The presentation of postoperative hemorrhage is the same for bariatric patients because it is for any patient following intra-abdominal surgery. The source of bleed may be extraluminal or intraluminal, particularly at any of the anastomoses or staple lines.

b. Workup

    i. The same hemorrhagic workup used for other postoperative patients may be used following bariatric surgery. In general, a more thorough workup can be considered for a stable patient but emergent return to the operating room is necessary for an unstable patient.

c. Management

    i. Unstable patients must return to the operating room immediately for exploration and control of bleeding. Of note, endoscopy can be a useful adjunct, particularly if an extraluminal bleed is not found.

    ii. For stable patients with a slow bleed, nonoperative management can be considered:

        1. Fluid resuscitation and/or blood products with trended hemoglobin to assess response.

        2. Correction of any coagulopathies and reversal of anticoagulants.

        3. Upper endoscopy for the evaluation and control of bleeding at the GJ. If an intraluminal bleed is suspected and there is no bleed seen in the gastric pouch, bleeding from the gastric remnant should be suspected. Access to the lumen of the gastric remnant can be obtained via the following techniques. Of note, these techniques are also useful for endoscopic retrograde cholangiopancreatography (ERCP) access:

            a. Laparoscopic-assisted transgastric endoscopy—A laparoscopic trocar is surgically placed into the gastric remnant and serves as a conduit for an endoscope.[86]

            b. Percutaneous endoscopic gastrostomy—Access the stomach as if you were placing a gastrostomy tube but then pass an endoscope through the hole. When endoscopy is complete, a G tube is placed.[87]

            c. Retrograde double balloon endoscopy—A very technically challenging procedure, which requires a specially trained advanced endoscopist.

    iii. Interventional radiology may be consulted for control of bleeding if endoscopy is ineffective.

iv. If the above interventions are unsuccessful in controlling the bleed, operative intervention is indicated.

SUMMARY

Bariatric surgery is a common and effective treatment of obesity but it is not without complications. Acute care surgeons should be aware of the most common complications of bariatric surgery including bowel obstruction, enteric leaks, MUs, LAGB complications, and bleeding. Early recognition and management of these complications is critical for optimal patient outcomes, and may involve a combination of medical management, endoscopic interventions, and surgical interventions. In addition, acute care surgeons should be aware of the unique anatomy of bariatric surgery patients. Overall, a multidisciplinary approach to the management of bariatric surgery complications is recommended, involving collaboration between surgeons, endoscopists, radiologists, nutritionists, and other specialists.

CLINICS CARE POINTS

- Internal hernias are one of the most common causes of SBO after RYGB and DS. However, they can have minimal symptoms and about 20% of internal hernias have negative CT scans.
- Management of internal hernias always requires operative intervention. Diagnostic laparoscopy and laparoscopic reduction of internal hernia with closure of the mesenteric defect is required. If surgeons encounter necrotic bowel and are not able to reduce it with a laparoscopic approach, conversion to an open approach and reduction of the hernia, with or without small bowel resection, is an acceptable alternative.
- The most common location of marginal ulcers is at GJ anastomosis. MUs can present with bleeding or perforation. Most bleeding from marginal ulcers can be managed with an endoscopic approach or a nonoperative approach. The management of perforated marginal ulcers is similar to that of perforated peptic ulcer disease. Laparoscopic exploration and omental pedicle flap closure of the perforated marginal ulcer is the most common initial approach.

DISCLOSURE

The authors have nothing to disclose.

REFERENCES

1. ASMBS. Estimate of bariatric surgery numbers, 2011-2020. American Society for Metabolic and Bariatric Surgery. Available at: https://asmbs.org/resources/estimate-of-bariatric-surgery-numbers. Published June 27, 2022. Accessed February 17, 2023.
2. Seeras K, Acho RJ, Prakash S. Laparoscopic Gastric Band Placement. [Updated 2022 Nov 23]. In: StatPearls [Internet]. Treasure Island (FL): StatPearls Publishing; 2022 Jan-. Available at: https://www.ncbi.nlm.nih.gov/books/NBK526062/. Accessed February 17, 2023.
3. Ramaswamy A. Laparoscopic sleeve gastrectomy - A sages wiki article. SAGES. Available at: https://www.sages.org/wiki/laparoscopic-sleeve-gastrectomy/. Published August 14, 2016. Accessed February 17, 2023.
4. Shouhed D, Fernandez-Ranvier G. Chapter 1: introduction and overview of current and emerging operations. In: Herron D, editor. Bariatric surgery complications and

emergencies. Springer International Publishing Switzerland; 2016. p. 1–15. https://doi.org/10.1007/978-3-319-27114-9_12.

5. Mitchell BG, Gupta N. Roux-en-Y Gastric Bypass. [Updated 2022 Jul 25]. In: Stat-Pearls [Internet]. Treasure Island (FL): StatPearls Publishing; 2022 Jan-. Available at: https://www.ncbi.nlm.nih.gov/books/NBK553157/. Accessed February 17, 2023.

6. Conner J, Nottingham JM. Biliopancreatic Diversion With Duodenal Switch. [Updated 2022 Sep 19]. In: StatPearls [Internet]. Treasure Island (FL): StatPearls Publishing; 2022 Jan-. Available at: https://www.ncbi.nlm.nih.gov/books/NBK563193/. Accessed February 17, 2023.

7. Sánchez-Pernaute A, Herrera MA, Pérez-Aguirre ME, et al. Single anastomosis duodeno-ileal bypass with sleeve gastrectomy (SADI-S). One to three-year follow-up. Obes Surg 2010;20(12):1720–6.

8. Simoni AH, Ladebo L, Christrup LL, et al. Chronic abdominal pain and persistent opioid use after bariatric surgery. Scand J Pain 2020;20(2):239–51.

9. Geubbels N, Lijftogt N, Fiocco M, et al. Meta-analysis of internal herniation after gastric bypass surgery. Br J Surg 2015;102(5):451–60.

10. Ahmed AR, Rickards G, Husain S, et al. Trends in internal hernia incidence after laparoscopic Roux-en-Y gastric bypass. Obes Surg 2007;17(12):1563–6.

11. Corey B, Grams J. Chapter 10: internal hernias: prevention, diagnosis, and management. In: Herron D, editor. Bariatric surgery complications and emergencies. Springer International Publishing Switzerland; 2016. p. 133–45. https://doi.org/10.1007/978-3-319-27114-9_12.

12. Al Harakeh AB, Kallies KJ, Borgert AJ, et al. Bowel obstruction rates in antecolic/antegastric versus retrocolic/retrogastric Roux limb gastric bypass: a meta-analysis. Surg Obes Relat Dis 2016;12(1):194–8.

13. Apostolou KG, Lazaridis II, Kanavidis P, et al. Incidence and risk factors of symptomatic Petersen's hernias in bariatric and upper gastrointestinal surgery: a systematic review and meta-analysis. Langenbeck's Arch Surg 2023;408(1):49.

14. Geubbels N, Röell EA, Acherman YI, et al. Internal herniation after laparoscopic roux-en-Y Gastric bypass surgery: pitfalls in diagnosing and the introduction of the AMSTERDAM classification. Obes Surg 2016;26(8):1859–66.

15. Nandipati KC, Lin E, Husain F, et al. Counterclockwise rotation of Roux-en-Y limb significantly reduces internal herniation in laparoscopic Roux-en-Y gastric bypass (LRYGB). Gastrointest Surg 2012;16(4):675–81.

16. Gandhi AD, Patel RA, Brolin RE. Elective laparoscopy for herald symptoms of mesenteric/internal hernia after laparoscopic Roux-en-Y gastric bypass. Surg Obes Relat Dis 2009;5(2):144–9 [discussion: 149].

17. Ahmed AR, Rickards G, Johnson J, et al. Radiological findings in symptomatic internal hernias after laparoscopic gastric bypass. Obes Surg 2009;19(11):1530–5.

18. Dilauro M, McInnes MD, Schieda N, et al. Internal hernia after laparoscopic roux-en-Y gastric bypass: optimal CT signs for diagnosis and clinical decision making. Radiology 2017;282(3):752–60.

19. Nawas MA, Oor JE, Goense L, et al. The diagnostic accuracy of abdominal computed tomography in diagnosing internal herniation following roux-en-Y gastric bypass surgery: a systematic review and meta-analysis. Ann Surg 2022;275(5):856–63.

20. Obeid A, McNeal S, Breland M, et al. Internal hernia after laparoscopic Roux-en-Y gastric bypass. J Gastrointest Surg 2014;18(2):250–5 [discussion: 255-6].

21. Yamamoto A, Nishida M, Muranaka T, et al. Usefulness of magnetic resonance imaging for the diagnosis of bowel obstruction after gastric bypass surgery. Obes Surg 2008;18(6):643–8.

22. Wang Y, Aslam R, Riaz M, et al. The role of magnetic resonance imaging in the diagnosis of internal hernias after laparoscopic Roux-en-Y gastric bypass surgery. Obes Surg 2019;29(9):2888–94.

23. McBride CL, Petersen A, Sudan D, et al. Short bowel syndrome following bariatric surgical procedures. Am J Surg 2006;192(6):828–32.

24. Cho M, Carrodeguas L, Pinto D, et al. Diagnosis and management of partial small bowel obstruction after laparoscopic antecolic antegastric Roux-en-Y gastric bypass for morbid obesity. J Am Coll Surg 2006;202(2):262–8.

25. Koppman JS, Li C, Gandsas A. Small bowel obstruction after laparoscopic Roux-en-Y gastric bypass: a review of 9,527 patients. J Am Coll Surg 2008;206(3): 571–84.

26. Shimizu H, Maia M, Kroh M, et al. Surgical management of early small bowel obstruction after laparoscopic Roux-en-Y gastric bypass. Surg Obes Relat Dis 2013;9(5):718–24.

27. Daellenbach L, Suter M. Jejunojejunal intussusception after Roux-en-Y gastric bypass: a review. Obes Surg 2011;21(2):253–63.

28. Hocking MP, McCoy DM, Vogel SB, et al. Antiperistaltic and isoperistaltic intussusception associated with abnormal motility after Roux-en-Y gastric bypass: a case report. Surgery 1991;110(1):109–12. PMID: 1866683.

29. Caputo V, Facchiano E, Soricelli E, et al. Small bowel obstruction after laparoscopic roux-en-Y Gastric bypass caused by hemobezoar: a case series and review of literature. Surg Laparosc Endosc Percutan Tech 2021;31(5):618–23.

30. Ben-Porat T, Sherf Dagan S, Goldenshluger A, et al. Gastrointestinal phytobezoar following bariatric surgery: systematic review. Surg Obes Relat Dis 2016;12(9): 1747–54.

31. Elnahas A, Okrainec A. Chapter 12: gastrointestinal obstruction in the bypass patient. In: Herron D, editor. Bariatric surgery complications and emergencies. Springer International Publishing Switzerland; 2016. p. 161–71. https://doi.org/10.1007/978-3-319-27114-9_12.

32. Lewis CE, Jensen C, Tejirian T, et al. Early jejunojejunostomy obstruction after laparoscopic gastric bypass: case series and treatment algorithm. Surg Obes Relat Dis 2009;5(2):203–7.

33. Parikh M, Issa R, McCrillis A, et al. Surgical strategies that may decrease leak after laparoscopic sleeve gastrectomy: a systematic review and meta-analysis of 9991 cases. Ann Surg 2013;257(2):231–7.

34. Aboueisha MA, Freeman M, Allotey JK, et al. Battle of the buttress: 5-year propensity-matched analysis of staple-line reinforcement techniques from the MBSAQIP database. Surg Endosc 2022. https://doi.org/10.1007/s00464-022-09452-y. Epub ahead of print. PMID: 35927350.

35. Aurora AR, Khaitan L, Saber AA. Sleeve gastrectomy and the risk of leak: a systematic analysis of 4,888 patients. Surg Endosc 2012;26(6):1509–15.

36. D'Ugo S, Gentileschi P, Benavoli D, et al. Comparative use of different techniques for leak and bleeding prevention during laparoscopic sleeve gastrectomy: a multicenter study. Surg Obes Relat Dis 2014;10(3):450–4.

37. Knapps J, Ghanem M, Clements J, et al. A systematic review of staple-line reinforcement in laparoscopic sleeve gastrectomy. J Soc Laparoendosc Surg 2013; 17(3):390–9.

38. Gagner M, Kemmeter P. Comparison of laparoscopic sleeve gastrectomy leak rates in five staple-line reinforcement options: a systematic review. Surg Endosc 2020;34(1):396–407.

39. Wang Z, Dai X, Xie H, et al. The efficacy of staple line reinforcement during laparoscopic sleeve gastrectomy: a meta-analysis of randomized controlled trials. Int J Surg 2016;25:145–52.

40. Al Zoubi M, Khidir N, Bashah M. Challenges in the diagnosis of leak after sleeve gastrectomy: clinical presentation, laboratory, and radiological findings. Obes Surg 2021;31(2):612–6.

41. Sakran N, Goitein D, Raziel A, et al. Gastric leaks after sleeve gastrectomy: a multicenter experience with 2,834 patients. Surg Endosc 2013;27(1):240–5.

42. Sethi M, Parikh M. Chapter 7: enteric leaks after sleeve gastrectomy: prevention and management. In: Herron D, editor. Bariatric surgery complications and emergencies. Springer International Publishing Switzerland; 2016. p. 91–105. https://doi.org/10.1007/978-3-319-27114-9_12.

43. Gjeorgjievski M, Imam Z, Cappell MS, et al. A Comprehensive review of endoscopic management of sleeve gastrectomy leaks. J Clin Gastroenterol 2021;55(7):551–76.

44. Gumbs AA, Duffy AJ, Bell RL. Incidence and management of gastrocutaneous fistulas after laparoscopic sleeve gastrectomy. Surg Obes Relat Dis 2013;9(6):941–6.

45. Ritter LA, Wang AY, Sauer BG, et al. Healing of complicated gastric leaks in bariatric patients using endoscopic clips. J Soc Laparoendosc Surg 2013;17(3):481–3.

46. Leeds SG, Burdick JS. Management of gastric leaks after sleeve gastrectomy with endoluminal vacuum (E-Vac) therapy. Surg Obes Relat Dis 2016;12(7):1278–85.

47. Archid R, Bazerbachi F, Abu Dayyeh BK, et al. Endoscopic negative pressure therapy (ENPT) is superior to stent therapy for staple line leak after sleeve gastrectomy: a single-center cohort study. Obes Surg 2021;31(6):2511–9.

48. Robert M, Pasquer A. Laparoscopic roux-en-Y fistulo-jejunostomy for a chronic gastric leak after sleeve gastrectomy. Obes Surg 2021;31(11):5100–1.

49. Nedelcu M, Danan M, Noel P, et al. Surgical management for chronic leak following sleeve gastrectomy: Review of literature. Surg Obes Relat Dis 2019;15(10):1844–9.

50. Degrandi O, Nedelcu A, Nedelcu M, et al. Roux-en-Y gastric bypass for the treatment of leak following sleeve gastrectomy. Obes Surg 2021;31(1):79–83.

51. Vidarsson B, Sundbom M, Edholm D. Incidence and treatment of leak at the gastrojejunostomy in Roux-en-Y gastric bypass: a cohort study of 40,844 patients. Surg Obes Relat Dis 2019;15(7):1075–9.

52. Durak E, Inabnet WB, Schrope B, et al. Incidence and management of enteric leaks after gastric bypass for morbid obesity during a 10-year period. Surg Obes Relat Dis 2008;4(3):389–93 [Erratum in: Surg Obes Relat Dis. 2008 Sep-Oct;4(5):689. PMID: 18407803].

53. Gonzalez R, Bowers SP, Venkatesh KR, et al. Preoperative factors predictive of complicated postoperative management after Roux-en-Y gastric bypass for morbid obesity. Surg Endosc 2003;17(12):1900–4.

54. Edholm D, Sundbom M. Comparison between circular- and linear-stapled gastrojejunostomy in laparoscopic Roux-en-Y gastric bypass–a cohort from the Scandinavian Obesity Registry. Surg Obes Relat Dis 2015;11(6):1233–6.

55. Alizadeh RF, Li S, Inaba C, et al. Risk factors for gastrointestinal leak after bariatric surgery: MBASQIP analysis. J Am Coll Surg 2018;227(1):135–41.
56. Afeneh C, Dakin G. Chapter 6: enteric leaks after gastric bypass: prevention and management. In: Herron D, editor. Bariatric surgery complications and emergencies. Springer International Publishing Switzerland; 2016. p. 81–90. https://doi.org/10.1007/978-3-319-27114-9_12.
57. Haddad A, Tapazoglou N, Singh K, et al. Role of intraoperative esophagogastroenteroscopy in minimizing gastrojejunostomy-related morbidity: experience with 2,311 laparoscopic gastric bypasses with linear stapler anastomosis. Obes Surg 2012;22(12):1928–33.
58. Lee S, Carmody B, Wolfe L, et al. Effect of location and speed of diagnosis on anastomotic leak outcomes in 3828 gastric bypass cases. J Gastrointest Surg 2007;11(6):708–13.
59. Ballesta C, Berindoague R, Cabrera M, et al. Management of anastomotic leaks after laparoscopic Roux-en-Y gastric bypass. Obes Surg 2008;18(6):623–30.
60. Jacobsen HJ, Nergard BJ, Leifsson BG, et al. Management of suspected anastomotic leak after bariatric laparoscopic Roux-en-y gastric bypass. Br J Surg 2014;101(4):417–23.
61. Bartell N, Bittner K, Kaul V, et al. Clinical efficacy of the over-the-scope clip device: a systematic review. World J Gastroenterol 2020;26(24):3495–516.
62. Joo MK. Endoscopic approach for major complications of bariatric surgery. Clin Endosc 2017;50(1):31–41.
63. Yang J, Zeng X, Cao Y, et al. Endoscopic stent placement for the management of gastric bypass leaks: a retrospective study. Surg Endosc 2021;35(2):747–54.
64. Coblijn UK, Goucham AB, Lagarde SM, et al. Development of ulcer disease after Roux-en-Y gastric bypass, incidence, risk factors, and patient presentation: a systematic review. Obes Surg 2014;24(2):299–309.
65. El-Hayek K, Timratana P, Shimizu H, et al. Marginal ulcer after Roux-en-Y gastric bypass: what have we really learned? Surg Endosc 2012;26(10):2789–96.
66. Azagury DE, Abu Dayyeh BK, Greenwalt IT, et al. Marginal ulceration after Roux-en-Y gastric bypass surgery: characteristics, risk factors, treatment, and outcomes. Endoscopy 2011;43(11):950–4.
67. Rodrigo DC, Jill S, Daniel M, et al. Which Factors Correlate with Marginal Ulcer After Surgery for Obesity? Obes Surg 2020;30(12):4821–7 [Erratum in: Obes Surg. 2020 Oct 12;: PMID: 32939660].
68. Sapala JA, Wood MH, Sapala MA, et al. Marginal ulcer after gastric bypass: a prospective 3-year study of 173 patients. Obes Surg 1998;8(5):505–16.
69. Huang CS, Forse RA, Jacobson BC, et al. Endoscopic findings and their clinical correlations in patients with symptoms after gastric bypass surgery. Gastrointest Endosc 2003;58(6):859–66.
70. Tansel A, Graham DY. New insight into an effective treatment of marginal ulceration after roux-en-Y gastric bypass. Clin Gastroenterol Hepatol 2017;15(4):501–3.
71. Barola S, Magnuson T, Schweitzer M, et al. Endoscopic suturing for massively bleeding marginal ulcer 10 days post roux-en-Y gastric bypass. Obes Surg 2017;27(5):1394–6.
72. Martinino A, Bhandari M, Abouelazayem M, et al. Perforated marginal ulcer after gastric bypass for obesity: a systematic review. Surg Obes Relat Dis 2022;18(9):1168–75.
73. Crawford CB, Schuh LM, Inman MM. Revision gastrojejunostomy versus suturing with and without omental patch for perforated marginal ulcer treatment after roux-en-Y gastric bypass. J Gastrointest Surg 2023;27(1):1–6.

74. Rogers A, Kennedy A, O'Rourke RW. Management of acute bleeding after gastric bypass surgery. Surg Clin North Am 2016;96(4):861–71.

75. Krikhely A, Gluzman E, Sherwinter D. Chapter 16: gastrointestinal obstruction in the bypass patient. In: Herron D, editor. Bariatric surgery complications and emergencies. Springer International Publishing Switzerland; 2016. p. 203–14. https://doi.org/10.1007/978-3-319-27114-9_12.

76. Fielding GA, Duncombe JE. Clinical and radiological follow-up of laparoscopic adjustable gastric bands, 1998 and 2000: a comparison of two techniques. Obes Surg 2005;15(5):634–40.

77. O'Brien PE, Dixon JB, Laurie C, et al. A prospective randomized trial of placement of the laparoscopic adjustable gastric band: comparison of the perigastric and pars flaccida pathways. Obes Surg 2005;15(6):820–6.

78. Mizrahi S, Avinoah E. Technical tips for laparoscopic gastric banding: 6 years' experience in 2800 procedures by a single surgical team. Am J Surg 2007; 193(2):160–5.

79. Lunca S, Vix M, Rikkers A, et al. Late gastric prolapse with pouch necrosis after laparoscopic adjustable gastric banding. Obes Surg 2005;15(4):571–5.

80. Kicska G, Levine M, Raper S, et al. Gastric volvulus after laparoscopic adjustable gastric banding for morbid obesity. Am J Roentgenol 2007;189(6):1469–72.

81. Sonavane SK, Menias CO, Kantawala KP, et al. Laparoscopic adjustable gastric banding: what radiologists need to know. Radiographics 2012;32(4):1161–78.

82. Pieroni S, Sommer EA, Hito R, et al. The "O" sign, a simple and helpful tool in the diagnosis of laparoscopic adjustable gastric band slippage. AJR Am J Roentgenol 2010;195(1):137–41.

83. Egberts K, Brown WA, O'Brien PE. Systematic review of erosion after laparoscopic adjustable gastric banding. Obes Surg 2011 Aug;21(8):1272–9.

84. Heneghan HM, Meron-Eldar S, Yenumula P, et al. Incidence and management of bleeding complications after gastric bypass surgery in the morbidly obese. Surg Obes Relat Dis 2012;8(6):729–35.

85. Dick A, Byrne TK, Baker M, et al. Gastrointestinal bleeding after gastric bypass surgery: nuisance or catastrophe? Surg Obes Relat Dis 2010;6(6):643–7.

86. Roberts KE, Panait L, Duffy AJ, et al. Laparoscopic-assisted transgastric endoscopy: current indications and future implications. J Soc Laparoendosc Surg 2008;12(1):30–6.

87. Gill KR, McKinney JM, Stark ME, et al. Investigation of the excluded stomach after Roux-en-Y gastric bypass: the role of percutaneous endoscopy. World J Gastroenterol 2008;14(12):1946–8.

Management of Colonic Emergencies

Haddon Pantel, MD[a], Vikram B. Reddy, MD, PhD, MBA[a],*

KEYWORDS

- Malignancy • Diverticulitis • Obstruction • Perforation • Abscess • Fistula
- Hemorrhage • Inflammatory bowel disease

KEY POINTS

- The etiology of colonic emergencies includes a wide-ranging and diverse set of pathologic conditions.
- The nuanced complexity in these situations usually revolves around the nonsurgical and/or endoscopic options and deciding when to proceed to the operating room.
- The primary principle of surgery will be to control the offending pathology, reestablish bowel continuity (only in a stable patient while minimizing any untoward complications) or provide an ostomy (diversion or end-stoma), and mitigate any long-term adverse outcomes.

INTRODUCTION

The etiology of colonic emergencies includes a wide-ranging and diverse set of pathologic conditions. Fortunately, for the surgeon treating a patient with one of these emergencies, the surgical management of these various causes is limited to choosing among proximal diversion, segmental colectomy with or without proximal diversion, or a total abdominal colectomy with end ileostomy (or rarely, an ileorectal anastomosis). The nuanced complexity in these situations usually revolves around the nonsurgical and/or endoscopic options and deciding when to proceed to the operating room.

MALIGNANCY

Malignancies of the colon and rectum can present as surgical emergencies due to obstruction, perforation, or bleeding. Such acute presentations account for 1 in 5 newly diagnosed colon cancers,[1] and management should be individually tailored. Clinical decision-making and treatment planning should stabilize the problem, either

a Colon and Rectal Surgery, Yale University School of Medicine, 450 George Street, New Haven, CT 06510, USA
* Corresponding author.
E-mail address: vikram.reddy@yale.edu

Surg Clin N Am 103 (2023) 1133–1152
https://doi.org/10.1016/j.suc.2023.06.006
0039-6109/23/© 2023 Elsevier Inc. All rights reserved.
surgical.theclinics.com

sepsis or bleeding, then attempt to achieve optimal oncologic control and maximize the opportunity for additional oncologic treatment[2] (**Fig. 1**).

Obstruction

Preoperative management of a patient with an obstructing colon or rectal cancer starts with correcting hypovolemia, electrolyte abnormalities, and anemia resulting from the underlying malignancy. In patients with an incompetent ileocecal valve and/or significant distention of the small bowel and stomach, a nasogastric tube should be inserted for decompression to mitigate any risk of aspiration during the induction of anesthesia. If resources and time permit, these patients also benefit from evaluation by an enterostomal therapy or wound ostomy continence nurse for preoperative stoma marking and education. If time or resources do not permit this, marking in the perioperative area by the surgeon in the infraumbilical fat mound or the upper abdomen while avoiding any creases, pant lines, or bony prominences. Patients with signs of systemic illness, concern for perforation, or impending perforation should be immediately taken to the operating room. Patients who do not require an immediate operation should complete appropriate staging with a computed tomography (CT) scan with IV contrast of the chest, abdomen, and pelvis and a baseline carcinoembryonic antigen. An MRI of the pelvis is also needed for staging rectal cancers. The surgical approach to these patients and intraoperative decision-making is described below. However, endoscopic stent placement may be a temporizing measure in select patients.

A self-expanding endoscopic stent can be placed for decompression in patients with obstructing left-sided colon cancer with potentially curable disease. Although, traditionally, patients with an obstructing tumor within range of an extended right colectomy were not considered a candidate for endoscopic stenting, current recommendations, although based on weaker retrospective data, support the selective use of decompressive endoscopic stents with interval colectomy.[2] It is important to note that outside of a palliative setting, a stent is a bridge to surgery instead of a destination.[3] This is due to the potential risk of stent erosion, migration, or tumor regrowth. The interval from stent to surgery is not well defined but the risk of stent complication

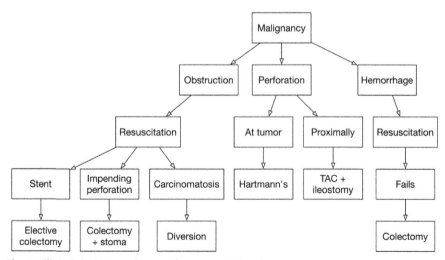

Fig. 1. Clinical decision-making and treatment planning.

increases after 6 days, and this is an often-cited interval-to-interval colectomy.[4] The technical consideration and details of endoscopic stent placement are outside the realm of this article. However, when considering endoscopic stent placement, the patient's clinical condition, surgical and endoscopic expertise, and goals of care should all be factored into decision-making.

Patients with signs of systemic illness, concern for perforation, or impending perforation should be expeditiously taken to the operating room. The operative choice is usually between a proximal diverting loop stoma or segmental colectomy with or without diversion. In certain situations, such as synchronous cancers or a distal tumor with proximal colonic ischemia or perforation, an extended resection, such as a subtotal colectomy, may be needed. When selecting the extent of the resection, the surgeon must consider the location of the tumor or tumors, the curative or palliative intent of surgery, and the patient's overall clinical stability.

Proximal diversion should be undertaken in several clinical scenarios. Locally advanced tumors that may be challenging to resect in the unstable patient should undergo proximal diverting loop stoma.[5] If, at the time of exploration or on preoperative workup, the patient is found to have diffuse metastatic disease with an unlikely path to cure, a proximal loop colostomy or loop ileostomy will be sufficient. Patients with obstruction due to extraperitoneal rectal cancer should undergo the creation of a diverting loop colostomy.[6] Although the loop colostomy can be situated in the transverse colon or sigmoid, we prefer to create a sigmoid loop colostomy. This facilitates an easier elective low anterior resection if the patient improves to undergo curative surgery. The efferent limb of the stoma can become the specimen's proximal extent, and an end to end anastomosis (EEA) stapler's anvil can be placed in the afferent limb of the stoma to create the anastomosis. A distal stoma may also preserve colonic reach to create a low pelvic anastomosis if required. A midtransverse loop colostomy is technically more straightforward and can be left in situ to serve as a proximal diversion during a later low anterior resection. The stoma location hinges on surgeon preference and patient habitus but, regardless, a well-constructed stoma is essential. A loop stoma can be created via an open or minimally invasive approach depending on the surgeon's comfort and visualization with pneumoperitoneum. The advantages of a minimally invasive procedure in this setting include the usual well-established benefits and a faster time to recovery with smaller incisions to facilitate a shorter interval between surgery and initiation of systemic treatment. Regardless of approach, the assessment of the proximal dilated colon and cecum should be undertaken to ensure no signs of ischemia or perforation, which would require resection.

Resection should be undertaken for most patients with obstructing colon cancer, apart from those scenarios mentioned above, where a proximal diverting loop stoma is preferred. When considering resection in this emergent setting, surgeons should ensure a safe resection without compromising oncologic principles while minimizing any untoward morbidity, which could delay or even prevent adjuvant oncologic treatment. A segmental colectomy using oncologic principles with adequate margins and high vascular ligation should be performed. Following resection, a decision to create either an end stoma or an anastomosis with or without proximal diversion is required following the same principles that guide any colorectal resection: the condition of the bowel, the condition of the peritoneal cavity, and the condition of the patient. Patients who are hemodynamically unstable during surgery or are medically frail should undergo an end stoma. Patients who are stable and otherwise fit can be considered for anastomosis. The anastomotic leak rate is significantly higher in emergency surgery for obstructing cancer and can be roughly 3 times higher than those reported in elective cases.[7] When creating an anastomosis in the setting of obstruction, we prefer to perform an end-to-side colorectal anastomosis or side-to-side ileocolonic anastomosis, given the relative size mismatch encountered between the proximal obstructed bowel and the decompressed distal bowel. Special consideration should be given in the setting of malignancy due to the higher likelihood of needing adjuvant chemotherapy, and proximal diversion should be strongly considered if an anastomosis is undertaken to mitigate any potential septic complications of anastomotic leak and ensure the timely administration of chemotherapy.

Perforation

Perforation is the natural progression of untreated, obstructing colorectal cancer. Perforation occurs either directly from tumor erosion through the colonic wall or, more commonly, proximal to the obstruction due to distention commonly affecting the cecum due to its thinner wall.[8] Surgical management is as outlined for malignant obstruction, with several notable exceptions. In the setting of perforation, preoperative management should include standard therapy for intra-abdominal infection, including resuscitation, empiric antibiotic coverage for intestinal flora, and other evidence-based practices following sepsis guidelines.[9] There is no role for endoscopic stent placement in the setting of perforation. Additionally, in the free perforation of colon cancer, proximal diverting loop stoma is not recommended without control of the perforation. A segmental resection, including the perforating cancer, should be undertaken with a stoma. In the setting of a perforation proximal to an obstructing tumor, resection of the tumor and the perforated segment should be undertaken.[2]

Bleeding

Chronic anemia due to slow, low-volume bleeding is common in patients with colon cancer. However, significant bleeding requiring emergent operation is uncommon.[10] In the rare case of a large-volume lower GI bleed from colon cancer, the initial approach should be similar to any significant GI bleed. This includes adequate intravenous access with large bore IV, resuscitation and transfusion as needed, correction of any coagulopathy, and close clinical monitoring.[11] In the setting of continual bleeding, current guidelines from the American Society of Colorectal Surgeons recommend management with nonsurgical approaches when possible.[2] However, with persistent bleeding, segmental colectomy following oncologic principles is recommended.

Intussusception

Intussusception is a rare cause of large bowel obstruction in adults compared with the pediatric population.[12] The classic triad of abdominal pain, emesis, and red-currant stools seen in children is rarely encountered but most adults present in a nonspecific manner. In the adult population, the most common cause for the lead point of the intussusception is a malignancy but benign processes, including polyps, gastrointestinal stromal tumors, and lipomas, have been implicated. Intussusception is often identified on cross-sectional imaging such as CT, which has a high diagnostic accuracy.[13] Colonoscopy can be used to determine the malignant potential of a lead point but colonoscopic decompression is not recommended.[14] Surgical intervention requiring oncologic resection of the affected segment with or without diversion is the recommended management given the malignant potential.

DIVERTICULITIS

Diverticulitis encompasses a wide range of pathology and clinical problems ranging in severity and management approaches. Although the underlying pathophysiology of diverticulitis is not well understood, the medical and surgical management of the disease continues to evolve and change. Regardless of severity and symptoms, diverticulitis involves symptomatic segmental colitis in the presence of diverticulosis. When evaluating and treating patients with presumed diverticulitis, it is crucial to consider and rule out alternative causes of segmental colitis, such as Crohn disease (CD), infectious colitis, ischemic colitis, or inflammation associated with underlying colon cancer (**Fig. 2**).

Uncomplicated diverticulitis

Uncomplicated diverticulitis is limited to inflammation of the colon only, with no free perforation, stricture, or fistula. The initial management of uncomplicated diverticulitis and subsequent recurrent attacks is outside the scope of this article because it does not represent a colonic emergency. However, an initial evaluation in patients with suspected diverticulitis should include a CT of the abdomen and pelvis as the most appropriate imaging study.[15] Once the diagnosis is made, the initial management is nonoperative in the acute setting. This includes either empiric antibiotic coverage for gastrointestinal flora or observation without antibiotics in selected patients. Omission of antibiotics in acute uncomplicated diverticulitis can be considered in select patients with minimal comorbid conditions and with limited signs of inflammation and/or infection.[16–19] Of these, a select few can be managed with observation without antibiotics as an outpatient.[17–19] After resolution, a colonoscopy should be performed if one has not been performed recently to rule out other causes of segmental colitis such as CD, infectious colitis, ischemic colitis, or inflammation associated with an underlying colon cancer.[15] The rate of misdiagnosis of an underlying malignancy after an episode of presumed uncomplicated diverticulitis ranges from 0.7%[20] to 1.3%.[21]

Complicated Diverticulitis

Complicated diverticulitis includes free perforation, stricture, or fistula. Free perforation and stricture with large bowel obstruction constitute situations where emergent

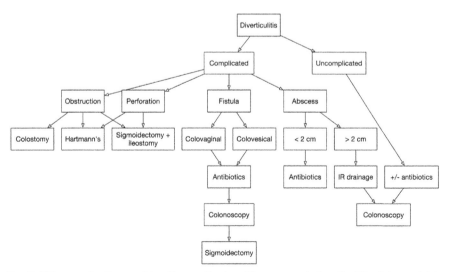

Fig. 2. When evaluating and treating patients with presumed diverticulitis, it is crucial to consider and rule out alternative causes of segmental colitis.

surgical intervention is warranted. Free perforation, diffuse peritonitis, or failure to respond to medical therapy are indications for surgery.[15] Surgical options are limited to a segmental colectomy or proximal diversion in rare cases. However, intraoperative decision-making following segmental colectomy can be nuanced regarding the creation of end colostomy or primary anastomosis with proximal loop stoma or primary anastomosis alone.

Proximal diverting loop colostomy is primarily of historical significance in the emergent surgical management of diverticulitis but there are rare instances where it may still be used. Historically, proximal loop colostomy was the first stage of 3 planned operations, followed by resection of the inflamed colon, and finally, stoma closure with the restoration of intestinal continuity.[22] Segmental colectomy involving the affected colon is the recommended operative approach to diverticulitis.[15] Yet, diversion and drainage can be used in highly selective circumstances. With a clinically unstable patient, proximal loop colostomy and wide drainage can allow for damage control and ongoing resuscitation while controlling sepsis. Additionally, this approach can be considered if the surgeon lacks the expertise, comfort, or available resources to deal with a hostile pelvis or retroperitoneum.[23]

Segmental colectomy is the recommended procedure for urgent management of diverticulitis.[15] Preoperatively, patients should be counseled and marked for colostomy and ileostomy, even when considering an anastomosis without diversion, to provide more flexibility in intraoperative decision-making. If time permits, ureteral stent placement, if available, can be performed to aid in identifying the ureter. The surgical approach, whether open, laparoscopic, or robotic-assisted, depends on surgeon expertise, patient stability, and resource availability. Regardless of the approach, the goal is to resect the diseased colon safely. Following colonic mobilization, proximal transection should be at an area of normal and healthy inflammation-free colon. Resection of all colonic diverticulosis is unnecessary and may hinder future attempts to reestablish continuity. The site of distal division may vary depending on whether an anastomosis is being created. If an anastomosis (with or without proximal diversion) is planned, distal transection should include all the sigmoid to the top of the rectum. This can be confirmed by visualizing the splaying out of the individual taenia coli because they form the outer layer of the muscularis propria of the rectum as a longitudinal full-thickness smooth muscle layer.[24] This can sometimes be misleading, and it is our practice to perform intraoperative flexible sigmoidoscopy before distal transection to ensure the planned site is truly at the rectum, free of diverticula while ensuring no major folds in the rectum, which may inhibit passage of a stapler. Transection at the upper rectum is essential as creating a colorectal instead of a colocolonic anastomosis is associated with a significant reduction in recurrent diverticulitis.[25] If considering an end colostomy, distal transection can be just distal to the perforation with resection of the remaining sigmoid and the creation of a colorectal anastomosis at the time of stoma closure.

The decision to create an anastomosis should follow the same safe principles of anastomotic decision-making outlined in this article. The advantages of creating an end colostomy following resection are the elimination of risk for anastomotic leak and reduced operative time, which is beneficial in an unstable patient. Although this may be the safest option at the time of index operation, there are several long-term drawbacks to this approach. Rates of restoration of intestinal continuity are much lower in the setting of end colostomy as opposed to anastomosis with proximal diversion.[26,27] Additionally, rates of postoperative complications are much higher for closure of end colostomy as compared with loop ileostomy.[26,27] In the appropriate clinical setting, when an end colostomy is created, it is often beneficial to place long tagging sutures of a nonabsorbable suture to aid in identifying the rectum at the time of stoma closure. When creating an end colostomy, achieving adequate reach for an everted colostomy may be challenging in someone with an obese abdominal wall, obese mesentery, or an immobile thickened mesentery from chronic inflammation. If this is the case, a loop-end colostomy can be used. Splenic flexure mobilization can also be performed but this should be undertaken cautiously because this may make the closure of an end colostomy more challenging by hindering the reach needed for an eventual anastomosis. If creating an everted suitable end colostomy is challenging, an anastomosis can be made in a stable patient, and a loop ileostomy can be used as an alternative because this may be easier to mobilize out of the abdominal wall.

Creation of a colorectal anastomosis can be performed safely after emergent sigmoidectomy for diverticulitis in select patients.[26,27] This is often performed with a proximal diverting stoma. When an anastomosis is created in this setting, a colon to rectal anastomosis should be fashioned to reduce the risk of recurrent diverticulitis.[25] Patients undergoing anastomosis, compared with nonrestorative resection, have been shown to have similar morbidity rates and organ space infection.[28,29] There are also increased long-term stoma-free rates and less morbidity associated with stoma closure.[28,29] Data are limited for the safety of creating an unprotected colorectal anastomosis—of the 3 randomized control trials, which included primary anastomosis with or without proximal diversion in the test arm, only 2 had significant numbers of patients who underwent primary anastomosis without proximal diversion.[27,30] In subgroup analysis, these patients' outcomes were no worse but these findings are likely confounded by selection bias as proximal diversion was not part of the randomization scheme.

INFLAMMATORY BOWEL DISEASE

The management of colonic emergencies due to inflammatory bowel disease (IBD) has evolved in recent times with the advent of biologics but surgery remains a mainstay. Most IBD emergencies are best addressed in a multidisciplinary approach with surgeons, gastroenterologists, radiologists, interventional radiologists, enterostomal therapy nurses, and nutritional services.

IBD includes a group of chronic inflammatory disorders including, but not limited to, ulcerative colitis (UC) and CD (**Fig. 3**). UC is characterized by mucosal inflammation, which typically starts distally in the rectum and progresses proximally to involve

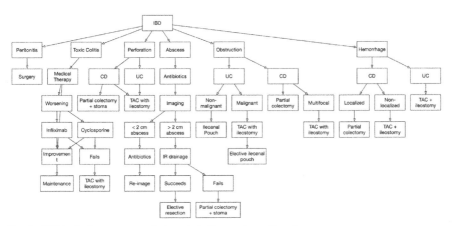

Fig. 3. IBD includes a group of chronic inflammatory disorders.

varying segments of the colon or the entire colon in pancolitis. Terminal ileal inflammation can often mimic CD but is secondary to backwash ileitis. CD is characterized by transmural inflammation that can affect any location from the mouth to the anus. The transmural nature of the inflammation accounts for abscesses and fistulae.

The incidence of IBD is increasing worldwide, even though most studies report stability or even decreasing incidence in North America and Europe.[31] The pathogenesis of IBD may be related to an overexcessive mucosal immune response triggered by luminal bacteria (environment) in a genetically susceptible individual.

Management of IBD is individualized and depends on several factors, including type, distribution, disease severity, comorbidities, and patient preferences. The nonsurgical management of IBD is beyond the scope of this article, and the information will focus on surgical management. However, medical management with immunomodulators and biologics has altered the need for surgical intervention. Colectomy rates in UC have also decreased since the introduction of biologics but the risk of a colectomy increases with time from diagnosis.[32] The risk of surgery for CD also has decreased,[33–35] and may be multifactorial but biologics, early diagnosis, and early treatment have been found to be helpful. However, patients with CD still show a progression toward a stricturing (stenosis) or penetrating (fistula/abscess) phenotype. Patients who do not progress to these phenotypes are considered to have an inflammatory phenotype and usually avoid surgery. The progression toward a stricturing or penetrating phenotype compounded by the failure of biologic therapy often leads to hospitalization and emergency surgery.

Acute complications requiring surgery include severe colitis, toxic megacolon, uncontrolled bleeding, perforation, and rarely obstruction.[36] The acute complications requiring surgery for CD include obstruction, abscess/fistula, severe colitis, toxic megacolon, bleeding, and perforation.[36]

Toxic Colitis

Toxic or fulminant colitis can be a potentially life-threatening manifestation of both UC and CD. It can be the initial presentation of the underlying disease in up to 30%. Toxic colitis has been noted in up to 10% of patients with UC,[37] whereas 50% of all toxic colitis cases may be secondary to Crohn colitis.[38] The presentation can be similar to a disease flare with fever, colicky abdominal pain, anorexia, and the sudden onset of bloody diarrhea. Diagnostic criteria as defined by Truelove and Witts[39] are described in **Table 1** below. Megacolon is a rare complication of toxic colitis with radiographic evidence of segmental or total colonic dilation to at least 6 cm.[40]

Patients with signs and symptoms of toxic colitis require admission, resuscitation, close monitoring, and an attempt at medical management if they are not in extremis. Intravenous fluid resuscitation to correct hypovolemia, serial laboratory testing, and

Table 1 Ulcerative colitis diagnostic criteria as defined by Truelove and Witts		
Symptoms	**Severe Colitis**	**Mild Colitis**
Diarrhea	≥ 6	≤ 4
Blood in stool	Large	Small
Fever	≥ 37.5 C	None
Tachycardia	≥ 90 bpm	None
Anemia	≤ 10.5 g/dL hemoglobin	None
Erythrocyte sedimentation rate	≥ 30 mm/h	Normal

correction of serum electrolytes are necessary. Nutritional assessment with prealbumin and albumin levels is undertaken. In the absence of ileus or toxic megacolon, attempts at enteral nutrition are preferred and effective compared with parenteral nutrition.[41] Imaging such as an abdominal radiograph or CT may assess the degree of inflammation and dilation or the presence of pneumoperitoneum. Discontinuation and further avoidance of opioids, anticholinergics, and antidiarrheals should be undertaken to minimize impaired intestinal motility and further dilation. Cautious use of opioids for pain can be entertained. Barium enemas should also be avoided. Nonsteroidal anti-inflammatory drugs may worsen mucosal damage and are generally avoided during an exacerbation.[42] Initiation of prophylactic low-molecular-weight heparin is essential in this population because they carry a 3 to 6 times higher incidence of venous thromboembolism.[43] Serial abdominal examinations, close monitoring of vitals, and serial abdominal imaging (especially when on high-dose steroids) should be instituted.

A multidisciplinary approach to the assessment of the emergency is warranted. Hepatitis B serologies and interferon-gamma release assays are obtained in anticipation of salvage with biologic therapy. Superinfection with Cytomegalovirus (CMV) and *Clostridium difficile* should be ascertained because they can worsen the presentation of colitis in patients with IBD. Stool studies for *C difficile* toxin and biopsy of ulcers for CMV via a flexible sigmoidoscopy should be entertained. Flexible sigmoidoscopy may also reveal the extent of the disease. *C difficile* infection is a risk factor for colectomy but can be treated with oral vancomycin and intravenous metronidazole.[44] CMV colitis responds to intravenous ganciclovir followed by oral valganciclovir. CMV coinfection has been noted in 25% to 36% of patients with steroid-refractory colitis.[45] Stool testing for other pathogens and treatment, if present, may also be warranted. Prophylactic antibiotics in the setting of toxic colitis have not been shown to increase the odds of remission or protection from a colectomy.[46,47]

If the patient has no peritonitis or pneumoperitoneum on imaging, medical management with steroids is initiated. Methylprednisolone (60 mg/d) and hydrocortisone (300 mg/d) in divided doses are the medications of choice.[48] Higher doses of intravenous steroids have not shown higher remission or colectomy-avoidance rates and should be avoided.[49] Patients should be observed closely during the next 3 to 5 days for an improvement, and if noted, can be transitioned to maintenance steroids. Failure should prompt rescue therapy with biologics or consideration of colectomy. Cyclosporine,[50] a calcineurin inhibitor, and infliximab,[51] a chimeric monoclonal antibody to human tumor necrosis factor-α, are the most commonly used agents for rescue, with 2 randomized controlled trials showing no difference in colectomy-free survival and adverse events.[52,53] Ustekinumab, a monoclonal antibody targeting interleukin-12 and -23, has also been successfully used for inducing remission.[54] Tofacitinib is a newer Janus Kinase inhibitor that has shown some efficacy in inducing remission in biologic-experienced patients.[55] Infliximab remains the agent of choice due to its reduced toxicity profile, ease of administration, and conversion to a maintenance regimen.[56]

Patients who clinically deteriorate or fail to respond within the first 72 hours of initiation of treatment require surgery. Delay in surgical care increases postoperative morbidity.[57] Postoperative mortality rates can increase to 40% with perforation.[40,58] The surgical option is a total or subtotal colectomy with ileostomy.[59,60] The distal rectal stump may be stapled off, oversewn, or brought to the lower midline skin and matured as a mucous fistula. An intraperitoneal distal rectal stump dehiscence with a pelvic abscess is a concern and can be managed with a pelvic drain or a rectal catheter to decompress the rectum.[61] Segmental resections will not address the entire diseased colon. A proctocolectomy should be avoided due to its higher postoperative morbidity and mortality in the emergent setting due to increased operative time, higher risk of blood loss, pelvic sepsis, risk of pelvic nerve damage, and prevention of future reconstruction via an ileorectal anastomosis or ileoanal pouch.[38] However, rectal perforation and unremitting rectal bleeding may warrant a proctocolectomy.

Perforation

Free perforation occurs in 2% of patients with UC and 1% to 3% with CD.[36] In UC, perforations are usually associated with toxic colitis or megacolon, and perforations in the absence of megacolon should raise suspicion for CD. Perforations in CD may occur in any part of the gastrointestinal tract and are usually due to a distal stricture causing proximal bowel dilation and perforation or due to penetrating disease where the perforation occurs at the site of inflammation. Rarely, free perforation can occur at the site of an abscess or due to a previously undiagnosed malignancy. Iatrogenic perforation can also occur due to colonoscopic surveillance. Immunosuppression and high-dose steroids can mask peritonitis, and keen clinical acumen and imaging studies such as an abdominal radiograph or a CT scan are needed. Intravenous fluid resuscitation, broad-spectrum antibiotics, and emergent surgical intervention are required.

The extent of surgery is tailored to the underlying IBD and individualized in patients with CD. The recommended procedure for managing perforation in UC is a total or subtotal colectomy with end ileostomy as described for toxic colitis or megacolon. Proctocolectomy should be avoided to decrease morbidity and mortality while preserving the option for a restorative proctocolectomy with an ileoanal pouch.

Perforations in CD can occur anywhere in the intestines, and the location and cause of the perforation define the operative management. Proximal diversion should be considered for all patients with malnutrition, steroid use, abscess or fistula,[62] and multiple earlier resections.[63] Perforation due to a terminal ileal stricture can be managed with an ileocecectomy with end ileostomy or anastomosis with proximal diversion. Perforations associated with toxic colitis are best served with a total colectomy with ileostomy. A perforation due to bowel dilation from an isolated colonic stricture will require resection of the stricture and the proximal dilated bowel with the perforation and creation of a stoma with or without a mucous fistula. Perforation of the cecum with a left-sided stricture may even require a subtotal colectomy with ileostomy. Management of perforation in a diseased segment of bowel is more straightforward and will require a resection of the diseased portion with anastomosis with or without proximal diversion or a Hartmann procedure. Although a segmental resection is associated with a higher recurrence of CD than a subtotal colectomy,[64,65] the functional outcomes after a segmental resection are better,[66] and should be entertained unless there is more than one segment involved.

Abscess and Fistula

Abscesses and fistulae are more common in CD, with an incidence of 10% to 28%,[67,68] and their presence in a patient with UC should raise suspicion of CD. Abscesses, more so than perforations, are the more frequent indication for intervention in CD.

The transmural inflammation of the bowel wall can lead to ulceration, which causes secondary adhesions with the adjacent tissues. Microperforation of the affected ulcerated wall can lead to a contained area of inflammation (phlegmon), which can then coalesce into an abscess contained within these adhesions. Abscesses occur most commonly in the right lower quadrant from terminal ileal inflammation. Abscesses can be intraperitoneal, retroperitoneal, or mesenteric. Imaging modalities such as CT and MRI are helpful in the diagnosis and may aid in management.

Intravenous antibiotics with coverage of enteric gram-negative bacteria and anaerobes are initiated along with fluid resuscitation. Smaller abscesses can be managed with antibiotics alone. Percutaneous drainage is feasible in collections larger than 2 cm in size.[69] Successful drainage carries less morbidity than surgical intervention and can decrease the overall complication rate after eventual surgery.[70] Clinical improvement should be noted in 3 to 5 days; if not, reimaging should be performed to assess progression, fistula development, inadequate drainage, or displacement of the preexisting catheter. Percutaneous drainage alone resolves the emergency in more than 90% of patients.[71] It also allows prompt resumption of biologic therapy and facilitates an elective resection, if needed, with a lower risk of an ostomy. The inability to percutaneously drain the abscess or clinical worsening warrants surgical intervention: resection with proximal diversion is the gold standard. Closed suction drainage of the abscess cavity may also be beneficial.

Even with successful percutaneous drainage, 20% to 77% will require elective bowel resection. Indications for surgery should be individualized but the development of a nonhealing fistula or a stricture at the area of the inflammation are the most common reasons. A trial of infliximab in biologic-naive patients or one of the newer agents in those already on biologic therapy should be entertained to attempt closure of the fistula before proceeding with a resection.

Obstruction

Similar to abscesses, obstructions are more common in CD than in UC. An obstruction in a patient with UC should raise the suspicion of malignancy or misdiagnosed CD. Small bowel obstructions are more common in CD, while isolated colonic obstructions account for 5% to 17%.[72] Colonic strictures in CD can be malignant in 6.8%, and biopsies may be essential to guide surgical management.[72] In CD, obstructions can be secondary to active inflammation or fibrostenotic disease due to chronic inflammation. The transmural nature of the inflammation in CD can cause edema of a segment of bowel wall with resultant luminal compromise. The affected segment may or may not have preexisting narrowing due to fibrostenotic disease. Rarely, an adjacent phlegmon or abscess can cause compression and obstruction but this is more likely in the small bowel rather than in the colon. Management of a patient with obstruction begins with intravenous fluid hydration. Cross-sectional imaging such as CT or MRI is usually obtained and can aid in identifying the location and cause of the obstruction. MRI may be more useful in differentiating active versus chronic versus acute-on-chronic inflammation, especially in CD. Endoscopic evaluation to assess for malignancy is warranted.

If there is no evidence of malignancy in patients with UC, a proctocolectomy with an ileoanal pouch is reasonable. However, if there is concern about malnutrition, other comorbidities, immunosuppression, or rectal sparing, a total colectomy with ileostomy should be undertaken, preserving the option for a future restorative proctocolectomy. If there is a malignancy or suspicion of malignancy, oncologic guidelines for resection should be followed. If the stricture is in the rectum, a proctocolectomy with ileostomy should be undertaken rather than a restorative proctocolectomy to prevent any ileoanal pouch damage should adjuvant radiation therapy be necessary. A malignant stricture in the colon can be managed with a proctocolectomy with an ileoanal pouch unless there is evidence of locally advanced disease or carcinomatosis, where a total colectomy with ileostomy is more appropriate.

In the absence of malignancy, medical management is a reasonable initial attempt with underlying CD, and surgical intervention is reserved for failure of medical management. Steroids and biologic therapy (initiation of infliximab in biologic-naive patients or change to a different biologic agent) are often successful in ameliorating the luminal compromise associated with active inflammation. However, 75% will go on to require some intervention, most commonly a dilation or surgical resection.

Endoscopic approaches, including dilation of the stricture or stricturotomy, have been successful for primary and anastomotic strictures. Most patients have excellent short-term success but long-term results decline, requiring the need for further redilation or some requiring surgical intervention within 2 years. Endoscopic stricturotomy is a newer option gaining popularity, and higher success rates have been noted. Failure of medical or endoscopic management requires surgery.

Surgery for managing CD strictures includes segmental resection with anastomosis with or without proximal diversion, segmental resection with end colostomy, and subtotal colectomy with ileostomy or proximal diversion in cases where resection of the stricture increases morbidity.

Hemorrhage

Although IBD can be characterized by mild bleeding, life-threatening hemorrhage requiring surgery is rare in IBD and has an incidence of less than 10%.[36] The cause of the bleeding is different in UC and CD and is related to the underlying pathologic condition. Although bleeding in UC is due to the underlying diffuse mucosal ulceration, with an increased risk of bleeding noted in pancolitis, CD is characterized by focal erosion into an intestinal vessel at the site of a transmural ulcer.

The initial approach to management in both CD and UC is similar: large-bore intravenous access, resuscitation with fluids or blood products as needed, and an attempt at localization of the bleeding. Nasogastric decompression and lavage to identify any upper gastrointestinal bleed is needed as 30% of patients with CD can have a bleeding duodenal ulcer as the cause. Localization of the bleeding is far more critical in CD than in UC due to the segmental nature of the disease in CD. Localization can be performed with CT angiography or interventional angiography with or without provocation.[73] Surgical intervention is reserved for severe hemorrhage with an ongoing transfusion requirement of greater than 6 units of packed red blood cells or an inability to manage the disease.

Surgical treatment of UC involves a total colectomy with ileostomy. A proctectomy should be avoided because it increases morbidity. Persistent rectal bleeding can be noted in up to 12% of patients despite a colectomy. However, this can be managed by packing the rectal stump with epinephrine-soaked gauze or saline enemas with epinephrine. Rarely a proctectomy is needed to control unremitting hemorrhage from the rectal stump.

In CD, a segmental disease, localization is necessary and can guide the surgical options. The small bowel (65%) is the most likely bleeding site, whereas the colon accounts for only 12%. The increased prevalence of CD in the small bowel likely explains this difference rather than any difference in the underlying pathophysiology. If the source is localized to a segment of colon, and the patient is healthy, a segmental colectomy is reasonable. If the source cannot be localized in patients with Crohn colitis, a subtotal colectomy with ileostomy is warranted. In a hemodynamically stable patient with rectal sparing, consideration should be given to a total colectomy with ileorectal anastomosis.

FUNCTIONAL EMERGENCIES

Unlike mechanical or inflammatory causes leading to obstruction or perforation, disordered motility of the colon can lead to emergencies requiring intervention. Functional abnormalities arise due to the luminal milieu, as in volvulus, or due to irregular colonic activity, as seen in Ogilvie syndrome.

Volvulus

Colonic volvulus is caused by a torsion of a mobile segment of the colon on a broad mesentery around its narrow pedicle, which can lead to luminal obstruction and progressive vascular compromise of the affected part of bowel with ensuing ischemia, infarction, and perforation. It accounts for about 2.5% of the large bowel obstruction (LBO) in developed countries but increases to about 80% elsewhere. In the USA, sigmoid volvulus accounts for 60%, cecal volvulus accounts for nearly 40%, and transverse colon volvulus is rare, accounting for about 2% to 4% (**Fig. 4**).

Sigmoid volvulus is frequently endemic in the "volvulus belt," which extends across Latin America, sub-Saharan Africa, the Middle East, Pakistan, India, Scandinavia, and Russia. A high-fiber diet and longer sigmoid colon lengths explain this geographic distribution.[74] In nonendemic areas, chronic constipation and dysmotility are predisposing factors.[74] In the United States, although sigmoid volvulus is common in elderly men who are institutionalized or have neuropsychiatric disorders, cecal volvulus is more common in young women.[74]

Patients with volvulus usually present with abdominal distention, obstipation, nausea, and pain. An incompetent ileocecal valve can lead to small bowel distention also. With advanced volvulus, where there are signs of ischemia and perforation, patients can present in extremis. Given the nonspecific presentation, imaging (historically radiographs but currently CT) will confirm the diagnosis and often show "coffee bean" or "bent inner tube" signs indicating the volvulized segment of the colon along with swirling of the mesenteric vessels of the affected segment.[75] If the patient has peritonitis, sepsis, or clinical deterioration, volvulus is often diagnosed at exploration.

In the absence of perforation, ischemia, or sepsis, an attempt at detorsion of the volvulus should be undertaken with a rigid proctoscope, or preferably, a colonoscope. With air insufflation, the scope can be advanced to the point of torsion. The scope should be advanced into the proximal colon with gentle manipulation, and the obstructed segment of colon is decompressed if the mucosa is viable. A rectal tube is placed to continue the decompression and to allow bowel preparation in anticipation of a semielective segmental resection. The success rate of endoscopic decompression is 60% to 95%[76,77] and carries low morbidity but the morbidity can be as high as 3%, reflecting the underlying comorbidities of the patient.[75] The risk of recurrence after endoscopic decompression can be as high as 70%, with a majority

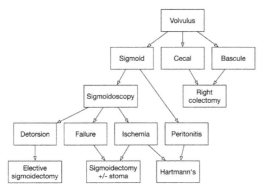

Fig. 4. Volvulus UC.

recurring within the first few months,[75,77,78] and an elective or semielective sigmoid resection should be undertaken.[76] Unfortunately, due to the multiple medical comorbidities of the patient presenting with a volvulus, surgical resection should be individualized.

The mortality of sigmoid volvulus presenting with perforation or ischemia can be as high as 33%.[74,75] Surgical resection of the gangrenous colon requires a resection without detorsion of the mesentery to prevent the release of bacteria, endotoxin, and potassium sequestered in the diseased colon. Midmesenteric division should be undertaken with an energy device to facilitate this type of resection. An end colostomy, rather than an anastomosis, is fashioned. If the proximal colon or cecum is compromised from the volvulus, a subtotal colectomy with ileostomy may be preferred to multiple segmental resections.

A sigmoid colectomy is the operation of choice for an elective or semielective surgical management.[74,76,78,79] Nonresectional options such as sigmoidopexy, mesenteroplasty, or operative detorsion carry a higher recurrence rate and are not recommended.[74,75,79] A sigmoidectomy can be performed laparoscopically or through a limited open incision. The redundant sigmoid colon is resected. Scarring over the peritoneal lining of the mesentery is encountered. Neither splenic flexure mobilization is needed nor does any other segment of redundant colon need to be removed. Due to the dilated lumen of the proximal colon, an end-to-side Baker anastomosis to the rectum is preferred. An end colostomy or a diverting loop ileostomy may be needed depending on the clinical status and comorbidities of the patient.

In contrast to a sigmoid volvulus, endoscopic detorsion has a low success rate and no role in managing a cecal volvulus. The procedure of choice is a right colectomy.[76] In a clinically unstable patient, an end ileostomy should be considered. The procedure can be performed open or laparoscopically. A cecopexy has a higher risk of recurrence and is not the procedure of choice.[76]

A cecal bascule is a variant of cecal volvulus where there is no torsion around the mesenteric pedicle—the cecum folds anteriorly over the ascending colon akin to a bascule bridge.[80] In the setting of a competent ileocecal valve, a bascule can precipitate a closed-loop obstruction. Management is similar to a cecal volvulus.[76]

Acute Colonic Pseudo-obstruction

Acute colonic pseudo-obstruction, or Ogilvie syndrome, is a nonmechanical, functional obstruction of the colon. Elderly patients are at risk, and several precipitating factors have been noted that cause disturbances of the autonomic input to the colon.[81] Abdominal distention is the most common presenting symptom with associated discomfort or mild pain. There is a 2:1 male preponderance, and the typical patient is elderly with a severe systemic illness or an unrelated surgical problem (gynecologic, orthopedic, or cardiothoracic) or trauma. Nausea and vomiting can also be present. Constipation precedes distention but 40% can have diarrhea. Diagnosis is usually clinical but can be aided by imaging such as a radiograph or CT. Characteristic findings are colonic dilation without a transition point. Severe pain, especially on the right, could be a sign of ischemia or perforation. The risk of perforation increases with cecal diameter: 0%, 7%, and 23% with diameters of less than 12 cm, 12 to 14 cm, and greater than 14 cm.[81] A cecal diameter greater than 12 cm warrants more invasive management.

In patients without a threatened cecum, conservative management with correction of fluid and electrolyte abnormalities, nasogastric and rectal tube decompression, mobilization, ambulation, and cessation of opioids, anticholinergics, and neuroleptics can be successful in more than 70%.[82] Endoscopic decompression with or without a decompression tube can be successful in 61% to 95%[83] but a third can require serial decompressions.[84] Endoscopy can also identify any distal obstruction. Once a distal obstruction has been ruled out with colonoscopy or fluoroscopic studies, intravenous neostigmine in a monitored unit can be successful in 90%.[85,86] Subcutaneous administration[87] or combination with glycopyrronium[88] can negate the cardiac side effects.

Surgery is reserved for patients with ischemia, perforation, or refractory disease. Surgical options include a cecostomy or segmental resection. A cecostomy could be performed through an open, laparoscopic, endoscopic, or percutaneous approach. However, complications associated with a cecostomy tube include leakage, sepsis, and catheter displacement. The perioperative mortality is high but this may reflect the medical condition of the patient rather than the cecostomy itself. A segmental resection, usually a right colectomy with ileostomy, is required if there are concerns for ischemia or perforation of the cecum.

SUMMARY

Although the pathophysiologies of colonic emergencies can be daunting, the principles of surgical management are relatively straightforward. A patient in extremis needs exploration. Else, after an initial attempt at nonoperative management, failure to achieve clinical improvement warrants some surgical management. The primary principle of surgery will be to control the offending pathologic condition, reestablish bowel continuity (only in a stable patient while minimizing any untoward complications) or provide an ostomy (diversion or end-stoma), and mitigate any long-term adverse outcomes.

CLINICS CARE POINTS

- In an emergency limited to a segment of colon, a limited resection is preferable to a total colectomy.

- While preservation of intestinal continuity is desirable, a prudent approach would involve preserving an option for re-establishing intestinal continuity and minimizing any post-surgical complications associated with an anastomotic leak while decreasing the operative time.

- In a relatively "stable" patient, when selective re-establishment of continuity is undertaken, a proximal diverting loop ileostomy or colostomy should be liberally applied.

- In emergencies requiring a total or subtotal colectomy, a proctectomy should be avoided to minimize pelvic dissection, sexual dysfunction, and pelvic bleeding.

- Even if it is temporary, a well-constructed stoma is paramount to patient well-being in the post-operative period and in maintaining long-term quality of life.

DISCLOSURE

No Disclosures.

REFERENCES

1. Hogan J, Samaha G, Burke J, et al. Emergency Presenting Colon Cancer Is an Independent Predictor of Adverse Disease-Free Survival. Int Surg 2015;100(1): 77–86.

2. Vogel JD, Felder SI, Bhama AR, et al. The American Society of Colon and Rectal Surgeons Clinical Practice Guidelines for the Management of Colon Cancer. Dis Colon Rectum 2022;65(2):148–77.

3. Tejero E, Mainar A, Fernandez L, et al. New procedure for the treatment of colorectal neoplastic obstructions. Dis Colon Rectum 1994;37(11):1158–9.

4. Lauro A, Binetti M, Vaccari S, et al. Obstructing Left-Sided Colonic Cancer: Is Endoscopic Stenting a Bridge to Surgery or a Bridge to Nowhere? Dig Dis Sci 2020;65(10):2789–99.

5. Hsu J, Sevak S. Management of Malignant Large-Bowel Obstruction. Dis Colon Rectum 2019;62(9):1028.

6. You YN, Hardiman KM, Bafford A, et al. The American Society of Colon and Rectal Surgeons Clinical Practice Guidelines for the Management of Rectal Cancer. Dis Colon Rectum 2020;63(9):1191–222.

7. De Simone B, Davies J, Chouillard E, et al. WSES-AAST guidelines: management of inflammatory bowel disease in the emergency setting. World J Emerg Surg WJES 2021;16:23.

8. Saegesser F, Chapuis G, Rausis C, et al. [Intestinal distension and colonic ischemia: occlusive complications and perforations of colo-rectal cancers. A clinical application of Laplace's law]. Chir Memoires Acad Chir 1974;100(7):502–16.

9. Evans L, Rhodes A, Alhazzani W, et al. Surviving Sepsis Campaign: International Guidelines for Management of Sepsis and Septic Shock 2021. Crit Care Med 2021;49(11):e1063–143.

10. Vernava AM, Moore BA, Longo WE, et al. Lower gastrointestinal bleeding. Dis Colon Rectum 1997;40(7):846–58.

11. Strate LL, Gralnek IM. ACG Clinical Guideline: Management of Patients With Acute Lower Gastrointestinal Bleeding. Am J Gastroenterol 2016;111(4):459–74.

12. Gore RM, Silvers RI, Thakrar KH, et al. Bowel Obstruction. Radiol Clin North Am 2015;53(6):1225–40.

13. Lindor RA, Bellolio MF, Sadosty AT, et al. Adult intussusception: presentation, management, and outcomes of 148 patients. J Emerg Med 2012;43(1):1–6.

14. Yalamarthi S, Smith RC. Adult intussusception: case reports and review of literature. Postgrad Med J 2005;81(953):174–7.

15. Hall J, Hardiman K, Lee S, et al. The American Society of Colon and Rectal Surgeons Clinical Practice Guidelines for the Treatment of Left-Sided Colonic Diverticulitis. Dis Colon Rectum 2020;63(6):728–47.

16. for the AVOD Study Group, Chabok A, Påhlman L, Hjern F, et al. Randomized clinical trial of antibiotics in acute uncomplicated diverticulitis13. Br J Surg 2012; 99(4):532–9.

17. Daniels L, Ünlü Ç, de Korte N, et al. Randomized clinical trial of observational *versus* antibiotic treatment for a first episode of CT-proven uncomplicated acute diverticulitis. Br J Surg 2016;104(1):52–61.

18. Mora-López L, Ruiz-Edo N, Estrada-Ferrer O, et al. Efficacy and Safety of Nonantibiotic Outpatient Treatment in Mild Acute Diverticulitis (DINAMO-study): A Multicentre, Randomised, Open-label, Noninferiority Trial. Ann Surg 2021;274(5): e435–42.

19. Jaung R, Nisbet S, Gosselink MP, et al. Antibiotics Do Not Reduce Length of Hospital Stay for Uncomplicated Diverticulitis in a Pragmatic Double-Blind Randomized Trial. Clin Gastroenterol Hepatol 2021;19(3):503–10.e1.

20. Sharma PV, Eglinton T, Hider P, et al. Systematic Review and Meta-analysis of the Role of Routine Colonic Evaluation After Radiologically Confirmed Acute Diverticulitis. Ann Surg 2014;259(2):263–72.

21. Meyer J, Orci LA, Combescure C, et al. Risk of Colorectal Cancer in Patients With Acute Diverticulitis: A Systematic Review and Meta-analysis of Observational Studies. Clin Gastroenterol Hepatol 2019;17(8):1448–56.e17.
22. Classen JN, Bonardi R, O'mara CS, et al. Surgical Treatment of Acute Diverticulitis by Staged Procedures. Ann Surg 1976;184(5):582–6.
23. Baxter NN. Emergency Management of Diverticulitis. Clin Colon Rectal Surg 2004;17(3):177–82.
24. Young B, O'Dowd G, Woodford P. Wheater's functional Histology: a Text and Colour Atlas. 6th edition. London, England: Churchill Livingston/Elsevier; 2014.
25. Thaler K, Baig MK, Berho M, et al. Determinants of Recurrence After Sigmoid Resection for Uncomplicated Diverticulitis. Dis Colon Rectum 2003;46(3):385–8.
26. Oberkofler CE, Rickenbacher A, Raptis DA, et al. A Multicenter Randomized Clinical Trial of Primary Anastomosis or Hartmann's Procedure for Perforated Left Colonic Diverticulitis With Purulent or Fecal Peritonitis. Ann Surg 2012;256(5): 819–27.
27. Bridoux V, Regimbeau JM, Ouaissi M, et al. Hartmann's Procedure or Primary Anastomosis for Generalized Peritonitis due to Perforated Diverticulitis: A Prospective Multicenter Randomized Trial (DIVERTI). J Am Coll Surg 2017;225(6): 798–805.
28. Gachabayov M, Oberkofler CE, Tuech JJ, et al. Resection with primary anastomosis *vs* nonrestorative resection for perforated diverticulitis with peritonitis: a systematic review and meta-analysis. Colorectal Dis 2018;20(9):753–70.
29. Ryan OK, Ryan ÉJ, Creavin B, et al. Systematic review and meta-analysis comparing primary resection and anastomosis versus Hartmann's procedure for the management of acute perforated diverticulitis with generalised peritonitis. Tech Coloproctology 2020;24(6):527–43.
30. Lambrichts DPV, Vennix S, Musters GD, et al. Hartmann's procedure versus sigmoidectomy with primary anastomosis for perforated diverticulitis with purulent or faecal peritonitis (LADIES): a multicentre, parallel-group, randomised, open-label, superiority trial. Lancet Gastroenterol Hepatol 2019;4(8):599–610.
31. Ng SC, Shi HY, Hamidi N, et al. Worldwide incidence and prevalence of inflammatory bowel disease in the 21st century: a systematic review of population-based studies. Lancet Lond Engl 2017;390(10114):2769–78.
32. Dai N, Haidar O, Askari A, et al. Colectomy rates in ulcerative colitis: A systematic review and meta-analysis. Dig Liver Dis 2023;55(1):13–20.
33. Ma C, Moran GW, Benchimol EI, et al. Surgical Rates for Crohn's Disease are Decreasing: A Population-Based Time Trend Analysis and Validation Study. Am J Gastroenterol 2017;112(12):1840–8.
34. Jeuring SFG, van den Heuvel TRA, Liu LYL, et al. Improvements in the Long-Term Outcome of Crohn's Disease Over the Past Two Decades and the Relation to Changes in Medical Management: Results from the Population-Based IBDSL Cohort. Off J Am Coll Gastroenterol ACG 2017;112(2):325.
35. Burr NE, Lord R, Hull MA, et al. Decreasing Risk of First and Subsequent Surgeries in Patients With Crohn's Disease in England From 1994 through 2013. Clin Gastroenterol Hepatol 2019;17(10):2042–9.e4.
36. Berg DF, Bahadursingh AM, Kaminski DL, et al. Acute surgical emergencies in inflammatory bowel disease. Am J Surg 2002;184(1):45–51.
37. Marion JF, Present DH. The modern medical management of acute, severe ulcerative colitis. Eur J Gastroenterol Hepatol 1997;9(9):831.
38. Fazio VW. Toxic megacolon in ulcerative colitis and Crohn's colitis. Clin Gastroenterol 1980;9(2):389–407.

39. Truelove SC, Witts LJ. Cortisone in Ulcerative Colitis. Br Med J 1955;2(4947): 1041–8.
40. Sheth SG, LaMont JT. Toxic megacolon. Lancet 1998;351(9101):509–13.
41. González-Huix F, Fernández-Bañares F, Esteve-Comas M, et al. Enteral versus Parenteral Nutrition as Adjunct Therapy in Acute Ulcerative Colitis. Am J Gastroenterol 1993;88(2):227–32.
42. Kvasnovsky CL, Aujla U, Bjarnason I. Nonsteroidal anti-inflammatory drugs and exacerbations of inflammatory bowel disease. Scand J Gastroenterol 2015; 50(3):255–63.
43. Cheng K, Faye AS. Venous thromboembolism in inflammatory bowel disease. World J Gastroenterol 2020;26(12):1231–41.
44. Chen Y, Furuya-Kanamori L, Doi SA, et al. Clostridium difficile Infection and Risk of Colectomy in Patients with Inflammatory Bowel Disease: A Bias-adjusted Meta-analysis. Inflamm Bowel Dis 2017;23(2):200–7.
45. Lawlor G, Moss AC. Cytomegalovirus in inflammatory bowel disease: Pathogen or innocent bystander? Inflamm Bowel Dis 2010;16(9):1620–7.
46. Chapman RW, Selby WS, Jewell DP. Controlled trial of intravenous metronidazole as an adjunct to corticosteroids in severe ulcerative colitis. Gut 1986;27(10): 1210–2.
47. Mantzaris GJ, Petraki K, Archavlis E, et al. A prospective randomized controlled trial of intravenous ciprofloxacin as an adjunct to corticosteroids in acute, severe ulcerative colitis. Scand J Gastroenterol 2001;36(9):971–4.
48. Kornbluth A, Sachar DB. Gastroenterology and TPPC of the AC of. Ulcerative Colitis Practice Guidelines in Adults: American College of Gastroenterology, Practice Parameters Committee. Off J Am Coll Gastroenterol ACG 2010;105(3):501.
49. Turner D, Walsh CM, Steinhart AH, et al. Response to Corticosteroids in Severe Ulcerative Colitis: A Systematic Review of the Literature and a Meta-Regression. Clin Gastroenterol Hepatol 2007;5(1):103–10.
50. Lichtiger S, Present DH, Kornbluth A, et al. Cyclosporine in severe ulcerative colitis refractory to steroid therapy. N Engl J Med 1994;330(26):1841–5.
51. Järnerot G, Hertervig E, Friis-Liby I, et al. Infliximab as rescue therapy in severe to moderately severe ulcerative colitis: a randomized, placebo-controlled study. Gastroenterology 2005;128(7):1805–11.
52. Williams JG, Alam MF, Alrubaiy L, et al. Infliximab versus ciclosporin for steroid-resistant acute severe ulcerative colitis (CONSTRUCT): a mixed methods, open-label, pragmatic randomised trial. Lancet Gastroenterol Hepatol 2016;1(1): 15–24.
53. Laharie D, Bourreille A, Branche J, et al. Long-term outcome of patients with steroid-refractory acute severe UC treated with ciclosporin or infliximab. Gut 2018;67(2):237–43.
54. Sands BE, Sandborn WJ, Panaccione R, et al. Ustekinumab as Induction and Maintenance Therapy for Ulcerative Colitis. N Engl J Med 2019;381(13):1201–14.
55. Berinstein JA, Sheehan J, Dias M, et al. Tofacitinib for Biologic-Experienced Hospitalized Patients with Acute Severe Ulcerative Colitis: A Retrospective Case-Control Study. Clin Gastroenterol Hepatol Off Clin Pract J Am Gastroenterol Assoc 2021;19(10):2112–20.e1.
56. Singh S, Murad MH, Fumery M, et al. First- and Second-Line Pharmacotherapies for Patients With Moderate to Severely Active Ulcerative Colitis: An Updated Network Meta-Analysis. Clin Gastroenterol Hepatol 2020;18(10):2179–91.e6.

57. Bartels SaL, Gardenbroek TJ, Bos L, et al. Prolonged preoperative hospital stay is a risk factor for complications after emergency colectomy for severe colitis. Colorectal Dis 2013;15(11):1392–8.

58. Heppell J, Farkouh E, Dubé S, et al. Toxic megacolon. An analysis of 70 cases. Dis Colon Rectum 1986;29(12):789–92.

59. Strong SA, Koltun WA, Hyman NH, et al. Standards Practice Task Force of The American Society of Colon and Rectal Surgeons. Practice parameters for the surgical management of Crohn's disease. Dis Colon Rectum 2007;50(11):1735–46.

60. Ross H, Steele SR, Varma M, et al. Practice Parameters for the Surgical Treatment of Ulcerative Colitis. Dis Colon Rectum 2014;57(1):5.

61. Arnell TD. Surgical Management of Acute Colitis and Toxic Megacolon. Clin Colon Rectal Surg 2004;17(1):71–4.

62. Yamamoto T, Allan RN, Keighley MR. Risk factors for intra-abdominal sepsis after surgery in Crohn's disease. Dis Colon Rectum 2000;43(8):1141–5.

63. Johnston WF, Stafford C, Francone TD, et al. What Is the Risk of Anastomotic Leak After Repeat Intestinal Resection in Patients With Crohn's Disease? Dis Colon Rectum 2017;60(12):1299.

64. Tekkis PP, Purkayastha S, Lanitis S, et al. A comparison of segmental vs subtotal/total colectomy for colonic Crohn's disease: a meta-analysis. Colorectal Dis 2006; 8(2):82–90.

65. Kiran RP, Nisar PJ, Church JM, et al. The Role of Primary Surgical Procedure in Maintaining Intestinal Continuity for Patients With Crohn's Colitis. Ann Surg 2011;253(6):1130.

66. Andersson P, Olaison G, Hallböök O, et al. Segmental resection or subtotal colectomy in Crohn's colitis? Dis Colon Rectum 2002;45(1):47–53.

67. Steinberg DM, Cooke WT, Alexander Williams J. Abscess and fistulae in Crohn's disease. Gut 1973;14(11):865–9.

68. Nagler SM, Poticha SM. Intraabdominal abscess in regional enteritis. Am J Surg 1979;137(3):350–4.

69. Cinat ME, Wilson SE, Din AM. Determinants for Successful Percutaneous Image-Guided Drainage of Intra-abdominal Abscess. Arch Surg 2002;137(7):845–9.

70. He X, Lin X, Lian L, et al. Preoperative Percutaneous Drainage of Spontaneous Intra-Abdominal Abscess in Patients With Crohn's Disease: A Meta-Analysis. J Clin Gastroenterol 2015;49(9):e82.

71. Gervais DA, Hahn PF, O'Neill MJ, et al. Percutaneous Abscess Drainage in Crohn Disease: Technical Success and Short- and Long-term Outcomes during 14 Years. Radiology 2002;222(3):645–51.

72. Yamazaki Y, Ribeiro MB, Sachar DB, et al. Malignant colorectal strictures in Crohn's disease. Am J Gastroenterol 1991;86(7):882–5.

73. Browder W, Cerise EJ, Litwin MS. Impact of emergency angiography in massive lower gastrointestinal bleeding. Ann Surg 1986;204(5):530–6.

74. Halabi WJ, Jafari MD, Kang CY, et al. Colonic volvulus in the United States: trends, outcomes, and predictors of mortality. Ann Surg 2014;259(2):293–301.

75. Perrot L, Fohlen A, Alves A, et al. Management of the colonic volvulus in 2016. J Visc Surg 2016;153(3):183–92.

76. Alavi K, Poylin V, Davids JS, et al. The American Society of Colon and Rectal Surgeons Clinical Practice Guidelines for the Management of Colonic Volvulus and Acute Colonic Pseudo-Obstruction. Dis Colon Rectum 2021;64(9):1046–57.

77. Naveed M, Jamil LH, Fujii-Lau LL, et al. American Society for Gastrointestinal Endoscopy guideline on the role of endoscopy in the management of acute

colonic pseudo-obstruction and colonic volvulus. Gastrointest Endosc 2020; 91(2):228–35.

78. Swenson BR, Kwaan MR, Burkart NE, et al. Colonic volvulus: presentation and management in metropolitan Minnesota, United States. Dis Colon Rectum 2012;55(4):444–9.

79. Kasten KR, Marcello PW, Roberts PL, et al. What are the results of colonic volvulus surgery? Dis Colon Rectum 2015;58(5):502–7.

80. Lung BE, Yelika SB, Murthy AS, et al. Cecal bascule: a systematic review of the literature. Tech Coloproctology 2018;22(2):75–80.

81. Vanek VW, Al-Salti M. Acute pseudo-obstruction of the colon (Ogilvie's syndrome). An analysis of 400 cases. Dis Colon Rectum 1986;29(3):203–10.

82. De Giorgio R, Barbara G, Stanghellini V, et al. Review article: the pharmacological treatment of acute colonic pseudo-obstruction. Aliment Pharmacol Ther 2001; 15(11):1717–27.

83. Saunders MD, Kimmey MB. Systematic review: acute colonic pseudo-obstruction. Aliment Pharmacol Ther 2005;22(10):917–25.

84. Jetmore AB, Timmcke AE, Gathright BJ, et al. Ogilvie's syndrome: Colonoscopic decompression and analysis of predisposing factors. Dis Colon Rectum 1992; 35(12):1135–42.

85. Valle RGL, Godoy FL. Neostigmine for acute colonic pseudo-obstruction: A meta-analysis. Ann Med Surg (Lond) 2014;3(3):60–4.

86. Vogel JD, Feingold DL, Stewart DB, et al. Clinical Practice Guidelines for Colon Volvulus and Acute Colonic Pseudo-Obstruction. Dis Colon Rectum 2016; 59(7):589.

87. Frankel A, Gillespie C, Lu CT, et al. Subcutaneous neostigmine appears safe and effective for acute colonic pseudo-obstruction (Ogilvie's syndrome). ANZ J Surg 2019;89(6):700–5.

88. Adiamah A, Johnson S, Ho A, et al. Neostigmine and glycopyrronium: a potential safe alternative for patients with pseudo-obstruction without access to conventional methods of decompression. Case Rep 2017;2017. bcr.

Anorectal Emergencies

Melissa K. Drezdzon, MD[a], Carrie Y. Peterson, MD, MS[b],*

KEYWORDS

- Anorectal • Hemorrhoid • Fissure • Abscess • Rectal prolapse
- Rectal foreign bodies • Complications

KEY POINTS

- Diagnosis and management of anorectal disease frequently seen in the emergency room.
- Management and treatment of rectal foreign bodies.
- Management of emergent complications of anorectal surgery.

INTRODUCTION

Benign anorectal disease is extremely common, although its exact prevalence is difficult to ascertain. The most prevalent anorectal disorder in the United States is hemorrhoid disease, which is estimated to affect about 4% of the population.[1] Other benign anorectal disorders include anorectal abscesses, anal fissures, and rectal prolapse. Most anorectal emergencies are acute presentations of these benign anorectal disorders. Not all patients affected by anorectal disease will present with an anorectal emergency; nonetheless, they are often encountered in general surgery practice and typically in an emergency department setting.

ANATOMY

Accurate diagnosis and appropriate management of anorectal emergencies starts with a good understanding of normal anorectal anatomy. Although full review of normal anatomy is beyond the scope of this article, key anatomic landmarks are described. For further reading the authors would direct you to *Anus* in *Sabiston Textbook of Surgery*, or the appropriate article in your textbook of choice.[2]

Two important landmarks on examination of the anus are the anal verge and the top of the anorectal ring (**Fig. 1**). The anal verge marks the distal-most portion of the anal canal, and its location is classically defined as coinciding with the intersphincteric groove, the palpable plane between the internal and external anal sphincter muscles.[3] The proximal aspect of the sphincter complex, or anorectal ring, creates a palpable and often visible

[a] Division of Colorectal Surgery, Department of Surgery, Medical College of Wisconsin;
[b] Division of Colorectal Surgery, Medical College of Wisconsin, HCM A6303, 8701 Watertown Plank Road, Milwaukee, WI 53226, USA
* Corresponding author.
E-mail address: cypeterson@mcw.edu

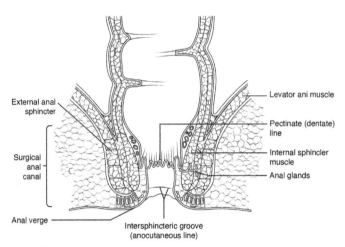

Fig. 1. Anatomy of anal canal.

boundary of the upper aspect of the anal canal. Noting where masses or lesions are in relation to the anal verge and top of the anorectal ring helps communicate the extent of lesions and is often more relevant than size measurements. Within the anal canal is the dentate line, which marks the transition from columnar epithelium proximally to squamous epithelium distally.[4] The dentate line is visible as a discrete, irregular demarcation at the midanal canal, and its identification can aid in the evaluation of anal fistulas, as well as differentiating between internal and external hemorrhoids.

PRINCIPLES OF EXAMINATION IN THE EMERGENCY DEPARTMENT

When evaluating a patient with severe anal pain, a well-taken history will often reveal the diagnosis. A focused medical history should include symptom onset and duration, presence of associated bleeding, incontinence, or itching and a review of normal bowel habits. Anticoagulant use should be delineated, as well as any history of prior anorectal disease or surgery, incontinence, and pregnancy.[5]

All patients presenting with anorectal complaints must receive a focused physical examination that includes an anorectal examination. This examination can be extremely sensitive, and a discussion with the patient that outlines the reason for the examination and what it entails can ensure a more comfortable experience for the patient and physician. Patients should be reassured that the examination can be stopped at any time and for any reason, and an examination chaperone is advised.

Examination in the emergency department can be challenging due to pain and other patient concerns. Ideal positioning for the anorectal examination includes both knees to the chest while the patient lays on their side or the Sims position, where patients lay on their left side with left leg straight and right hip and knee bent (**Fig. 2**). Be sure to adjust the bed height, arrange the lighting, use appropriate personal protective equipment, and have lubricating jelly and gauze available. Lastly, it is helpful to ensure privacy by asking for a private room, pulling the curtain, and having the patient face toward any doors, thus the examinaiton area is protected from accidental exposure.

The examination begins with a visual inspection of the perineum, anal margin (the skin surrounding the anus), and anal verge, noting skin breaks, fissures, or other abnormalities. Gentle palpation of any lesions can clarify if they are painful, and further examination can be deferred if needed. Asking the patient to bear down will cause the anal sphincter complex to relax and may allow for visualization of hemorrhoids

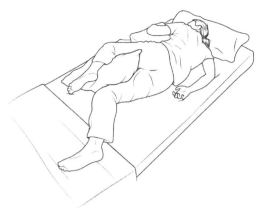

Fig. 2. Sims position for anorectal examination in the emergency department.

or rectal prolapse. If the patient can tolerate a digital rectal examination, this should follow by applying gentle pressure and allowing the sphincter complex to relax. A circumferential sweep allows for palpation of the canal and assessment of the anorectal ring. In men, the prostate will be slightly proximal and anterior. If tolerable, the patient should also be asked to Valsalva and squeeze their sphincter to assess function.[1] If the patient tolerates this and an abnormality is not appreciated, anoscopy can be considered. The anoscope should be gently inserted with adequate lubrication and the obturator removed. The anal canal structures can be evaluated by slowly pulling the scope distally, reinserting the obturator and gently rotating one-third circumference and repeating the process. In this way, the entire circumference of the anal canal can be evaluated. Any masses or areas of irregularity should be noted by anterior-posterior and lateral location.

Depending on the patient's presenting complaints, it may not be possible or reasonable to conduct a digital examination or anoscopy. If the surgeon remains uncertain about the diagnosis, an examination under anesthesia may be necessary.

THROMBOSED EXTERNAL HEMORRHOIDS

Hemorrhoid tissue is a normal part of anorectal anatomy, and hemorrhoidal disease represents one of the oldest known and most common anorectal pathologies, accounting for millions of outpatient visits per year.[5] The prevalence of hemorrhoids peaks between age 45 and 65 years and affects men and women equally.[6] Hemorrhoid complaints can range from negligible to excruciating, depending on the location

Table 1 Classification of internal hemorrhoids	
Grade	**Description**
I	Visible bulge without prolapse. Possible bleeding.
II	Prolapse with Valsalva, spontaneous reduction. Possible bleeding and pruritis.
III	Prolapse that must be manually reduced. Possible bleeding, mucous drainage, and pruritis.
IV	Prolapse that is unable to be reduced. Possible bleeding, mucous drainage, incontinence, pruritis. Risk of thrombosis and strangulation.

and presentation. Although medically and surgically there is a clear definition of hemorrhoid disease and anatomy, to many patients "hemorrhoid problems" can include any number of anal complaints. Internal hemorrhoids most often present with painless bleeding and are classified by degree of prolapse (**Table 1**).[7] Common symptoms of external hemorrhoids include itching and mucoid drainage. Sudden onset, severe anal pain that is not associated with bowel movements should prompt suspicion for thrombosed external hemorrhoids, which occur when a clot forms in an external hemorrhoid vessel, leading to local edema and venous congestion.

Diagnosis

Physical examination in patients with thrombosed external hemorrhoids may be limited by pain. On examination, the perianal skin should be inspected for external hemorrhoids, which if thrombosed, are not subtle. Findings of external thrombosed hemorrhoid include a firm blue or purple nodule near the anal verge with possible overlying ulceration that is tender to palpation[8] (**Fig. 3**). In the setting of hemodynamic instability or suspicion of strangulated or gangrenous hemorrhoids, emergent examination under anesthesia should be performed. In general, a digital rectal examination is extremely painful and should be deferred unless clinically indicated and performed under sedation. The diagnosis of thrombosed external hemorrhoids is clinical, and there is no indication for any laboratory tests or imaging unless there is suspicion of associated infection.

Management

Thrombosed external hemorrhoids are severely painful at onset but symptoms usually begin to improve spontaneously within about 72 hours, as the clot dissolves.[9] Patients presenting after 72 hours of symptom onset should be offered nonoperative management, aimed at symptom relief and future hemorrhoid prevention. Nonoperative management includes the following:

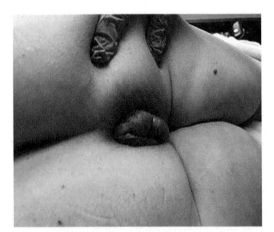

Fig. 3. Thrombosed external hemorrhoids. In this photo, multiple columns of external hemorrhoids are thrombosed, which is noted by the presence of keratinized epithelium characteristic of external hemorrhoids. On palpation these are exquisitely tender and often hard to the touch, with a distinct purple appearance. Excision of the largest with clot extraction is indicated to allow the edema to improve. Smaller thrombosed hemorrhoids can be left to resolve on their own. Excision of all columns can lead to stricturing and should be avoided in the emergent setting.

- Pain control with oral over-the-counter analgesia, such as nonsteroidal antiinflammatory drugs or acetaminophen. Opioid medication should be avoided, as constipation exacerbates the pain.
- Topical nifedipine may improve sphincter relaxation and reduce spasm.[10]
- Application of heating or cooling pads.
- Sitz baths for 10 to 15 minutes after bowel movements.[5,11]
- Addition of a fiber supplement to bulk stool accompanied by increased water intake.[12]

Patients with thrombosed external hemorrhoids who present within 72 hours of symptom onset may be candidates for excision, which can provide immediate relief. Compared with conservative management, surgical excision has been shown to have decreased rates of recurrence, a longer interval to recurrence, and faster symptom resolution.[9] Thrombosed external hemorrhoid excision can be performed quickly at the bedside in the emergency department with local anesthesia alone or with conscious sedation, if needed. A scalpel, fine scissor, or cautery device is used to create an elliptical incision around the thrombosed hemorrhoid, and the clot is excised. The principles of conservative hemorrhoid management apply after hemorrhoid excision, including nonopioid analgesia, sitz baths, a high-fiber diet or fiber supplement, and drinking plenty of water.

INCARCERATED AND GANGRENOUS HEMORRHOIDS

Strangulated and gangrenous hemorrhoids are rare presentations of hemorrhoidal disease although they represent true anorectal emergencies in which expeditious diagnosis and treatment are necessary for good patient outcomes. Prolapse of hemorrhoid tissue occurs in patients with grade II, grade III, and grade IV internal hemorrhoids; however, only grade IV internal hemorrhoids are considered incarcerated (see **Table 1**). Because prolapsed internal hemorrhoids traverse the anal sphincter complex, the anal sphincter exerts pressure on the hemorrhoid tissue, leading to impaired venous outflow.[13] Increased venous pressure in the prolapsed tissue leads to fluid extravasation and edema, and blood flow may become compromised. In this situation, grade IV hemorrhoid incarceration progresses to strangulation. If left untreated, hemorrhoid strangulation can lead to necrosis or gangrene.

Diagnosis

Patients presenting with incarcerated or strangulated hemorrhoids will often present with extreme pain, rectal pressure, and mucous discharge or bleeding. A prior history of hemorrhoids and their grades should be delineated, as well as any recent events that may have resulted in acute prolapse. Signs of sepsis including fever, tachycardia, or leukocytosis should be noted, as these findings will guide the choice of intervention.

On examination, patients with incarcerated internal hemorrhoids will have evidence of hemorrhoid tissue prolapsing through the anus (**Fig. 4**). Unlike prolapsed rectum, prolapsed hemorrhoids have radial creases in the visualized anoderm extending from the orifice outward. Incarcerated internal hemorrhoids may look like normal hemorrhoid tissue or may seem edematous and erythematous. Suspicion for strangulated or gangrenous hemorrhoids should be raised if the prolapsed tissue seems dusky or violaceous or has ulcerations or mucosal sloughing (**Fig. 5**).

Management

For patients with incarcerated internal hemorrhoids and without signs of ischemia, reduction can be attempted. In the emergency department setting, intravenous

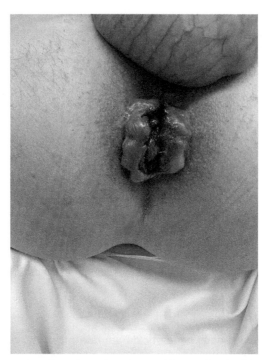

Fig. 4. Nonincarcerated prolapsed grade III internal hemorrhoid. Although these external hemorrhoids look edematous due to the patient's dependent position, the internal component is not incarcerated and they are soft and nontender on examination. Note the exposed mucosa in the right posterior column protruding from the anal canal.

analgesia and anxiolytics should be used to optimize patient comfort and relaxation. When attempting reduction, Trendelenburg position is most helpful. Applying ample table sugar (cups, not packets) to the prolapsed hemorrhoids may also reduce swelling and ease reduction.[14] If sugar is applied, it will need some time, at least 1 hour, to work. Manual reduction should be attempted by externally applying gentle steady pressure.

If reduction is successful, patients should be advised that the likelihood of recurrence is high and interval surgical hemorrhoidectomy is indicated.[15] After reduction, patients can use the same principles of hemorrhoid management as discussed earlier, including sitz baths, high-fiber diet with fiber supplementation, and ice packs and non-opioid analgesia for pain control.

Emergent excisional hemorrhoidectomy in the operating room is indicated in most cases of strangled and gangrenous hemorrhoids due to significant patient discomfort or signs of sepsis. Depending on surgeon experience, either the closed Ferguson technique or open Milligan-Morgan technique for hemorrhoid excision should be used.[5] Stapled hemorrhoidopexy or Doppler-assisted hemorrhoid artery ligation is not recommended for strangulated or gangrenous hemorrhoids. Care should be taken to limit the excision of hemorrhoid columns to only those that are ischemic or largely prolapsed. Once the remaining hemorrhoid tissue is reduced, additional excision should be undertaken cautiously; it is far too easy to excise a large portion of anoderm and cause stenosis in the emergent setting. Similarly, due to tissue edema and distortion, it is easy to inadvertently injure the anal sphincter muscles during excision and

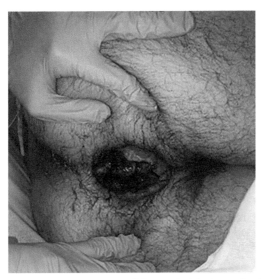

Fig. 5. Strangulated and gangrenous internal hemorrhoids. Note the ischemic-appearing mucosa and mucosal sloughing. Also note the radial folds in the tissue that is characteristic of prolapsed internal hemorrhoids (even when not ischemic). This requires emergent surgical intervention to avoid progression to gangrene and pelvic sepsis. Incarcerated prolapsed hemorrhoids (inability to reduce) without ischemia often also require emergent intervention due to excessive pain. If left prolapsed, incarcerated hemorrhoids can progress to ischemia and strangulation.

cause incontinence, so extra care should be taken to minimize this risk. Postoperative care should entail similar principles as listed earlier.

ACUTE ANAL FISSURE

Approximately 342,000 new cases of anal fissure are reported each year in the United States, and among differential diagnoses for severe anorectal pain, anal fissure often tops the list.[16] Anal fissures are linear tears in the anal mucosa, and the vast majority (75%–90%) are located in the posterior midline of the anal canal; however, they can also be seen in the anterior midline, especially in women.[17,18] Although most fissures are benign, lateral anal fissures or multiple synchronous anal fissures should raise suspicion for associated conditions such as human immunodeficiency virus, Crohn disease, tuberculosis, or syphilis and prompt additional evaluation.[16] Acute anal fissures are defined as fissures that have been present for fewer than 8 weeks and are usually adequately treated with nonoperative management.[16,17]

Diagnosis

The classic presentation of anal fissure is sharp, cutting pain with defecation and blood streaking on stool or toilet tissue.[18,19] Patients may describe the sensation as "passing a shard of glass," or "being cut with a knife." The pain or burning may persist for minutes to hours after having a bowel movement and may improve in the time between.

Examination of the area may be challenging due to significant pain; however, the diagnosis of anal fissure may be suspected on history alone, given the unique sharp pain that is classically described. Examination is limited to gently spreading the buttocks or anal margin skin to expose the distal aspect of the anal canal. An elliptical tear at the posterior or anterior midline is most consistent with an acute anal fissure, and the presence of a fibrotic skin tag at the radial end is suggestive of a chronic fissure[19,20] (**Fig. 6**). A digital rectal examination is not necessary to establish a diagnosis of anal fissure when one is seen on inspection. An examination under anesthesia may be necessary if a patient cannot tolerate an examination due to pain and no other cause is identified.

Management

First-line treatment of patients with acute anal fissures is nonoperative management directed at stool bulking and anal sphincter relaxation.[17,19,20] Patients should be given a goal of 25 to 30 g of dietary fiber per day, which will likely require the addition of a fiber supplement such as psyllium, methylcellulose, or dextran, all of which are available over the counter.[19] Increased water intake should always accompany an increase in fiber. Topical nitrates, such as nitroglycerin have been found to improve rates of fissure healing compared with placebo; however, headaches are a common side effect and affect compliance.[17,21] Topical calcium channel blockers, such as diltiazem and nifedipine, have similar efficacy to nitrates with significantly lower reported rates of side effects and lower rates of fissure recurrence, making them the first-line topical therapy for acute anal fissure.[17] These medications are prepared in a compounding pharmacy, and patients are instructed to apply a pea-sized amount to the outside

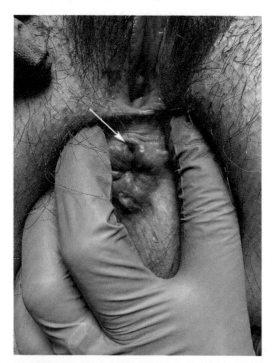

Fig. 6. Anal fissure. Note the disruption in the anoderm that is a characteristic of fissure (*arrow*). This is located just proximal to the anal verge in the distal aspect of the anal canal. Often, gentle traction (as seen in this photo) is needed to clearly see the fissure. Such a maneuver often reproduces pain, so care is warranted. This patient also has a small sentinel pile (skin tag) at the distal aspect of the fissure, which is fibrous and associated with chronicity.

of the anus 3 times daily. Other aspects of treatment include oral, nonopioid analgesia with ibuprofen or acetaminophen and sitz baths after bowel movements.[22] If medical therapy fails, surgical treatment is offered; however, this is not necessary in the emergent setting. Surgical treatment options include Botox injection into the anal sphincters or lateral internal sphincterotomy.[17]

ACUTE ANORECTAL ABSCESS

An estimated 100,000 new patients are treated for anorectal abscesses each year in the United States.[23] Anorectal abscess is more common in men (2:1 male-to-female diagnosis ratio), and peak incidence is between ages 20 to 40.[24,25] The most common anorectal abscesses are cryptoglandular in origin and arise from the anal glands near the dentate line.[25] Obstruction of the anal crypts results in infection of the anal gland and subsequent abscess formation.[26] Anorectal abscesses can also occur due to other infection, autoimmune conditions, trauma, or prior surgery (**Table 2**).[25,27–31]

There are several potential spaces in the pelvis in which anorectal abscesses develop and extend into, including the perianal, intersphincteric, submucosal ischiorectal, and supralevator spaces[32] (**Fig. 7**). Anorectal abscesses are named for the space they occupy, with perianal abscesses being the most common, followed by ischiorectal, intersphincteric, then supralevator abscesses. Associated fistula tracts may be present in approximately 34% of patients at their initial presentation.[33]

Diagnosis

Anorectal abscesses, similar to many anorectal emergencies, are diagnosed clinically. Patient history should include any reports of unusual rectal drainage, incontinence, perirectal swelling or sensations of fullness, and pain in the perineum, back, or buttocks, which might suggest a rare supralevator abscess. Information about prior anorectal surgery, obstetric history, malignancy or pelvic radiation, personal or family history of inflammatory bowel disease, and baseline continence is also important to elucidate (**Box 1**).

Table 2 Causes for anorectal abscess	
Nonspecific Etiology	**Cryptoglandular Abscess**
Infection	HIV Tuberculosis Lymphogranuloma venereum
Inflammatory condition	Crohn disease Sarcoidosis
Trauma	Rectal foreign body Anal fissure Iatrogenic injury
Prior surgery	Episiotomy Hemorrhoidectomy Prostatectomy Lateral internal sphincterotomy
Malignancy	Rectal carcinoma Leukemia Lymphoma Pelvic radiation

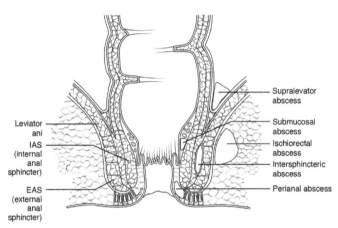

Supralevator abscess

Submucosal abscess

Ischiorectal abscess

Intersphincteric abscess

Perianal abscess

Leviator ani

IAS (internal anal sphincter)

EAS (external anal sphincter)

Fig. 7. Classification of anorectal abscesses by location. EAS, external anal sphincter; IAS, internal anal sphincter.

Physical examination should begin with a visual inspection, looking specifically for erythema, swelling, and evidence of cellulitis. Palpation of the buttock and anal margin may reveal an area of fluctuance and/or significant tenderness. If tolerated, a digital rectal examination and anoscopy is performed, with attention paid to areas of fullness or swelling and inspection for any fistula tracts or purulent drainage. Diagnostic imaging is not necessary to establish the diagnosis of anorectal abscesses in most cases, if the location of the abscess is apparent on examination.[34] Certain situations warrant pelvic imaging, including inability to locate abscess, recurrent or suspected complex abscesses such as horseshoe abscesses, immunosuppressed patients, or those with Crohn disease. Computed tomography (CT) scans have a 77% sensitivity for detecting anorectal abscesses, although they are less likely to identify fistula tracts compared with MRI.[35,36] CT scans will also have difficulty identifying small intersphincteric abscesses, which can be extremely painful, and these are best diagnosed on physical examination in the operating room.

Management

The cornerstone of anorectal abscess management is adequate incision and drainage (I&D). Antibiotic therapy alone is insufficient and not generally recommended.[23] Neutropenic patients with absolute neutrophil counts less than 500/mm^3 are an exception, as they may not mount a suppurative response to infection and will have a difficult time healing an incision, thus a trial of antibiotics before attempting I&D is recommended.[37]

Box 1
Indications for imaging for diagnosis of anorectal abscess

Occult anorectal abscess

Recurrent anal fistula

Complex anal fistula

Immunosuppression

Crohn disease

Perianal and ischiorectal abscesses can often be drained at the bedside under local anesthesia. Once the area has been prepped, fluctuance should be identified and a radial or cruciate incision is made close to the anal verge, avoiding the sphincter complex.[25] Making an incision close to the anal sphincter ensures that if a fistula does develop, the tract will be as short as possible. Packing the abscess cavity is not recommended and may increase patient discomfort without reducing recurrence rates.[38,39] If the cavity is large, a Pezzar or Malecot drain can be used to allow for adequate drainage and prevent premature skin healing. It is held in place by its wide tip within the cavity but can also be secured by suturing to the skin. This suture can be removed in outpatient clinic after 3 to 5 days. For patients with uncomplicated anorectal abscesses who undergo adequate I&D, adjuvant antibiotics have not been shown to improve outcomes, nor have they been found to reduce the risk of subsequent fistula formation.[40,41] Post-I&D antibiotics are indicated for patients with neutropenia, diabetes, or for those who are immunosuppressed.[25]

Postprocedure instructions should include the following:

- Sitz baths twice a day and after bowel movements
- Oral analgesia with acetaminophen and ibuprofen; opioid medications may be needed for large abscesses but should be used sparingly
- Dry gauze at the site of drainage, as needed
- Outpatient follow-up with a surgeon to ensure proper healing and evaluation of recurrent abscess or fistula

If the abscess is large, difficult to reach (proximal in the pelvis or deep in the ischiorectal space), or has horseshoe appearance, the incision and drainage should take place in the operating room under anesthesia.[42] If this is done, careful inspection for fistula tracts can be undertaken, and if found, a draining seton can be placed or fistulotomy performed depending on the location of the fistula tract and sphincter muscle involved.

RECTAL PROLAPSE

Rectal prolapse is the full-thickness protrusion and intussusception of the rectum through the anal canal. External, full-thickness rectal prolapse is characterized by concentric circumferential folds of tissue protruding from the anus, unlike hemorrhoidal prolapse that presents with radial folds[43] (**Fig. 8**). Prevalence of external rectal

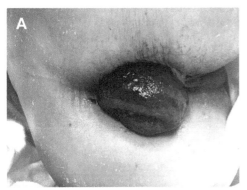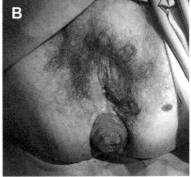

Fig. 8. Rectal prolapse. (*A*) Smaller prolapse. (*B*) Larger prolapse. Note the circumferential folds of mucosa that is characteristic of rectal prolapse (compared with the radial folds of hemorrhoids seen in **Figs. 3–5**).

prolapse is rare, affecting less than 0.5% of people, and most of the rectal prolapse patients (>90%) are women older than 50 years with a history of vaginal childbirth.[44,45] Although the pathophysiology of rectal prolapse is unclear, risk factors for prolapse development include connective tissue disorders, constipation with repeated straining, multiparity, and intestinal motility disorders.[43]

Patients with rectal prolapse may present with sensations of rectal pressure, mucous discharge, rectal bleeding, and pain.[43] Patients presenting with incarceration or strangulation of their rectal prolapse will present with a large, painful rectal mass.[44]

Diagnosis

Rectal prolapse is a clinical diagnosis and usually easily identifiable on physical examination. A focused patient history should include duration of prolapse, presence of associated symptoms, history of fecal incontinence and constipation, and history of other pelvic organ prolapse.

Physical examination includes visual inspection of the prolapsed rectum and evaluation for strangulation, which may present as dusky, ischemic-appearing tissue, ulceration, or mucosal sloughing. The patient should also be assessed for signs and symptoms of sepsis. Imaging is not routinely indicated for external rectal prolapse, and laboratory testing can be limited to patients presenting with concerns for sepsis.

Management

Although surgical intervention in the elective setting is the ideal and definitive management for patients with rectal prolapse, the primary goal of managing rectal prolapse in the emergency department setting is reduction of prolapse or identifying an indication for emergent surgery.[43] If mucosa seems pink and well perfused, manual reduction with gentle external pressure can be attempted. As was mentioned in the discussion of incarcerated hemorrhoids, intravenous analgesia and anxiolytics can be used to improve patient comfort and success. Placing the patient in Trendelenburg and coating the rectal mucosa in ample amounts of table sugar may also help with manual reduction.[14] After successful reduction, the patient should be scheduled for close interval follow-up with a surgeon for further workup and surgical planning. The patient should also be counseled to ensure adequate fiber and fluid intake, including 30 grams of fiber and 2 liters of water per day, and to avoid straining.[46]

If the prolapse cannot be reduced in the emergency department or if the prolapsed rectum seems gangrenous, the patient should proceed to the operating room. In some cases, the patient will relax after the induction of anesthesia, and the rectum is able to be reduced without any surgical intervention. For patients with true incarceration or strangulation with gangrene, a perineal rectosigmoidectomy, or Altemeier procedure, with coloanal anastomosis should be performed.[2]

ACUTE PILONIDAL ABSCESS

Pilonidal disease is a chronic condition that involves the sacrococcygeal natal cleft. Acute pilonidal abscess occurs in the setting of an infected pilonidal cyst or sinus tract. It is suspected that pilonidal disease develops due to repeated friction and moisture in the natal cleft, and a foreign body reaction occurs due to the presence of hair trapped in sinus tracts, leading to an abscess cavity.[2,47] Patients with pilonidal abscesses usually present with pain and pressure that is localized at the natal cleft, and they may report purulent drainage. Pilonidal disease typically affects younger patients and affects males and females equally.[48] Risk factors for development of pilonidal disease include obesity, poor hygiene, hirsutism, sitting for long periods, and family history of the disease.[49,50]

Diagnosis

Pilonidal abscess may be a patient's initial presentation of pilonidal disease. Patients with pilonidal abscesses will report pain, drainage, and may even report rectal bleeding, mistaking their presentation for hemorrhoid disease. On physical examination, an area of erythema, induration, tenderness, and fluctuance will be found lateral to the midline. Pilonidal pits or sinuses with protruding tufts of hair and associated drainage may also be present. The pits will likely be located along the midline and may be at some distance from the acute abscess itself.[47] Diagnosis of pilonidal abscess is clinical, and there is no indication for further laboratory testing. Imaging is also not routinely indicated.

Management

For patients presenting with acute pilonidal abscess, I&D is standard of care and can be performed at the bedside in the emergency department with local analgesia. Important principles of I&D for pilonidal abscesses include making an off-midline incision over the area of maximum fluctuance.[47] Packing the wound is not indicated; however, making a cruciate or elliptical incision to avoid skin edge approximation can help prevent early recurrence due to premature healing. In addition to drainage of the abscess, removal of hair and debris is also important to reduce the risk of recurrence. Postprocedure pain control can be achieved with ibuprofen and acetaminophen; opioid medications are not routinely prescribed. Antibiotics are not indicated for most of the patients with pilonidal abscess but should be considered in special circumstances, including patients with extensive erythema, signs of sepsis, immunocompromised patients, or patients with prosthetic heart valves.[51] After I&D, patients should also be educated on risk factor reduction, which includes good hygiene and hair removal with shaving, waxing, or laser hair removal. Patients may also benefit from follow-up in surgery clinic to discuss definitive management of their pilonidal disease once the acute infection has resolved.

UNIQUE SITUATIONS
Complications of Anorectal Surgery

Anorectal procedures are extremely common and well tolerated. Major postoperative complications after anorectal surgery are rare, but these procedures are not without risk. Postprocedure bleeding may prompt an emergency department visit and can be delayed, occurring 5 to 7 days after surgery. Bleeding may be painless, but quite perfuse, and can present as bright red blood per rectum or passage of clots. The surgical wound should be inspected, although visualization will likely be limited due to bleeding and patient discomfort. If examination in the emergency department is limited or bleeding is severe, patients will require an examination under anesthesia for thorough examination and identification of the offending vessel. If a bleeding vessel is seen, cautery, silver nitrate, or a small figure-of-eight stitch using absorbable suture may be needed.[8]

Pelvic sepsis is a rare, but dreaded, complication following anorectal procedures. Case reports of perirectal sepsis after rubber band ligation, stapled hemorrhoidectomy, and open hemorrhoidectomy suggest that rectal perforation may occur during these procedures, resulting in fecal contamination and subsequent infection of the perirectal space.[52] Patients who report postoperative pelvic pain radiating to the abdomen that is accompanied by fever, swelling, or fullness, and urinary retention should be promptly evaluated for pelvic sepsis. Management includes emergent surgical debridement for infectious source control, drain placement or surgical washout, admission to the ward or intensive care unit, fluid resuscitation, and broad-spectrum antibiotics.

Rectal Foreign Bodies

Occasionally, surgeons are called to consult on patients who present with retained rectal foreign bodies. An open, focused medical history should be obtained along with an abdominal radiograph to evaluate for perforation or the presence of a sharp object that could injure the examining surgeon.[53] After abdominal radiograph, a digital rectal examination can be performed, and manual extraction can be attempted. If extraction is not possible in the emergency department due to patient discomfort or difficulty maneuvering the object, an examination under anesthesia and extraction in the operating room is indicated. If a vacuum seal has formed around the foreign body, insertion of a pneumatic dilation balloon past the object with inflation of the balloon can equalize the pressure.[54] Exploratory laparotomy is indicated if there is evidence of pneumoperitoneum on radiograph or if the patient has signs and symptoms of peritonitis.[55] For small rectal foreign bodies, laxatives or an enema can be used to attempt to flush out the object.[56] If it is suspected that the foreign bodies are drug packets, any maneuver that could disrupt the package should be avoided, the patient should be admitted for observation, and the objects should be allowed to pass on their own.[53]

Anorectal Sexually Transmitted Infections

General surgeons may also be called to evaluate patients with anorectal sexually transmitted infections (STIs), as they are often confused for more common pathologies such as hemorrhoids or anal fissures. Diagnosis of anorectal STIs require a high index of suspicion and an open, nonjudgmental discussion about patient risk factors. Symptoms of anorectal STIs are nonspecific and include anal pain, tenesmus, bleeding, and drainage.[57] Physical examination findings of painless or painful ulcers, condylomatous growths, or mucopurulent drainage may prompt provider's suspicion for anorectal STIs. Once anorectal STI is suspected, workup proceeds with laboratory testing that includes serology, nucleic acid amplification test, venereal disease research laboratory test, and Gram stain and culture. There is a limited role for surgical intervention for anorectal STIs in an emergency setting. For patients with anal condylomas due to human papilloma virus or with lesions due to molluscum contagiosum, elective examination under anesthesia with fulguration or cryotherapy or lesions may be indicated as part of their treatment.[58]

SUMMARY

Anorectal emergencies are uncommon presentations of extremely common diseases. A thorough understanding of anorectal anatomy and common pathology allows for expeditious diagnosis and management. Most anorectal emergencies can be managed nonoperatively or with a bedside procedure performed in the emergency department. Indications for operative intervention include signs and symptoms of systemic infection or evidence of strangulation in cases of prolapse. Most patients diagnosed with anorectal pathology in the emergent setting benefit from outpatient surgical clinic follow-up for further evaluation and definitive treatment planning.

CLINICS CARE POINTS

- Diagnosis and management of anorectal disease is frequently seen in the emergency room.
- Diagnosis of anorectal disease can often be made with focused history and physical examination.
- Most anorectal emergencies can be managed nonoperatively or with a bedside procedure under local anesthesia.

DISCLOSURE

The authors have nothing to disclose.

REFERENCES

1. Sun Z, Migaly J. Review of hemorrhoid disease: presentation and management. Clin Colon Rectal Surg 2016;29(1):22–9.
2. Hyman N, Umanskiy K. Anus. In: Townsend CM, Beauchamp RD, Evers BM, et al, editors. Sabiston textbook of surgery. 21 ed. Philadelphia, PA: Elsevier; 2022. p. 1401–24.
3. Milligan ETC, Morgan CN. Surgical anatomy of the anal canal: with special reference to anorectal fistulae. Lancet 1934;224(5804):1150–6.
4. Carmichael J, Mills S. Anatomy and embryology of the colon, rectum, and anus. In: Steele SR, Hull TL, Hyman N, et al, editors. *ASCRs textbook of colon and rectal surgery.* 4th edition. Switzerland: Springer Nature; 2022. p. 3–27.
5. Davids J and Ridolfi T. Hemorrhoids, In: Steele SR, Hull T, Hyman N, et al. *ASCRS textbook of colon and rectal surgery,* 4th edition, 2022, Springer Nature; Switzerland, 209-229.
6. Everhart JE, Ruhl CE. Burden of digestive diseases in the United States part I: overall and upper gastrointestinal diseases. Gastroenterology 2009;136(2): 376–86.
7. Davis BR, Lee-Kong SA, Migaly J, et al. The American society of colon and rectal surgeons clinical practice guidelines for the management of hemorrhoids. Dis Colon Rectum 2018;61(3):284–92.
8. Lohsiriwat V. Anorectal emergencies. World J Gastroenterol 2016;22(26): 5867–78.
9. Greenspon J, Williams SB, Young HA, et al. Thrombosed external hemorrhoids: outcome after conservative or surgical management. Dis Colon Rectum 2004; 47(9):1493–8.
10. Perrotti P, Antropoli C, Molino D, et al. Conservative treatment of acute thrombosed external hemorrhoids with topical nifedipine. Dis Colon Rectum 2001; 44(3):405–9.
11. Abcarian A, Abcarian H. Anorectal: management of hemorrhoids. In: Cameron JL, Cameron AM, editors. Current surgical therapy. 14 ed. Philadelphia: Elsevier; 2023. p. 287–95.
12. Alonso-Coello P, Mills E, Heels-Ansdell D, et al. Fiber for the treatment of hemorrhoids complications: a systematic review and meta-analysis. Am J Gastroenterol 2006;101(1):181–8.
13. Suwanabol P, Regenbogen S. Anorectal physiology. In: Steele SR, Hull T, Hyman N, et al, editors. *ASCRS textbook of colon and rectal surgery.* 4th edition. Switzerland: Springer Nature; 2022. p. 41–50.

14. Myers JO, Rothenberger DA. Sugar in the reduction of incarcerated prolapsed bowel. Report of two cases. Dis Colon Rectum 1991;34(5):416–8.
15. Rasmussen OO, Larsen KG, Naver L, et al. Emergency haemorrhoidectomy compared with incision and banding for the treatment of acute strangulated haemorrhoids. A prospective randomised study. Eur J Surg 1991;157(10):613–4.
16. Mapel DW, Schum M, Von Worley A. The epidemiology and treatment of anal fissures in a population-based cohort. BMC Gastroenterol 2014;14:129.
17. Stewart DB, Gaertner W, Glasgow S, et al. Clinical practice guideline for the management of anal fissures. Dis Colon Rectum 2017;60(1):7–14.
18. Hananel N, Gordon PH. Re-examination of clinical manifestations and response to therapy of fissure-in-ano. Dis Colon Rectum 1997;40(2):229–33.
19. Lu Y, Kwaan MR, Lin AY. Diagnosis and treatment of anal fissures in 2021. JAMA 2021;325(7):688–9.
20. Rosser R, Harikrishnan A. Benign anorectal conditions: perianal abscess, fistula in ano, haemorrhoids, fissures and pilonidal sinu. Surgery 2020;38(6):322–8.
21. Nelson RL, Thomas K, Morgan J, et al. Non surgical therapy for anal fissure. Cochrane Database Syst Rev 2012;2012(2):CD003431.
22. Gupta P. Randomized, controlled study comparing sitz-bath and no-sitz-bath treatments in patients with acute anal fissures. ANZ J Surg 2006;76(8):718–21.
23. Abcarian H. Anorectal infection: abscess-fistula. Clin Colon Rectal Surg 2011;24(1):14–21.
24. Adamo K, Sandblom G, Brannstrom F, et al. Prevalence and recurrence rate of perianal abscess–a population-based study, Sweden 1997-2009. Int J Colorectal Dis 2016;31(3):669–73.
25. Johnson E, Bernier G. Crytoglandular abscess and fistula. In: Steele SR, Hull T, Hyman N, et al, editors. *ASCRS textbook of colon and rectal surgery.* 4th edition. Switzerland: Springer Nature; 2022. p. 249–69.
26. Eisenhammer S. The internal anal sphincter and the anorectal abscess. Surg Gynecol Obstet 1956;103(4):501–6.
27. Marks CG, Ritchie JK, Lockhart-Mummery HE. Anal fistulas in Crohn's disease. Br J Surg 1981;68(8):525–7.
28. Culp CE. Chronic hidradenitis suppurativa of the anal canal. A surgical skin disease. Dis Colon Rectum 1983;26(10):669–76.
29. Miles RP. Rectal lymphogranuloma venereum. Br J Surg 1957;45(190):180–8.
30. North JH Jr, Weber TK, Rodriguez-Bigas MA, et al. The management of infectious and noninfectious anorectal complications in patients with leukemia. J Am Coll Surg 1996;183(4):322–8.
31. Johnston MJ, Robertson GM, Frizelle FA. Management of late complications of pelvic radiation in the rectum and anus: a review. Dis Colon Rectum 2003;46(2):247–59.
32. Robinson AM Jr, DeNobile JW. Anorectal abscess and fistula-in-ano. J Natl Med Assoc 1988;80(11):1209–13.
33. Ramanujam PS, Prasad ML, Abcarian H, et al. Perianal abscesses and fistulas. A study of 1023 patients. Dis Colon Rectum 1984;27(9):593–7.
34. Gaertner WB, Burgess PL, Davids JS, et al. The American society of colon and rectal surgeons clinical practice guidelines for the management of anorectal abscess, fistula-in-ano, and rectovaginal fistula. Dis Colon Rectum 2022;65(8):964–85.
35. Caliste X, Nazir S, Goode T, et al. Sensitivity of computed tomography in detection of perirectal abscess. Am Surg 2011;77(2):166–8.

36. Singh K, Singh N, Thukral C, et al. Magnetic resonance imaging (MRI) evaluation of perianal fistulae with surgical correlation. J Clin Diagn Res 2014;8(6):RC01–4.

37. Thorsen A. Aorectal: Management of anorectal abscess and fistula. In: Cameron JL, Cameron AM, editors. Current surgical therapy. Philadelphia: Elsevier; 2023. p. 298–307.

38. Newton K, Dumville J, Briggs M, et al. Postoperative packing of perianal abscess cavities (PPAC2): randomized clinical trial. Br J Surg 2022;109(10):951–7.

39. Tonkin DM, Murphy E, Brooke-Smith M, et al. Perianal abscess: a pilot study comparing packing with nonpacking of the abscess cavity. Dis Colon Rectum 2004;47(9):1510–4.

40. Seow-En I, Ngu J. Routine operative swab cultures and post-operative antibiotic use for uncomplicated perianal abscesses are unnecessary. ANZ J Surg 2017; 87(5):356–9.

41. Sozener U, Gedik E, Kessaf Aslar A, et al. Does adjuvant antibiotic treatment after drainage of anorectal abscess prevent development of anal fistulas? A randomized, placebo-controlled, double-blind, multicenter study. Dis Colon Rectum 2011;54(8):923–9.

42. Browder LK, Sweet S, Kaiser AM. Modified Hanley procedure for management of complex horseshoe fistulae. Tech Coloproctol 2009;13(4):301–6.

43. Murphy M, Vogler S. Rectal prolapse. In: Steele SR, Hull T, Hyman N, et al, editors. The ASCRS textbook of colon and rectal surgery. 4th edition. Springer Nature, Switzerland; 2022. p. 1019–33.

44. Bordeianou L, Hicks CW, Kaiser AM, et al. Rectal prolapse: an overview of clinical features, diagnosis, and patient-specific management strategies. J Gastrointest Surg 2014;18(5):1059–69.

45. Hori T, Yasukawa D, Machimoto T, et al. Surgical options for full-thickness rectal prolapse: current status and institutional choice. Ann Gastroenterol 2018;31(2): 188–97.

46. Ternent CA, Bastawrous AL, Morin NA, et al. Practice parameters for the evaluation and management of constipation. Dis Colon Rectum 2007;50(12):2013–22.

47. Bhama AR, Davis BR. Pilonidal disease and hidradenitis suppurativa. In: Steele SR, Hull T, Hyman NH, et al, editors. The ASCRS textbook of colon and rectal surgery. 4th edition. Switzerland: Springer Nature; 2022. p. 293–310.

48. Sondenaa K, Andersen E, Nesvik I, et al. Patient characteristics and symptoms in chronic pilonidal sinus disease. Int J Colorectal Dis 1995;10(1):39–42.

49. Yildiz T, Elmas B, Yucak A, et al. Risk factors for pilonidal sinus disease in teenagers. Indian J Pediatr 2017;84(2):134–8.

50. Doll D, Matevossian E, Wietelmann K, et al. Family history of pilonidal sinus predisposes to earlier onset of disease and a 50% long-term recurrence rate. Dis Colon Rectum 2009;52(9):1610–5.

51. Khanna A, Rombeau JL. Pilonidal disease. Clin Colon Rectal Surg 2011;24(1): 46–53.

52. Aldouri AQ, Alexander DJ. Presentation and management of perirectal sepsis. Ann R Coll Surg Engl 2008;90(5):W4–7.

53. Tarasconi A, Perrone G, Davies J, et al. Anorectal emergencies: WSES-AAST guidelines. World J Emerg Surg 2021;16(1):48.

54. Koornstra JJ, Weersma RK. Management of rectal foreign bodies: description of a new technique and clinical practice guidelines. World J Gastroenterol 2008; 14(27):4403–6.

55. Zhang Y, Han Y, Xu H, et al. A retrospective analysis of transanal surgical management of 291 cases with rectal foreign bodies. Int J Colorectal Dis 2022; 37(10):2167–72.
56. Grantham JP, Hii A, Bright T, et al. Successful expulsion of a golf ball from the sigmoid colon using volume laxatives. Case Rep Surg 2023;2023:5841246.
57. Cowan M, Schlussel AT. Sexually transmitted infections of the colon and rectum. In: Steele SR, Hull T, Hyman NH, et al, editors. *The ASCRS textbook of colon and rectal surgery*. 4th edition. Switzerland: Springer Nature; 2022. p. 323–42.
58. D'Ambrogio A, Yerly S, Sahli R, et al. Human papilloma virus type and recurrence rate after surgical clearance of anal condylomata acuminata. Sex Transm Dis 2009;36(9):536–40.

Non-Traumatic Hepatobiliary Emergencies

Christopher Decker, MD*, Dorothy Liu, MD

KEYWORDS

- Cholangitis • Liver cyst • Hepatic abscess • Cholecystitis • Pancreatitis
- Bile duct injury

KEY POINTS

- Non-traumatic hepatobiliary emergencies are a common general surgery consult and can be life threatening if left untreated.
- Symptomatology is often vague and nonspecific, often requiring expeditious workup combining physical exam, laboratory findings, and diagnostic imaging to quickly narrow differential diagnosis.
- While surgery is often the definitive treatment, endoscopic or percutaneous options exist for those patients that are poor surgical candidates.

INFLAMMATORY BILIARY DISEASE
Acute Calculous Cholecystitis

More than 200,000 people are diagnosed with acute cholecystitis each year.[1] It typically presents with right upper quadrant pain and tenderness, nausea, and fever. Oftentimes these symptoms are associated with the consumption of greasy or fatty foods. The arrest of inspiration with right upper quadrant palpation is known as the Murphy sign and is pathognomonic for acute cholecystitis. Acute calculous cholecystitis is the most common type of acute cholecystitis and it results from obstruction of the cystic duct by gallstones, resulting in inflammation, edema, and eventually necrosis of the bile ducts and the gallbladder. Cholelithiasis is present in 10-15% of adults in the United States, of whom only 20% will develop symptoms when followed for 15 years.[2] However, gallstones are responsible for 90-95% of all cases of acute cholecystitis.[1] Acute calculous cholecystitis can be differentiated from biliary colic based on its temporality–biliary colic is transient in nature (<3 hours) and persistence of pain beyond this timeframe is suggestive of acute cholecystitis.

Temple University Hospital Department of Surgery, 3401 N. Broad St., Philadelphia, PA 19104, USA
* Corresponding author. LKSOM, Temple University Hospital, 3401 N. Broad, Philadelphia, PA 19104.
E-mail address: christopher.decker@nyulangone.org
Twitter: @ChrisDeckerMD (C.D.)

Surg Clin N Am 103 (2023) 1171–1190
https://doi.org/10.1016/j.suc.2023.05.015
0039-6109/23/© 2023 Elsevier Inc. All rights reserved.
surgical.theclinics.com

Labs obtained should include a CBC, BMP, and LFTs. Labs may reveal a leukocytosis with a left shift, and LFTs may be normal or show a mild hyperbilirubinemia of <3 mg/dL, which results from inflammation of the biliary tract or compression of the biliary tree by the distended gallbladder.[1] Total bilirubin levels >3 mg/dL are suggestive of an obstruction in the common bile duct (such as Mirizzi syndrome or choledocholithiasis), making acute cholecystitis less likely.

Right upper quadrant ultrasound, which has a sensitivity of 81-88%, and a specificity of 80-83%[1,2] is often the first imaging study of choice as it is inexpensive, fast, and does not expose the patient to radiation. Features that support a diagnosis of acute calculous cholecystitis include the presence of cholelithiasis or sludge, gallbladder distension, gallbladder wall thickening >4 mm, pericholecystic fluid, and sonographic Murphy's sign. CT scan also has a 94% sensitivity and a 59% specificity for detecting acute cholecystitis and will demonstrate pericholecystic fat stranding and/or fluid, gallbladder distension, and mural thickening. CT has the added benefit of a more expansive view of pericholecystic involvement in instances of acute cholecystitis complicated by gangrene, hemorrhage, abscess, fistulization, or perforation. However, cholelithiasis is not always detectable with CT scans as this depends on their composition and the thickness of the CT slices.

Hepatobiliary iminodiacetic acid (HIDA) scan, or hepatobiliary scintigraphy, is often used if ultrasonography results are equivocal. It has a sensitivity of 96% and a specificity of 89%.[1]

Early laparoscopic cholecystectomy is the standard of care in the United States for uncomplicated, acute calculous cholecystitis.[1] Patients who have a dilated common bile duct (CBD) visualized on ultrasound or hyperbilirubinemia warrant an intraoperative cholangiogram to evaluate for possible obstruction. Patients who undergo laparoscopic cholecystectomy within 72 hours of presentation have been shown to have lower rates of complications, mortality, conversion to open cholecystectomy, and shortened length of hospital stay.[1,3]

Patients with mild acute cholecystitis and severe medical comorbidities can be considered for initial treatment with 7-14 days of antibiotics covering the most commonly involved organisms: enteric gram-negatives (*Escherichia coli, Klebsiella, and Enterobacter* species); anaerobes (*Clostridium, bacteroides*); enterococci; and streptococci. If these patients do not improve within 72 hours, consideration should be given to biliary drainage with a percutaneous cholecystostomy tube. Medical therapy has been reported to have a >85% response rate with no acute biliary events in most patients over the following 1-3 years.[4]

When left untreated, uncomplicated acute cholecystitis can progress to emphysematous cholecystitis, gangrene, and eventually gallbladder perforation. Operative management is necessary in complicated acute cholecystitis. In fact, gangrenous cholecystitis is considered a surgical emergency as it is associated with a 15% rate of sepsis and death.[2] If laparoscopic or open cholecystectomy cannot be safely performed, subtotal cholecystectomy should be considered, which involves removal of the gallbladder wall and/or ablation of remnant gallbladder mucosa, removal of gallstones, and closure of the cystic duct[5] to reduce the risk of bile leak. For patients with complicated acute cholecystitis who either refuse surgery or are at unacceptably high surgical risk, percutaneous cholecystostomy tube placement and initiation of broad-spectrum antibiotics is appropriate.

Surgical technique
Laparoscopic cholecystectomy is the standard treatment for acute calculous cholecystitis. Recall that if the patient has bilirubinemia or a dilated CBD on imaging, there

may be the presence of choledocholithiasis in which case an intraoperative cholangiogram is also indicated.[2]

- The patient should be positioned supine on the operating room table, and the table positioned in such a way that a fluoroscopic C-arm can access the upper abdomen easily. Arms should be abducted.
- The surgeon stands on the patient's left while an assistant stands on the patient's right. A second assistant who is holding the camera should position themselves standing behind the surgeon, on the patient's left side.
- The laparoscopic screens should be at 10 and 2 o'clock in relation to the patient's head.
- A total of 4 trocars are typically used, with one or two 10- or 12-mm trocars and two or three 5-mm trocars.
- Access into the abdomen should be achieved either using a Veress needle followed by placement of a 10- or 12-mm supraumbilical trocar, or using a Hasson technique to place a 10- or 12-mm trocar in the supraumbilical position. Carbon dioxide should be used to insufflate the abdomen until one reaches 15 mm Hg of pneumoperitoneum.
- Additional ports should be placed in the epigastrium (using a 10-mm trocar), in the right upper quadrant (5-mm trocar), and an assistant port in the right lateral abdomen in the anterior axillary line (5-mm trocar) as the assistant port.
- The patient should be positioned in the Reverse Trendelenburg position with slight rotation towards the patient's left to help with exposure.
- The assistant utilizes the assistant port to provide cephalad traction on the gallbladder fundus to expose the infundibulum and the porta hepatis. Adequate cephalad retraction is critical to successful exposure and dissection of the cystic duct and cystic artery during this procedure.
  - At times, if exposure is inadequate despite positioning the patient in steep Reverse Trendelenburg and adequate retraction, a fifth trocar can be placed on the patient's left side, and an instrument used to push the duodenum down out of your view.
  - Use of a 30-degree angled scope is also crucial for adequate exposure intraoperatively.
- The peritoneum of the gallbladder should be incised at the infundibulum at its junction with the cystic duct and the peritoneum opened laterally and medially while using a grasper to retract the gallbladder laterally (while performing medial dissection) and medially (while performing the lateral dissection).
- The peritoneum should be teased off of the cystic duct and the space between the cystic duct and cystic artery dissected to expose Calot's triangle. During this dissection it is also reasonable to dissect the peritoneal attachments between the gallbladder and liver bed at the inferior aspect of the gallbladder to aid in retraction. Ideally, the surgeon should achieve the critical view of safety before dividing the cystic duct or cystic artery, but in order to pedunculate the gallbladder, the cystic artery may have to be ligated with clips and transected. Exposure of the cystic duct only needs to proceed as far as is required to allow adequate length for placement of clips.
- Once the gallbladder is pedunculated, one clip can be placed on the cystic duct as close to the gallbladder infundibulum as possible. It is at this point a cholangiogram can be performed if necessary. If no cholangiogram is required, or once the cholangiogram is complete, 2 clips should be placed on the duct just below

its junction with the gallbladder and the duct divided. The same can be done for the cystic artery.

- The gallbladder should be dissected off of the liver bed. The gallbladder fossa should be checked for hemostasis just before removing the last bit of peritoneum connecting the gallbladder to the liver, as the gallbladder can be used as a handle for exposure of the fossa.
- Once the gallbladder is off of the liver, it can be placed in a sterile retrieval bag and removed from the abdomen through either the periumbilical or the epigastric port. This can prove to be challenging if there are large stones in the gallbladder; the fascia can be dilated with a kelly clamp to facilitate its removal.
- Once the gallbladder is removed, the surgeon should replace the trocar in the port that the gallbladder was removed from and the right upper quadrant should be irrigated and suctioned, making sure to remove fluid from the subphrenic space and Morison's pouch where it tends to collect.
- Once the abdomen is desufflated, the skin should be closed with subcuticular sutures and covered with sterile surgical glue or steri strips.

The most common complications of laparoscopic cholecystectomy include intra-abdominal or abdominal wall bleeding (1.8%), wound infection (1.0%), or extrahepatic bile duct injury (0.4%).[1] Less common complications include related to trocar placement, thermal injury to the duodenum, retained CBD stones, gallstone spillage, or intra-abdominal abscess.

Bile leak is one of the most feared complications and is both highly morbid and costly. Rates of bile leak are higher in laparoscopic cholecystectomy (0.1–0.5%) versus the open approach (0.2%) and often occurs due to misidentification of biliary tree anatomy or technical error. Use of intraoperative cholangiography (IOC) has been shown to reduce rates of CBD injury, from 0.58% without IOC to 0.39% with IOC.[6] To minimize the risk of bile duct injury, the Society of American Gastrointestinal and Endoscopic Surgeons (SAGES) recommends utilizing the following 6 strategies intraoperatively.

1. Using the critical view of safety to identify the cystic artery and cystic duct intraoperatively
2. Be aware of the potential for aberrant anatomy
3. Make liberal use of cholangiography intraoperatively to delineate biliary anatomy intraoperatively
4. Consider an intraoperative momentary pause prior to clipping, cutting, or transecting any ductal structures
5. Recognize when dissection is reaching an area of significant risk and halt dissection before entering this zone. If it appears to be too dangerous to continue then consider other methods to conclude the operation safely.
6. Get help from another surgeon when the dissection or conditions are difficult.

The management of bile duct injuries differs based on the location and severity of the injury and is visited in more detail later in this article.

Specific scenarios: pregnancy

Acute cholecystitis occurs in approximately 1 in 1600 pregnancies and is the second most common indication for surgery during pregnancy. Elevation in circulating estrogen and progesterone levels promote gallstone formation during pregnancy by increasing cholesterol secretion, decreasing bile acid production, and delaying gallbladder emptying. As a result, bile becomes supersaturated with cholesterol, leading to increased gallstone formation.

Symptoms of cholecystitis in pregnancy are similar to those in nonpregnant women–postprandial epigastric or right upper quadrant pain. After pregnancy-related causes for pain have been ruled out, workup can proceed similarly with lab work (including a CBC, BMP, LFTs, and a lipase) and a right upper quadrant ultrasound. If choledocholithiasis is suspected, MRCP is considered safe for use in pregnancy. If needed, ERCP can also be performed at radiation levels that are safe for the fetus.

Biliary colic in pregnancy can first be managed conservatively with bowel rest, intravenous fluids, and pain control. However, failure of conservative management should prompt consideration of laparoscopic cholecystectomy as the risk for recurrent symptoms can range as high as 38%-72%. Relapse of symptoms is also associated with a 27% chance of developing complicated disease, including acute cholecystitis, choledocholithiasis, or gallstone pancreatitis. Complicated gallstone disease can result in increased maternal and fetal morbidity or even fetal loss. Pregnant patients who undergo laparoscopic cholecystectomy have been shown to have significantly lower maternal complications (4.3% to 16.5%) and fetal complications (5.8% to 16.5%) than those who do not.[7]

Laparoscopic cholecystectomy can be performed in any trimester and has been shown to be associated with shorter operative time, shorter hospital stay, and lower rates of maternal and fetal adverse outcomes than an open approach. Intraoperative cholangiography exposes the mother and fetus to minimal radiation and is safe to use selectively in pregnancy. Efforts should be made to shield the fetus from any radiation.[8]

If the fetus is previable, evaluation of the fetal heart rate pre- and post-procedurally is sufficient. For viable fetuses, an obstetric professional should be involved with the administration of corticosteroids in the event of preterm labor. Intraoperative fetal heart monitoring is recommended as well. Pregnant patients are typically positioned with a bump under their right side to offload compression of the inferior vena cava by the gravid uterus with the rest of their positioning being the same as a laparoscopic cholecystectomy in a nonpregnant patient.[7]

SUMMARY

Acute calculous cholecystitis is a common consultation for the general surgeon. Standard management is with a laparoscopic cholecystectomy with or without an intraoperative cholangiogram, depending on specifics of the situation. One must always be wary of bile duct injuries when performing laparoscopic cholecystectomy as this can be one of the most feared complications of the surgery.

Acute Acalculous Cholecystitis

Approximately 5-10% of cases of patients presenting with acute cholecystitis have acute acalculous cholecystitis (AAC),[1] in which patients can develop acute gallbladder inflammation without any existing gallstones. The etiology of AAC is multifactorial and quite different from that of calculous cholecystitis–largely, it is secondary to bile stasis and ischemia in critically ill patients. It is also associated with risk factors including: trauma, shock, burn, fever, prolonged fasting, diabetes, HIV infection, atherosclerosis, congestive heart failure, leukemia, ESRD, and TPN. It is also the cause of cholecystitis in about 50-70% of cases of acute cholecystitis in children. Contributing factors in this population include dehydration, infection, and lymphadenopathy.[4]

Clinically, AAC can mimic calculous cholecystitis with right upper quadrant pain and fever. It should be suspected in all critically ill patients in which the etiology of their illness has not been identified. Since many patients with AAC are intubated and sedated, they are often unable to participate in the examination. Abnormal LFTs and leukocytosis may or may not be present. Overall, these findings are nonspecific and can make clinical diagnosis of acalculous cholecystitis difficult.

Imaging holds the key to the diagnosis of AAC. Ultrasound is recommended as the first choice and will demonstrate gallbladder wall thickening (>3.5 mm), pericholecystic fluid, intramural gas or edema, or a sloughed mucosal membrane. Note that abnormal gallbladder findings on ultrasound can also be present in critically ill patients without AAC, and that these findings may not be specific on their own and require consideration of the rest of the patient's clinical picture as well for diagnosis.[9]

CT and HIDA scans are also useful imaging modalities. CT scan has the added benefit of being able to evaluate the abdomen for other possible pathologies. HIDA scan has a high rate of false positives (ie, it does not demonstrate filling of the gallbladder with radionuclide marker after 60 minutes), and adding morphine (which causes contraction of the sphincter of Oddi and promotes gallbladder filling) can increase its sensitivity. Nonvisualization of the gallbladder 30 minutes after morphine administration is considered a positive test. Contraction and emptying of the gallbladder with the administration of cholecystokinin (CCK) would suggest against a diagnosis of AAC.[9]

Treatment of AAC relies on adequate source control. Broad-spectrum antibiotics to cover biliary organisms should be initiated. While cholecystectomy is the only definitive treatment option, oftentimes patients with AAC are unable to tolerate surgery. Cholecystostomy tubes can serve as either definitive treatment or as a temporizing measure until cholecystectomy can be safely performed. After the cholecystostomy tract has matured (about three weeks), if the patient's cholecystitis has improved, cholangiography should be performed to confirm a patent cystic duct and the cholecystostomy tube can be removed. Cholecystostomy tube placement has been shown to have reduced morbidity, hospital costs, and length of stay than cholecystectomy for AAC without a significant difference in mortality.[10] In patients who are at high surgical risk or poor surgical candidates, cholecystostomy tube placement can be definitive and has been shown to have low rates of recurrence as they do not have gallstones to cause cholecystitis.[11] If a patient fails to improve with cholecystostomy tube placement or if there is evidence of gallbladder perforation, cholecystectomy is indicated.

If surgery or cholecystostomy tube placement cannot be performed, endoscopic retrograde cholangiopancreatography (ERCP) can be attempted to decompress the biliary tree.

Surgical techniques

- Please refer to the section on acute calculous cholecystitis for laparoscopic cholecystectomy technique.
- The majority of cholecystostomy tubes are placed percutaneously under ultrasound or CT guidance using a transhepatic or transperitoneal approach.
- The transhepatic approach is often preferred to prevent peritoneal bile spillage. However, it does come with the risk of hepatic abscess formation or transient bacteremia from forming direct connections between the biliary system and the hepatic sinusoids.
- A transperitoneal approach is best used when the gallbladder is extremely inflamed and thickened as this has a higher likelihood to seal around the cholecystostomy tube and prevent spillage.
- The gallbladder is accessed with a sheathed needle and the bile aspirated to confirm the positioning of the needle tip in the gallbladder. Sometimes the bile

can be clear secondary to hydrops. Using the Seldinger technique a pigtail catheter is coiled into the gallbladder lumen and secured to the skin.[2]

The main complications of cholecystostomy tube placement include bile leakage, bleeding, or tube dislodgement. Bleeding can be prevented by making sure to correct any coagulopathy before tube placement, especially when using a transhepatic approach. Bile leakage can occur if the gallbladder is necrotic and does not form a good seal around the site of tube insertion into the gallbladder. This should be suspected if a patient has clinical worsening after tube placement or if they have initial improvement and subsequent clinical worsening after tube placement.[2]

SUMMARY

AAC is a disease process typically seen in the critically ill that should be suspected when other possible causes of critical illness have been ruled out. Signs and symptoms of AAC are often non-specific, and its diagnosis can prove to be elusive. Imaging is key to an accurate diagnosis. While cholecystectomy is recommended, often times patients are not well enough to tolerate a surgical procedure and may require biliary drainage with a cholecystostomy tube or endoscopically.

Acute Cholangitis

Acute cholangitis is a dreaded sequela of biliary tract obstruction that results from the ascension of bacteria into the biliary system. Bile is naturally sterile, but bacteria can ascend into the biliary system through the sphincter of Oddi and a gallstone or stent can serve as a nidus of infection, allowing for rapid bacterial proliferation. It is most common in patients 50-70 years old and occurs with the same frequency in men and women. Risk factors include prior biliary surgery and cholelithiasis. The most common cause of cholangitis is choledocholithiasis (30–70%),[4] but there are a myriad of other causes including malignancy causing extrinsic compression of the bile duct, Mirizzi syndrome, primary sclerosing cholangitis with stricturing, obstruction of existing stents, or previous biliary surgery leading to duct stricturing. Bacteremia and sepsis results when bacteria translocate from the biliary system into the portal vein and thus the systemic circulation. Acute cholangitis requires urgent management and can be life threatening if left untreated.

Acute cholangitis classically presents with right upper quadrant pain, fever, and jaundice–a constellation of signs known as Charcot's triad. Severe cholangitis and sepsis can also manifest as altered mental status and hypotension (Reynold's pentad).

Labs will demonstrate a leukocytosis and direct hyperbilirubinemia (obstructive pattern) with associated elevations in alkaline phosphatase and transaminases. Ca 19-9 can be elevated in the presence of biliary obstruction, but does not necessarily indicate malignancy. If the Ca 19-9 is found to be elevated at initial presentation it should be rechecked after resolution of the infection. 60-90% of bile cultures will be positive as well as 20-70% of blood cultures. *Escherichia coli* is the most commonly seen organism on bile or blood cultures followed by *klebsiella* and *pseudomonas* species.[4]

If there is a very high suspicion of acute cholangitis, a patient can undergo ERCP without preceding imaging so as to not delay treatment. However, if the diagnosis is not entirely clear, the first imaging study that should be obtained is an abdominal ultrasound. Ultrasound will typically demonstrate intra- and/or extra-biliary duct dilation, depending on the level of obstruction. Cholelithiasis and gallbladder sludge are also commonly visualized. Choledocholithiasis can be diagnosed only about 30% of the time with ultrasound but as much as 80% of choledocholithiasis can be identified with MRCP (with stones being >6 mm). MRCP is the best study for characterizing bile duct obstruction and its cause.[4] CT scan can identify biliary ductal dilation and the location of an obstruction but is unable to diagnose the cause of obstruction.

Any patient who is suspected to have acute cholangitis should be initiated on appropriate antibiotic coverage and have urgent drainage of the gallbladder. Ultimately, once the acute infection is addressed, the patient should have definitive treatment of the cause of obstruction. Per the 2018 Tokyo Guidelines, piperacillin-tazobactam or carbapenems are optimal single agents that can be used for empiric antibiotic coverage. Dual agents should include metronidazole combined with either a cephalosporin or a fluoroquinolone. If severe, vancomycin or antifungals should be considered as well. The patient should also be admitted to an ICU for fluid resuscitation and close monitoring.

Definitive treatment involves biliary drainage; this may result in slightly different procedures depending on the exact etiology of the cholangitis. In 90-95% of cases, ERCP with sphincterotomy and stent placement is sufficient. In patients who cannot undergo ERCP (ie, those with altered anatomy due to prior surgical reconstruction, a duodenal obstruction, or difficult access to the ampulla) and have intrahepatic biliary dilation, percutaneous transhepatic cholangiography (PTC) and percutaneous transhepatic biliary drainage (PTBD) is an effective option. When performed, it is successful 90% of the time. The presence of ascites is a contraindication to PTC and PTBD because it can have complications such as biliary fistulas, bleeding, recurrent cholangitis, and hepatic abscesses. Finally, in those who cannot undergo ERCP and also do not have intrahepatic biliary dilation that would make them candidates for PTBD, a third option is an EUS-guided biliary drainage (EUS-BD). EUS-BD can be used to place a covered metallic stent across a choledochoduodenostomy or hepaticogastrostomy; however, this technique is often limited to tertiary care centers with advanced endoscopic capabilities.

Surgical techniques

- Please refer to the section on acute acalculous cholecystitis for the technique of percutaneous cholecystostomy tube placement.
- In the open technique, the gallbladder should be located with an ultrasound and a transverse muscle-splitting incision made over the expected location of the gallbladder.
- A purse-string suture should be placed in the fundus of the gallbladder, followed by decompression of the gallbladder and removal of the stones (if present) with forceps or a scoop.
- Then, a #20 or #24 french foley catheter, malecot drain, or similar drainage catheter should be placed through a separate stab incision in the abdominal wall and secured within the fundus of the gallbladder using the previously placed purse-string suture. The transverse incision should then be closed.[2]
- Open cholecystostomy and cholecystolithotomy has been shown in a small case series to be a safe and effective option in patients who are severely ill or elderly.[12]

Please refer to the section on acute acalculous cholecystitis for complications and management of cholecystostomy tube placement.

SUMMARY

Acute cholangitis results from biliary obstruction and can be life-threatening. Appropriate management involves initiation of broad-spectrum antibiotics and urgent biliary drainage. This can be accomplished endoscopically, percutaneously, or with surgery.

Gallstone Pancreatitis

Gallstones are the most common cause of acute pancreatitis in the Western world and accounts for about 60% of cases (with alcoholic pancreatitis being the next most common underlying etiology). As of 2014, the incidence of gallstone pancreatitis (GSP) was estimated to be in approximately 20 of every 100,000 people.

Risk factors for GSP are similar to those that predispose patients to developing cholelithiasis. The incidence of developing GSP from symptomatic gallstones is about 3-8%. 80% of GSP cases are mild with a mortality of 1%–3%. The other 20% of GSP cases are severe and mortality is as high as 30%.[13] In the presence of cholelithiasis, GSP is thought to be a result of transient obstruction of the common bile or pancreatic duct by a passing stone. Another theory for the pathophysiology of GSP is biliary sludge causing cholestasis or irritating the sphincter of Oddi, thus causing edema of the sphincter and biliary outflow obstruction. In either instance, the obstructive process results in excessive activation of pancreatic enzymes and inappropriate inflammation and subsequently autodigestion of pancreatic tissue.

Patients who present with GSP will typically present with sudden-onset, constant epigastric or right upper quadrant pain radiating to the back with or without complaints of preceding biliary colic. It is associated with nausea, and vomiting. Oral intake exacerbates the pain. Patients will typically have exquisite abdominal tenderness upon examination. Bruising of the flanks (Grey Turner's sign), umbilicus (Cullen's sign) or inguinal regions are classically seen if hemorrhagic pancreatitis is present. Concomitant jaundice or alcoholic stools should raise suspicion of obstructive choledocholithiasis or cholangitis.

Peripancreatic inflammation can have deleterious effects on other parts of the body. Generalized ileus can result as a reaction to peripancreatic inflammation. Moderate or severe pancreatitis can incite a systemic inflammatory response and present with tachycardia, fevers, and tachypnea.

Laboratory analysis with a lipase and/or amylase level is helpful in the initial evaluation: a serum lipase or amylase level >3x the upper limit of normal is generally accepted as being diagnostic for pancreatitis. One should be mindful to consider the duration of symptoms when interpreting these laboratory values. Additionally, the lipase and amylase levels do not necessarily correlate with disease severity. Note that lipase is more specific than amylase, as amylase is also found in saliva. LFTs are also useful for determining whether or not the etiology of pancreatitis is related to gallstones or if there is biliary obstruction. Elevated alkaline phosphatase or gamma-glutamyl transpeptidase may reflect persistent cholestasis. In 10% of cases of GSP, LFTs will be normal.

All patients presenting with acute pancreatitis and no obvious cause should undergo initial evaluation with an abdominal ultrasound to detect the presence of sludge or gallstones. The gallbladder is usually not inflamed as GSP is a result of the migration of cholelithiasis or sludge rather than acute cholecystitis. Ultrasound is limited because it cannot assess the severity of pancreatitis, and so CT scan is often performed to evaluate the degree of peripancreatic inflammation and extent of disease. A pancreas protocol CT is the ideal study to evaluate the degree of inflammation as well as disruption of the pancreatic parenchyma and main duct. Up to 20% of patients with GSP will present with severe disease (with associated organ failure) and will require intensive care.[4,13]

In patients with mild gallstone pancreatitis, it is recommended to perform cholecystectomy within the same hospital admission to prevent future recurrence. In more severe disease, patients should undergo delayed cholecystectomy in order to avoid serious complications secondary to ongoing inflammation and scarring.[14] Patients can develop multi-organ system failure due to a hyperinflammatory systemic response. The resulting immunosuppression leaves them more susceptible to highly resistant infections that can lead to infected pancreatic necrosis, bacteremia, urinary tract infections, or pneumonia.

Infected pancreatic necrosis (IPN) is a dreaded complication that can be diagnosed when gas is seen within peripancreatic collections on CT scan or ultrasound. EUS with fine-needle aspiration can be used to confirm the presence of bacteria and guide antibiotic treatment, but it is not necessary for diagnosis. Clinical suspicion should be raised if the patient has a new onset of organ failure 2 weeks after admission with fever and rising inflammatory markers without an alternative source. IPN should be managed in specialty centers by experienced interdisciplinary teams including surgeons, gastroenterologists, and interventional radiologists. Mortality for patients with IPN is as high as 30%.

Based on the Pancreatitis, Necrosectomy versus Step Up Approach (PANTER) trial, the step-up approach is preferred over surgical management for IPN and has become the standard of care. This entails management with percutaneous catheter drainage, followed by video-assisted retroperitoneal debridement (VARD), and if that fails, then necrosectomy. The step-up approach has been shown to decrease associated morbidity and mortality as compared to aggressive, early surgical intervention.[4]

SUMMARY

Gallstones are the most common cause of pancreatitis in the Western world. Disease severity resulting from gallstone pancreatitis can range from mild disease to severe disease with associated multi-system organ failure. Cholecystectomy is recommended for mild disease but if severe pancreatitis develops, delayed cholecystectomy is preferred.

Iatrogenic bile duct injury

If a bile duct injury occurs and is recognized intraoperatively, the size of the injury and comfort level of the surgeon determine next management steps. Small injuries can be repaired over a T-tube. Major injuries (ie, transection) warrant consultation of a hepatobiliary surgeon for repair, or if one is not available, the surgeon should place a drain in the area and transfer the patient to a center with hepatobiliary expertise for definitive management. If there is no obvious identified leak intraoperatively but the dissection was particularly difficult and there is a concern for a possible leak, closed-suction drainage should be left in the gallbladder fossa.

About 75% of bile duct injuries are identified postoperatively. Patients with postoperative leaks typically present with abdominal pain and fever, and a mild hyperbilirubinemia. Patients who have stricture and occlusion of the biliary system without a leak typically present with jaundice with or without abdominal pain. They may also have abnormal liver function tests, recurrent cholangitis, or evidence of stricture on imaging.

The first proposed system of classifying bile duct injuries was proposed by H. Bismuth in 1982 and later modified by Strasberg, which identifies different types of bile duct injuries based on their location in the biliary tract.[15] Evaluation and subsequent management of a bile duct injury proceeds quite differently for a bile leak versus an obstructive injury (such as a stricture). If there is a concern for a bile leak, initial workup should include a hepatic function panel as well as an ultrasound or an abdominal CT scan. CT scans have a higher sensitivity for detecting fluid collections (96% to 70%) as compared to ultrasound.[4] If intraoperative drain placement was not performed, percutaneous drainage should be performed to drain the fluid or, if present, the biloma. Slow, low-volume leaks (<300 cc/day) can be managed with 5-7d of drainage alone. A patient with a high-volume leak (>300 cc/day) should undergo ERCP which can be both diagnostic and therapeutic. If the bile leak appears to be secondary to a duct of Luschka or cystic duct stump leak, endoscopic treatment with stent placement and/or sphincterotomy should be performed to decompress the biliary tree in addition to drainage. However, if the bile leak is a result of an injury to the common bile duct, definitive management with a hepaticojejunostomy should be performed.[2]

In patients who present postoperatively with jaundice, one must investigate an underlying obstructive process. MRCP is a useful initial test in evaluating the biliary tree for intrahepatic duct dilation, any associated fluid collections or abscesses, and level of injury. A normal postoperative CBD will demonstrate slow tapering in size–but an abrupt cutoff with associated intrahepatic biliary duct dilation should raise suspicion of a clipped hepatic duct or CBD. An ERCP has utility in visualizing the biliary anatomy proximal to the level of injury. PTC should be performed to define the proximal extent of the biliary injury followed by placement of a catheter to allow for drainage of the intrahepatic biliary system.[4]

All patients who present with a bile duct injury should undergo either an MR or CT angiography to identify any arterial or portal venous injury.[4]

The management of bile duct injuries, like their evaluation, is dependent on many factors including the timing of diagnosis, the level and extent of the injury, and the patient's baseline status. Leaks from the cystic duct or CBD or lateral injuries can be managed with ERCP and stent placement. Associated bilomas should be drained percutaneously. Noncircumferential strictures, as well as strictures of the hepatic duct and CBD can also be managed with ERCP, serial dilations, and stent placement.

For those with a completely occluded or transected bile duct, surgical intervention is required. Patients who present within days after their injury should undergo preoperative evaluation immediately followed by surgical intervention. Those who present weeks to months from their injury may benefit from decompression of the biliary tree for several months before proceeding with surgery, to allow any acute inflammatory changes to resolve.

Surgical management of occluded/transected bile ducts aims to create a tension-free, mucosa-to-mucosa biliary-enteric anastomosis. A Roux-en-Y hepaticojejunostomy with a 40 cm roux limb is preferred over a choledochojejunostomy, which is associated with more complications including reflux gastritis or sump syndrome.[16] Stents are often placed across the anastomosis and left in for several months postoperatively.

SUMMARY

Iatrogenic bile duct injury is one of the most feared complications of laparoscopic cholecystectomy; it can be identified intraoperatively but is more commonly diagnosed postoperatively. Any surgeon with intraoperative concern for a bile duct injury should place a drain in the gallbladder fossa; intraoperative repair should only be attempted in the hands of a surgeon experienced with the technique. The management of bile duct injury depends on its etiology.

HEPATIC DISEASE
Liver Abscess

The incidence of liver abscess has been on the decline as the diagnostic and treatment of intraabdominal infections continues to improve. The annual incidence is estimated to be 2.3 cases per 100,000 people however this varies based on country, age, and even sex of the patient[17] Current literature suggests that the incidence in Taiwan for example may be as high as 17.6 per 100,000. Overall, it is estimated that liver abscesses make up roughly 13% of intra-abdominal abscess.[18,19]

The etiology of the majority of liver abscesses can be attributed to biliary tract infections, malignancies, or interventions. In addition, other common sources include intra-abdominal infections such as appendicitis and diverticulitis with translocation of bacteria via portal vein or hepatic artery. Finally, direct trauma to the liver parenchyma may result in contamination, necrosis, bile leakage and subsequent resulting infection. More than half can result from biliary sources including cholangitis[20,21]

Classifications of these abscess are additionally separated by organism. The vast majority are pyogenic, however amoebic, echinococcal, and fungal also make up the milieu. Despite the over declining incidence, it is important to understand the severity of these abscesses as they continue to have high mortality risk in untreated patients.

Pyogenic liver abscess

While many pyogenic liver abscess are polymicrobial the most common organisms in the western countries are *Streptococcus*, *Staphylococcus*, *Escherichia coli,* and *Klebsiella* in the East.[20] Septic emboli from intra-abdominal sources can form larger intra-hepatic abscesses. Hematogenous spread is not limited to the portal system but can be from endocarditis or pyelonephritis as well.

The workup begins with a history and physical followed by imaging. Fever, chills, night sweats, malaise, right shoulder pain (due to phrenic nerve irritation), right upper quadrant pain, nausea, and vomiting.[22] Leukocytosis and abnormalities in liver functions tests are also expected. In a minority of cases, septic shock and peritonitis may be present in the presence of prolonged untreated course or rupture of abscess.

CT scan is considered the most useful imaging modality as it has high sensitivity in detecting the abscess but also to look for the underlying source. As with most infections, source control is the fundamental component of treatment. Antibiotic coverage is also important and must cover *Enterobacteriaceae*, anaerobes, *Streptococci*, and *Enterococci*.[17] Such antibiotic regimens may include a cephalosporin plus metronidazole or beta-lactam/beta-lactamase inhibitor plus metronidazole, or synthetic penicillins plus aminoglycosides and metronidazole as an example. Published data suggest a duration ranging from 2-6 weeks. The duration should depend on a clinical course and adequacy of source control.

The majority of the pyogenic liver abscesses occur in the right lobe which may allow ultrasound-guided aspiration. Percutaneous aspiration is often used for an abscess <5 cm. For those larger than 5 cm or multiloculated, a percutaneous catheter is preferred and will allow for continued drainage[23–25] In either case obtaining a gram stain and culture is important to guide antibiotic therapy and narrow broad-spectrum antibiotics whenever possible. Although ultrasound or CT-guided drainage has a reported success rate of over 80% surgical drainage continues to have a role.

Indications for surgical drainage include peritonitis, failure of the percutaneous drainage attempts to obtain adequate source control, or concomitant intra-abdominal process that requires surgical intervention.[4] Current literature suggests that a laparoscopic approach to drainage is both a safe and effective alternative to an open approach and may reduce post-operative recovery time and hospital length of stay.[26]

Amebic liver abscess

Entamoeba histolytica, although rare in the United States, should be considered in those with recent travel or immigration. *E. histolytica* is endemic in Africa, India,

Mexico, and Central and South America.[27,28] Some population studies estimate that more than 50% of the population in these endemic areas may be infected although most are not symptomatic. Patients found to have amebic cysts without recent travel or immigration should be considered for immunosuppression from HIV, infection, malnutrition etc.

The life cycle of this protozoan is important to understand the symptomatology of the disease. Ingestion of a cyst occurs through the fecal-oral route from the direct transmission, unwashed fruits, vegetables, or contaminated water. Passing into the intestinal tract the trophozoite is released from the cyst and can infiltrate the colonic mucosa. From here, they migrate via the portal system to the liver. Abdominal pain, fever, diarrhea, and hepatomegaly are a few of the most common symptoms that initially occur.[27] Stool studies should be obtained in those with high suspicion. In addition, serology for Echinococcus is needed.

CT or US imagine are typical components of the work up. However, a nuclear medicine gallium or technetium 99m liver scan may aid in differentiating amebic from pyogenic as there will be a lack of enhancement as there are no leukocytes present in amebic cysts.

In general, 10 days of oral metronidazole is the first-line treatment. This is curative in 90 percent of the patients. Chloroquine is less effective but remains a viable alternative. Needle aspiration is typically not indicated unless of failure of metronidazole which may be seen in large cysts >5 cm.[29]

Parasitic liver abscess

Echinococcus granulosus is a canine tapeworm which causes a hydatid cyst of the liver. More predominant in Africa, Middle Eastern countries, and Asia, this tapeworm's intermediate host is most often found in sheep. Patients typically present with symptoms that include abdominal pain, fever, RUQ pain or fullness, and hepatomegaly from cyst expansion. Laboratory tests may include eosinophilia seen on a complete blood count, and elevation in LFTs may be seen. Finally, enzyme-linked immunosorbent assay (ELISA) seems to be the most sensitive and specific for *Echinococcus*.[4,29]

Ultrasound (US) and CT scan, consistent with other liver cysts is the most widely used with high sensitivity and specificity in the diagnosis. US worldwide has a specificity of 90% and is often the first line given the availability. Thick walls, daughter cysts, calcifications are some of the classic ultrasound findings. CT scan offers further details that can help differentiate the type of cyst (**Fig. 1**).

A fundamental component of treatment is with Benzimidazoles, an antihelminthic drug. Albendazole 15 mg/kg twice daily for two to six months depending on clinical response is the standard regimen. This should be used in combination with surgical or percutaneous intervention as evidence suggests combination therapy is better than either alone.[4] There is a high risk of anaphylaxis if the cyst ruptures into the abdominal cavity. Therefore, early intervention remains the recommendation. Traditionally, an open surgical approach has been used, ensuring the abdomen is completely packed off to prevent spread diffuse seeding and anaphylaxis in case of rupture.[30] With improved interventional radiology capabilities the PAIR technique is gaining support in select patients: Puncture, Aspiration, Injection of a scolicidal agent, and Respiration.[31] The World Health Organization recommends using 20% hypertonic saline as the scolicidal agent. There has been encouraging evidence in both short- and long-term results that suggest this technique is a safe and viable alternative to surgical drainage in select patients.[32–34]

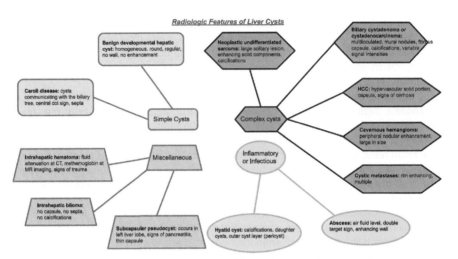

Fig. 1. Radiologic features of different types of liver abscesses. (Cameron's).

Fungal liver abscess

Fungal liver abscesses are typically seen in severely immunocompromised patients. As with pyogenic forms, fungal abscess formation is thought to be spread from the gastrointestinal tract or the biliary system. In addition to immunosuppression other risk factors include indwelling biliary stents in patients, multiple courses of antibiotics due to recurrent cholangitis, or known malignancy within the hepatobiliary system[4,27,30] Empiric antifungal therapy and source control are the mainstays of treatment as in pyogenic cysts.

Nontraumatic hemobilia

Hemobilia is defined as bleeding into the biliary tree from an abnormal connection between a blood vessel and a bile duct. It manifests as a gastrointestinal (GI) bleed and can often be difficult to distinguish from more common causes of GI bleeding. While the 2 most common causes of hemobilia are iatrogenic causes and trauma, the most common non-traumatic cause is malignancy (which accounts for approximately 10% of all hemobilia cases), which will be the focus of this section. Hemobilia has been associated with cholangiocarcinoma, pancreatic adenocarcinoma, gall bladder carcinoma, hepatocellular carcinoma (HCC), or liver metastases.[35]

The classic presentation of hemobilia is the constellation of signs known as Quincke's triad: abdominal pain, jaundice, and GI bleeding. Serum LFTs are often abnormal, most commonly demonstrating hyperbilirubinemia and an elevated alkaline phosphatase. The pathophysiology is not fully known but it is believed to develop as a result of the rich vascular supply and friable tissue that often accompanies malignancy, thus creating an environment that is at higher risk of spontaneous hemorrhage. In patients with HCC for example, while spontaneous rupture is rare (<3% reported), it is highly fatal (>50%).

Other, more rare causes of non-traumatic hemobilia include portal biliopathy, chronic ductal obstruction, and intraductal infection by organisms such as *Clonorchis sinensis* (Chinese river fluke), roundworms, or *Fasciola hepatica* (sheep river fluke).

Angiography remains the gold standard for both diagnosis and treatment of hemobilia; however, less invasive studies have arisen as alternatives before proceeding with angiography. A CT angiogram (CTA) of the abdomen is often the initial imaging study performed for suspected hemobilia. The benefit of a CTA is that it allows for the evaluation of other possible causes of GI bleeding and it is noninvasive. Upper endoscopy can also be used to evaluate the major papilla to assess for sources of blood and ERCP will help to visualize the biliary tree. EUS can detect vascular abnormalities, blood clots within the biliary tree, or choledochal varices that would suggest portal biliopathy as a cause of hemorrhage.

Treatment of hemobilia should factor in 2 important components: hemostasis; and maintaining bile flow, which prevents obstructive clot formation in the biliary system. Management of hemobilia differs based on the particular situation (**Fig. 2**). Mild hemobilia (ie, small volume of blood loss without hemodynamic instability) can be managed with the correction of coagulopathy and intravenous fluids. Patients with major hemorrhage and drop in hemoglobin despite supportive care should undergo endoscopic (for hemostatic techniques and/or stent placement), interventional radiologic, or surgical intervention. Patients who are hemodynamically unstable should undergo emergent hepatic angiography and embolization or surgical resection. Care must be taken when performing angiography and transarterial embolization as there is a risk of hepatic and biliary ischemia and necrosis.

Surgery is reserved for instances when endoscopic or interventional management has failed, except in the case of pseudoaneurysms that are infected or compressing vascular structures.

Complications of hemobilia are primarily related to obstruction of the biliary tree by blood clots, which can result in acute cholecystitis, cholangitis, acute pancreatitis, or obstructive jaundice. These can be managed medically or with ERCP. Biliary strictures can result from hepatic artery embolization and can also be managed either endoscopically or percutaneously with dilation of the strictured segment.[36]

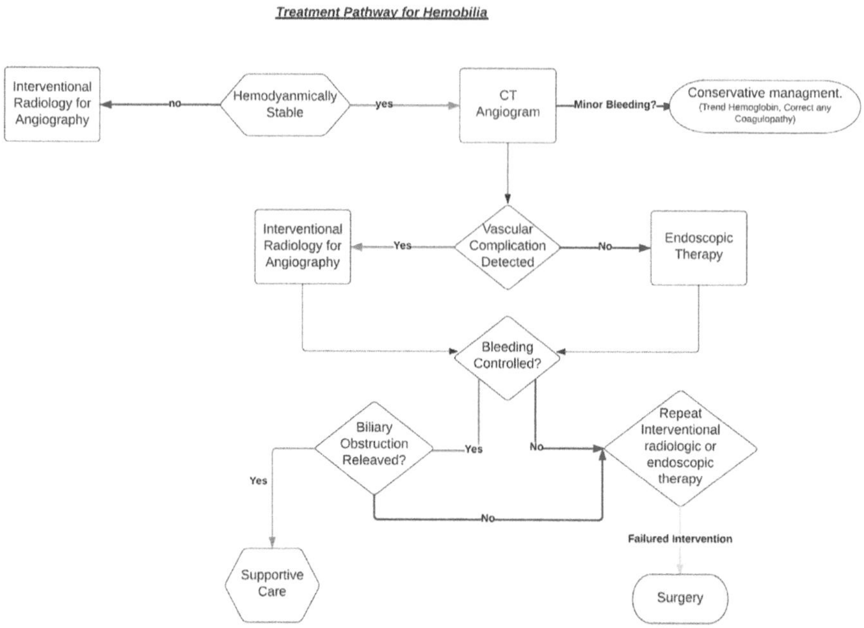

Fig. 2. A flowchart demonstrating the proposed management pathways of hemobilia.

Acute portal vein thrombosis

The major vascular supply to the liver is derived from the portal vein supplying 75% of its blood flow while the remaining 25% of inflow is from the hepatic artery. The portal vein forms from the confluence for the splenic and superior mesenteric veins draining the spleen and small bowel. The portal vein, approximately 6–8 cm long divides in the hilum of the liver into the left and right portal vein branches. Portal blood drains into hepatic sinusoids and eventually through the hepatic veins which empty into the inferior vena cava (IVC) (see **Fig. 2**).

In the non-cirrhotic liver, portal vein thrombosis (PVT) is rare. Thrombophillia is the most common reason cited for acute portal vein thrombosis in non-cirrhotics which requires workup if PVT is diagnosed.[37,38] Disorders of the coagulation cascade such as Factor V Leiden is the most common inherited hypercoagulable state in the United States. Deficiency in protein C or protein S, antiphospholipid syndrome may also be the underlying cause of a hypercoagulable state. Underlying malignancy must also be considered especially those hematologic in nature.

In the cirrhotic liver the prevalence varies widely with the degree of cirrhosis, however may be as high as 20% in those on the transplant waiting list.[39,40] The diminished hepatic synthetic function reduces circulating levels of coagulation factors, inhibitors of coagulation, and fibrinolytic factors. Platelet numbers are decreased because of a combination of decreased thrombopoietin synthesis and spleno-megaly with sequestration.[38]

The most common symptom is acute onset of abdominal pain and distention. Fever may be present and should prompt consideration of an intraabdominal infection which should be treated concurrently or ruled out. Nausea, vomiting. and splenomegaly may also be found depending on the extent of PVT.[37,38,41]

In patients with bowel ischemia, laboratory testing may reveal metabolic acidosis, signs of renal or respiratory failure, leukocytosis, and elevated lactate.

Diagnostic imaging is required to confirm the diagnosis. US findings consist of hyperechoic material within the lumen of the portal vein, dilation, and diminished blood flow. US sensitivity ranges from 73-90% and has a negative predictive value of 98%[42–44] CT scan however is preferred to assess the extent of the thrombus and any mesenteric or splanchnic involvement. Signs of mesenteric thrombus include mesenteric congestion and thickened bowel walls. In severe cases, indistinct bowel wall margins, and ascites raise suspicion for intestinal infarction or gangrene.[45]

Current guidelines divide treatment options between cirrhotic and non-cirrhotic patients.[37] Therapeutic anticoagulation however remains the mainstay of treatment in both groups. In the non-cirhottic patient therapeutic anticoagulation has been proven to increase portal vein patency rates as high 72%.[46] The goal of anticoagulation is to halt propagation of clot, reduce bowel ischemia from venous outflow obstruction and mesenteric congestion, reduce hospital length of stay, and improve survival.[37,41]

Current guidelines recommend anticoagulation for 3 to 6 months with low molecular weight heparin or warfarin as there is limited evidence of direct oral anticoagulants especially in cirrhotics. CT imaging should take place at three months after initiation of anticoagulation to assess recanalization. To date, it is not clear whether to continue anticoagulation beyond six months if complete recanalization has not occurred by that time[41,37,47,48]

Thrombolysis continues to emerge with observational studies among non-cirrhotic acute portal vein thrombosis. Two methods include indirect via superior mesenteric arterial infusion of tissue plasminogen activator, urokinase or streptokinase or directly into the portal vein via transhepatic approach,[49,50] This may considered for those patients with extensive mesenteric vein thrombosis, who have progressive thrombosis despite anticoagulation and are at risk of intestinal ischemia.[49,51,52]

Finally, in patients with a high suspicion or confirmed infarction or perforation of the intestines surgical resection must take place if the compromised bowel. Often because of the venous congestion a temporary closure and repeat trips to the operating room may warranted to ensure there is no progression of disease prior to anastomosis and closure.

CLINICS CARE POINTS

- Overall mortality is 10% but this increases in the presence of cirrhosis and malignancy which are often associated.

- Complications include portal hypertension, mesenteric ischemia leading to mesenteric infarction, worsneing hepatic function including coagulopathy.

- Treatment options range from systemic anticoagulation to cateter directed lysis. In addition attempt to determine and treat the underlying cause of the thrombus shoudl be made.

- Serial abdominal exams and monitoring laboratory such as white blood cell and lactate may suggest the bowel ischemia has progressed to perofration requiring exploratory laporotomy.

DISCLOSURE

The authors have nothing to disclose.

REFERENCES

1. Gallaher JR, Charles A. Acute cholecystitis: a review. JAMA 2022;327(10): 965–75.
2. Fischer J. Fischer's Mastery of Surgery. 7th ed. Wolters Kluwer Health. Available at: https://wolterskluwer.vitalsource.com/books/9781496399403.
3. Zafar SN, Obirieze A, Adesibikan B, et al. Optimal time for early laparoscopic cholecystectomy for acute cholecystitis. JAMA Surgery 2015;150(2):129–36.
4. Cameron J.L., Cameron A.M., Current Surgical Therapy. 9th ed. Elsevier - OHCE. Available at: https://bookshelf.health.elsevier.com/books/9780323640619.
5. Strasberg SM, Pucci MJ, Brunt LM, et al. Subtotal cholecystectomy–"fenestrating" vs "reconstituting" subtypes and the prevention of bile duct injury: definition of the optimal procedure in difficult operative conditions. J Am Coll Surg 2016; 222(1):89–96.
6. Flum DR, Dellinger EP, Cheadle A, et al. Intraoperative cholangiography and risk of common bile duct injury during cholecystectomy. JAMA 2003;289(13): 1639–44.
7. Schwulst SJ, Son M. Management of gallstone disease during pregnancy. JAMA Surgery 2020;155(12):1162–3.
8. Pearl JP, Price RR, Tonkin AE, et al. Guidelines for the Use of Laparoscopy during Pregnancy - A SAGES Publication. SAGES. https://www.sages.org/publications/guidelines/guidelines-for-diagnosis-treatment-and-use-of-laparoscopy-for-surgical-problems-during-pregnancy/. Accessed August 28, 2022.
9. Huffman JL, Schenker S. Acute acalculous cholecystitis: a review. Clin Gastroenterol Hepatol 2010;8(1):15–22.

10. Simorov A, Ranade A, Parcells J, et al. Emergent cholecystostomy is superior to open cholecystectomy in extremely ill patients with acalculous cholecystitis: a large multicenter outcome study. Am J Surg 2013;206(6):935–41.

11. Kirkegård J, Horn T, Christensen SD, et al. Percutaneous cholecystostomy is an effective definitive treatment option for acute acalculous cholecystitis. Scand J Surg 2015;104(4):238–43.

12. Slama EM, Hosseini M, Staszak RM, et al. Open cholecystostomy under local anesthesia for acute cholecystitis in the elderly and high-risk surgical patients. Am Surg 2022;88(3):434–8.

13. Cucher D, Kulvatunyou N, Green DJ, et al. Gallstone pancreatitis. Surg Clin 2014; 94(2):257–80.

14. Kimura Y, Takada T, Kawarada Y, et al. JPN Guidelines for the management of acute pancreatitis: treatment of gallstone-induced acute pancreatitis. J Hepato-Biliary-Pancreatic Surg 2006;13(1):56–60.

15. Chun K. Recent classifications of the common bile duct injury. Korean J Hepato-biliary Pancreat Surg 2014;18(3):69–72.

16. Schreuder AM, Franken LC, van Dieren S, et al. Choledochoduodenostomy versus hepaticojejunostomy – a matched case–control analysis. HPB 2021; 23(4):560–5.

17. Mischnik A, Kern WV, Thimme R. [Pyogenic liver abscess: changes of organisms and consequences for diagnosis and therapy]. Dtsch Med Wochenschr 2017; 142(14):1067–74.

18. Kaplan GG, Gregson DB, Laupland KB. Population-based study of the epidemiology of and the risk factors for pyogenic liver abscess. Clin Gastroenterol Hepatol 2004;2(11):1032–8.

19. Altemeier WA, Culbertson WR, Fullen WD, et al. Intra-abdominal abscesses. Am J Surg 1973;125(1):70–9.

20. Lardière-Deguelte S, Ragot E, Amroun K, et al. Hepatic abscess: diagnosis and management. J Visc Surg 2015;152(4):231–43.

21. Czerwonko ME, Huespe P, Bertone S, et al. Pyogenic liver abscess: current status and predictive factors for recurrence and mortality of first episodes. Oxford): HPB; 2016.

22. Mohsen AH, Green ST, Read RC, et al. Liver abscess in adults: ten years experience in a UK centre. QJM 2002;95(12):797–802.

23. Zerem E, Hadzic A. Sonographically guided percutaneous catheter drainage versus needle aspiration in the management of pyogenic liver abscess. AJR Am J Roentgenol 2007;189(3):W138–42.

24. Cai YL, Xiong XZ, Lu J, et al. Percutaneous needle aspiration versus catheter drainage in the management of liver abscess: a systematic review and meta-analysis. HPB (Oxford) 2015;17(3):195–201.

25. Domínguez-Guzmán DJ, Moreno-Portillo M, García-Flores C, Blas-Franco M. Drenaje laparoscópico de absceso hepático. Experiencia inicial [Laparoscopic drainage of liver abscess. Initial experience]. Cir Cir 2006;74(3):189–94.

26. Ndong A, Tendeng JN, Diallo AC, et al. Efficacy of laparoscopic surgery in the treatment of hepatic abscess: a systematic review and meta-analysis. Ann Med Surg (Lond). 2022;75:103308.

27. Townsend CM, Beauchamp RD, Evers BM. In: Mattox KL, editor. Sabiston textbook of surgery. 20th edition. Philadelphia, PA: Elsevier; 2016.

28. Hasan S, Fearn R. Fungal liver abscess in an immunocompetent patient who underwent repeated ERCPs and subtotal cholecystectomy. Case Reports 2018; 2018. bcr-2017.

29. Akhondi H., Sabih D.E., Liver Abscess. [Updated 2022 Jul 4]. In: StatPearls [Internet]. Treasure Island (FL): StatPearls Publishing; 2022 Jan-. Available at: https://www.ncbi.nlm.nih.gov/books/NBK538230/. Accessed December 2022.

30. Tamarozzi F, Vuitton L, Brunetti E, et al. Non-surgical and non-chemical attempts to treat echinococcosis: do they work? Parasite 2014;21:75.

31. Khuroo MS, Dar MY, Yattoo GN. Percutaneous drainage versus albendazole therapy in hepatic hydatidosis: a prospective, randomized study. Gastroenterology 1993;104:1452–9.

32. Khuroo M. Hydatid disease. Indian J Gastroenterol 2001;20:C39–43.

33. Khuroo M. Hydatid disease: current status and recent advances. Ann Saudi Med 2002;22:56–64.

34. Khuroo MS. Percutaneous drainage in hepatic hydatidosis-the PAIR technique: concept, technique, and results. J Clin Exp Hepatol 2021;11(5):592–602.

35. Cathcart S, Birk JW, Tadros M, et al. Hemobilia: an uncommon but notable cause of upper gastrointestinal bleeding. J Clin Gastroenterol 2017;51(9):796.

36. Zhornitskiy A, Berry R, Han JY, et al. Hemobilia: Historical overview, clinical update, and current practices. Liver Int 2019;39(8):1378–88.

37. Simonetto DA, Singal A, Garcia-Tsao G, et al. ACG Clinical Guideline: Disorders of the Hepatic and Mesenteric Circulation. Am J Gastroenterol 2020;115(1): 18–40.

38. Northup PG, Garcia-Pagan JC, Garcia-Tsao G, et al. Vascular liver disorders, portal vein thrombosis, and procedural bleeding in patients with liver disease: 2020 practice guidance by the american association for the study of liver diseases. Hepatology 2021;73:366–413.

39. Nery F, Chevret S, Condat B, et al. Causes and consequences of portal vein thrombosis in 1,243 patients with cirrhosis: results of a longitudinal study. Hepatology 2015;61:660–7.

40. Samant H., Asafo-Agyei K.O., Garfield K., Portal Vein Thrombosis. [Updated 2022 Sep 12]. In: StatPearls [Internet]. Treasure Island (FL): StatPearls Publishing; 2022 Jan-. Available at: https://www.ncbi.nlm.nih.gov/books/NBK534157/. Accessed December 2022.

41. de Franchis R. Evolving consensus in portal hypertension. Report of the Baveno IV consensus workshop on methodology of diagnosis and therapy in portal hypertension. J Hepatol 2005;43:167–76.

42. Bach AM, Hann LE, Brown KT, et al. Portal vein evaluation with US: comparison to angiography combined with CT arterial portography. Radiology 1996;201: 149–54.

43. Brunaud L, Antunes L, Collinet-Adler S, et al. Acute mesenteric venous thrombosis: case for nonoperative management. J Vasc Surg 2001;34:673–9.

44. Lee HK, Park SJ, Yi BH, et al. Portal vein thrombosis: CT features. Abdom Imaging 2008;33:72–9.

45. Lee SS, Ha HK, Park SH, et al. Usefulness of computed tomography in differentiating transmural infarction from nontransmural ischemia of the small intestine in patients with acute mesenteric venous thrombosis. J Comput Assist Tomogr 2008;32:730–7.

46. Plessier A, Darwish-Murad S, Hernandez-Guerra M, et al. Acute portal vein thrombosis unrelated to cirrhosis: a prospective multicenter follow-up study. Hepatology 2010;51:210–8.

47. Maldonado TS, Blumberg SN, Sheth SU, et al. Mesenteric vein thrombosis can be safely treated with anticoagulation but is associated with significant sequelae of portal hypertension. J Vasc Surg Venous Lymphat Disord 2016;4:400–6.

48. Amitrano L, Guardascione MA, Scaglione M, et al. Prognostic factors in noncirrhotic patients with splanchnic vein thromboses. SOAm J Gastroenterol 2007; 102(11):2464–70.
49. Hollingshead M, Burke CT, Mauro MA, et al. Transcatheter thrombolytic therapy for acute mesenteric and portal vein thrombosis. J Vasc Interv Radiol 2005;16: 651–61.
50. Wolter K, Decker G, Kuetting D, et al. Interventional treatment of acute portal vein thrombosis. Röfo 2018;190(8):740–6.
51. Smalberg JH, Spaander MVMCW, Jie KS, et al. Risks and benefits of transcatheter thrombolytic therapy in patients with splanchnic ve-nous thrombosis. Thromb Haemost 2008;100:1084–8.
52. Cao G, Ko GY, Sung KB, et al. Treatment of postoperative main portal vein and superior mes-enteric vein thrombosis with balloon angioplasty and/or stent placement. Acta Radiol 2013;54:526–32.

Diabetic Soft Tissue Infections

Christine Castater, MD, MBA[a],*, Elliot Bishop, MD[b],
Adora Santos, DO[b], Mari Freedberg, MD[b], Phillip Kim, MD[b],
Christopher Sciarretta, MD[c]

KEYWORDS

- Diabetic foot • Infection • Diabetes • Necrotizing soft tissue infection
- Soft tissue infections • Cellulitis

KEY POINTS

- Pathophysiology of diabetes is a risk factor for developing soft tissue infections as well as for wound healing.
- Surgical site infections are increased in poorly controlled diabetic patients.
- Cellulitis and abscesses are more common in diabetic patients because of bacterial colonization and decreased immune competence.
- Because necrotizing soft tissue infections (NSTIs) can progress rapidly and cause sepsis and even death, diagnosis and surgical debridement must be aggressive and prompt.
- Expedited diagnosis and management of all soft tissue infections associated with diabetes is paramount.

INTRODUCTION

Diabetes affects millions of adults worldwide and up to 10% of Americans, so it is important to understand the health sequelae associated with the disease. Hyperglycemia impairs the immune system and leads to a susceptibility to infections. These infections can range from cellulitis or abscesses to necrotizing soft tissue infections (NSTIs). In addition, increased vascular insufficiency and peripheral neuropathy lead to an increased risk of foot wounds. Most important to the general surgeon is the association between hyperglycemia and increased surgical site infections (SSIs). The workup and management of these infections vary, so it is important to understand them. It is important to have a high index of suspicion for soft tissue infections in diabetic patients.

[a] Morehouse School of Medicine, Grady Memorial Hospital 1C-144, 80 Jesse Hill Jr Drive Southeast, Atlanta, GA 30303, USA; [b] Emory University, Grady Memorial Hospital Glenn Building 69 Jesse Hill Jr Drive Southeast, Atlanta, GA 30303, USA; [c] University of Tennessee, University of Tennessee College of Medicine, 975 3rd Avenue, Chattanooga, TN 37403, USA
* Corresponding author. Morehouse School of Medicine, Grady Memorial Hospital, 80 Jesse Hill Jr Drive SE, Room 2C144, Atlanta, GA 30303.
E-mail address: ccastater@msm.edu
Twitter: @grannysurgeon (C.C.)

Surg Clin N Am 103 (2023) 1191–1216
https://doi.org/10.1016/j.suc.2023.06.002
0039-6109/23/© 2023 Elsevier Inc. All rights reserved.

surgical.theclinics.com

PATHOPHYSIOLOGY

Diabetes not only puts patients at risk of developing infection but also leads to delayed wound healing. In particular, this relates to poorly controlled diabetes with hyperglycemia.[1] Susceptibility to infection is caused by many factors, including impaired immune response, vascular insufficiency, peripheral neuropathy, increased asymptomatic colonization, and organism-specific factors.

Immunologic impairment occurs by multiple complex mechanisms, including decreased chemotaxis, opsonization, phagocytosis, and wound maturation.[2] Neutrophil function is reduced owing to decreased tumor necrosis factor-alpha (TNF-alpha) and interleukin-1 (IL-1) release from macrophages as well as decreased chemotaxin release.[3,4] Hyperglycemia diverts nicotinamide adenine dinucleotide phosphate from the opsonization pathway, thereby impairing it and decreasing bacterial and fungal clearance.[5] Increased gene induction leads to increased early apoptosis in wounds, thereby impairing intracellular bactericidal ability and normal wound maturation.[6] Reduction in major histocompatibility complex class 1 expression and reduced production of IL-10, interferon-gamma, and TNF-alpha significantly impair phagocytosis.[7] Hyperglycemic inhibition of oligosaccharide binding reduces the function of many aspects of cell-mediated immunity.[8]

Vascular disease is common in diabetic patients and can cause local tissue ischemia. This enhances the growth of certain bacteria while also impeding leukocyte function. It also impairs the inflammatory response and decreases antibiotic absorption. Peripheral neuropathy can cause unnoticed wounds to develop into serious infections. In addition, diabetic patients are more likely to be colonized with bacteria, such as *Staphylococcus aureus* including methicillin-resistant strains as well as with pseudomonal species.[9] Fungal colonization including with candida and rhizopus (mucor) is also common in diabetic patients.[10] Hyperglycemia causes glucose-induced proteins to assist *Candida* species in epithelial adherence and phagocytosis resistance.[11] Mucor species also thrive in these high-glucose, acidic environments.[12]

SURGICAL SITE INFECTIONS

SSIs and poor wound healing directly correlate with poor diabetes control and perioperative hyperglycemia.[13,14] This is due to many of the same cytologic factors that increase general infection risk. Growth factor production, angiogenic response, macrophage function, collagen accumulation, epidermal barrier function, quantity of granulation tissue, and keratinocyte and fibroblast migration and proliferation are all impaired.[15] After retrospectively controlling for other factors, postoperative hyperglycemia has been shown to be the sole risk factor for SSI[16] with increased levels of hyperglycemia directly correlating with increased SSI risk (**Fig. 1**). This is supported by both prospective and retrospective data as well as by data showing that perioperative glycemic control decreases SSI rates.[17–19]

DIABETIC FOOT WOUNDS
Epidemiology

According to the International Diabetes Federation, it is estimated that 537 million adults between the ages of 20 and 79 have been diagnosed with diabetes. The prevalence is predicted to increase to 643 million by 2030 and 783 million by 2045.[20] The global annual incidence of diabetic foot ulcers is estimated to be between 9.1 million and 26.1 million, with a lifetime incidence as high as 19% to 34%.[21] Among the reasons for hospital admission of a diabetic patient, foot wounds are the most common,[22] with an associated

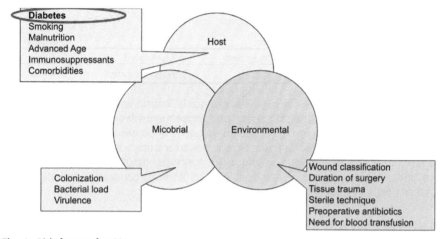

Fig. 1. Risk factors for SSI.

morbidity and mortality as high as 50% across a 5-year period.[23] In addition, diabetic foot ulcers are the leading cause of nontraumatic amputations in the United States,[24] and postamputation mortality increases to 39% to 80% over a 5-year period.[25]

Pathophysiology

The underlying pathophysiology that leads to the development of a diabetic foot wound is complex and multifactorial. Poor glycemic control leads to polyneuropathy and arterial insufficiency predisposing individuals to unrecognized trauma with poor perfusion, which then increases the risk for wounds, ulcerations, and infections.[26]

The polyneuropathy caused by diabetes mellitus is attributed to dysfunction of motor, sensory, and autonomic nerve fibers.[27] Dysfunction in peripheral motor fibers leads to muscle atrophy of the lumbricals and interosseous muscles, which results in anatomic changes to the arch of the foot. These changes can lead to "claw" deformities of the toes, hammertoe contractures of digits, and equine ankle deformity[28,29] (**Fig. 2**).

Neuropathy is further complicated by damage to sensory nerve fibers, specifically, damage to type A and type C fibers. Dysfunction in type A fibers results in loss of proprioception, pressure sensation, vibratory perception, and gait abnormalities. Damage to type C fibers decreases the ability to perceive painful stimuli[30] (**Table 1**). Changes in

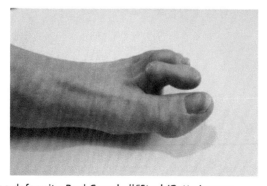

Fig. 2. Hammer toe deformity. Paul Campbell/iStock/Getty Images.

Table 1 Comparison of type A and type C nerve fibers			
Type of Nerve Fiber	**Function**	**Myelin**	**Diameter**
Type A	Proprioception	Myelinated	Large
Type C	Pain	Nonmyelinated	Small

peripheral autonomic nerve fibers cause changes in thermoregulation and anhidrosis, resulting in disruptions to the skin barrier and subsequent infection risk.[31,32] As previously discussed, unmanaged hyperglycemia leads to endothelial injury and combined with hyperlipidemia causes atherosclerosis, vascular compromise, and poor tissue perfusion.[33] Decreased perfusion affects immunologic function, leukocyte activity, and complement function.[34,35] Any infection that develops can lead to complications, such as hospitalization, amputation, and death.

Clinical Manifestation

On initial presentation of a patient with a suspected diabetic foot wound, it is important to identify what underlying risk factors or comorbidities exist. Pertinent details include glycemic control and regimen, prior ulcers, infections or surgeries, vascular disease, recent or past trauma causing foot deformity, systemic symptoms (ie, fevers), and tobacco use.[36]

Physical examination
Clinical examination should include visual inspection and assessment of the vascular, neurologic, and musculoskeletal systems.[37] Evaluation of the skin should pay particular attention to the dorsal aspect of the toes, plantar surface at the metatarsal heads, the heel, and the interdigital skin[38] (**Fig. 3**).

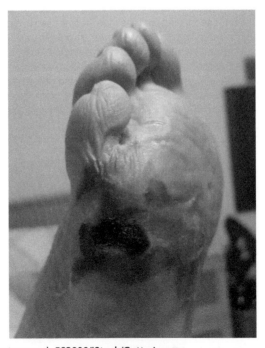

Fig. 3. Diabetic foot wound. PS3000/iStock/Getty Images.

Vascular compromise is highly prevalent among patients with diabetes mellitus and approximately two-thirds of patients presenting with foot ulcers will have peripheral arterial disease.[39] Providers should evaluate for palpable dorsalis pedis and/or posterior tibialis pedal pulses; if absent, further assessment with doppler, ankle-brachial index, or toe brachial pressure index is recommended.[40,41] The clinical examination is catered more toward identifying the presence of loss of protective sensation rather than neuropathy, although neuropathy can also be examined.[42] Evaluating neuropathy is done via 10-g monofilament, vibration, touch, and thermal sensation tests[21,42–48] (**Fig. 4**). The musculoskeletal examination should include assessment for gross deformities of both the arch and the toes.[49]

Not all diabetic foot wounds or ulcers are infected, but roughly 50% to 60% will lead to infection,[50] and 20% of moderate to severe infections will result in amputation.[51] Diagnosis typically involves clinical assessment, laboratory studies, and imaging. Diabetic foot infections (DFIs) present on a spectrum and can range from superficial skin infection to osteomyelitis.[52] Classic signs of inflammation include erythema, edema, tenderness, warmth, and purulence (**Fig. 5**).[53]

Laboratory workup

Blood tests, such as complete blood count, C-reactive protein, and erythrocyte sedimentation rate (ESR), lack sensitivity and specificity. Up to 50% of patients presenting with a deep wound infection do not have leukocytosis.[54,55]

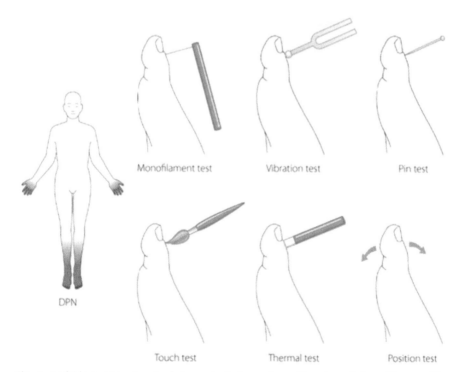

Monofilament test   Vibration test   Pin test

DPN

Touch test   Thermal test   Position test

Fig. 4. Bedside examination tools to evaluate large (type A) and small (type B) nerve fiber function. Large fibers are examined using 10-g monofilament, vibration with 128-Hz tuning fork, touch and joint position, and small fibers are examined using cold and warm sensation, and pinprick. (*From* Gylfadottir SS, Weeracharoenkul D, Andersen ST, Niruthisard S, Suwanwalaikorn S, Jensen TS. Painful and non-painful diabetic polyneuropathy: Clinical characteristics and diagnostic issues. J Diabetes Investig. 2019;10(5):1148-1157.)

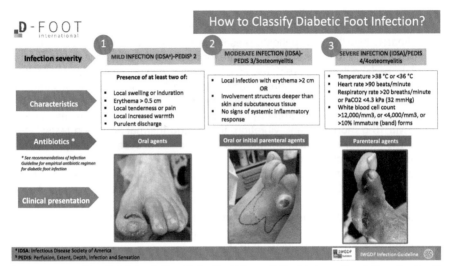

Fig. 5. How to Classify Diabetic Foot Infection? From D-Foot International How to classify diabetic foot infections. Available at https://d-foot.org/resources/resources/diabetic-foot-info-cards.

Radiography

Diagnostic imaging typically begins with plain radiographs to assess for fracture, foreign bodies, gas in soft tissues, or signs of osteolytic bone changes suggestive of osteomyelitis. Further evaluation can be done with computed tomography (CT) imaging or MRI, with the latter being the most sensitive and specific for diagnosis of osteomyelitis.[56–58]

Treatment

Antibiotic therapy

The Infectious Disease Society of America recommends initiating antibiotic treatment if 2 or more signs of inflammation exist (warmth, erythema, tenderness, pain, induration, or purulent discharge).[59,60] Many patients with mild to moderate infections can be managed in the outpatient setting with enteral antibiotics,[61] whereas those presenting with deeper wound infections will likely require parenteral antibiotics. Other considerations when determining inpatient versus outpatient management include compliance and health literacy.[62] Another important step in the management of a diabetic foot ulcer is staging and classification. The most common classification systems used are the Wagner and University of Texas Systems,[63] both of which assist in assessing the presence of infection, ulcer depth, and risk of amputation, while the University of Texas System also identifies the presence of ischemia[64] (**Tables 2** and **3**).

Table 2	
Wagner Diabetic Foot Ulcer Grade Classification System (sometimes referred to as Merritt-Wagner)	
0	Intact skin
1	Superficial ulcer
2	Deep ulcer
3	Ulcer with bone involvement
4	Forefoot gangrene
5	Full foot gangrene

Adapted from Wagner FW Jr. The dysvascular foot: a system for diagnosis and treatment. Foot Ankle. 1981;2(2):64-122; with permission.

Table 3
University of Texas diabetic foot ulcer classification system

Stage/Grade	0	1	2	3
A	Preulcerative or postulcerative lesion completely epithelialized	Superficial ulcer, noninvolving tendon capsule or bone	Ulcer penetrating to tendon or capsule	Ulcer penetrating to bone or joint
B	Infection	Infection	Infection	Infection
C	Ischemia	Ischemia	Ischemia	Ischemia
D	Infection & ischemia	Infection & ischemia	Infection & ischemia	Infection & ischemia

Score: Grade____ Stage____

Adapted from Lavery LA, Armstrong DG, Harkless LB. Classification of diabetic foot wounds. J Foot Ankle Surg. 1996;35(6):528-531; with permission.

Surgical management

For more severe infections, surgical intervention may be required and can range from basic incision and drainage to more extensive wound debridement or even amputation.[54] Even though 25% of diabetic foot ulcers that fail to heal will require amputation,[65] aggressive diagnosis and treatment reduce amputation rates.[66] Emergent operative management is indicated when signs of sepsis, ischemia, necrotizing fasciitis, or gas gangrene are present.[54] Overall management is centered on prevention with patient education being the most important preventive strategy.[67–70]

CELLULITIS AND ABSCESSES
Epidemiology

Cellulitis is an acute bacterial infection of the dermis and the subcutaneous tissue that can affect any part of the body, but most commonly occurs in the lower extremities.[71] The most common causes of cellulitis are the following: soft tissue trauma from puncture wounds or bites, burns, SSI, or secondary infection of existing skin conditions, such as eczema or venous stasis ulcers. These typically result from disruption of the skin by some exogenous factor. Less common causes are extension of a subjacent infection or hematogenous spread from a distant site of infection.

Risk factors for cellulitis[72] include the following:
- Diabetes mellitus
- Immunocompromise
- Peripheral vascular disease
- Lymphedema
- Interstitial edema
- History of irradiation to tissue

Because diabetic patients often develop peripheral vascular disease over time, their risk of developing cellulitis is increased.

Pathophysiology

Clinical manifestation

A skin abscess is a collection of pus within the dermis or subcutaneous space. It manifests as a painful, fluctuant, erythematous nodule without or without surrounding cellulitis. Spontaneous drainage of purulent material may occur, and regional adenopathy may be seen. Skin abscesses may develop via a deep infection of a hair follicle (furuncle), where purulent material has extended through the dermis into the subcutaneous tissue. Possible predisposing factors include increased friction and perspiration, corticosteroid use, diabetes mellitus, and inherited or acquired defects in neutrophil function.[73,74] Multiple furuncles can coalesce to form carbuncles, where destruction of fibrous tissue septa and interconnected abscesses are seen (**Fig. 6**). For both, *S aureus* is the most common causative organism. *S aureus* is frequently colonized on the skin of patients with diabetes, which contributes to their increased risk. Ultrasonography or radiographic examination can be useful to ascertain whether a skin or deeper abscess is present.

Signs and symptoms

Most patients with cellulitis will have the nonnecrotizing form of the disease process. Patients present with acute pain, erythema, and edema accompanied by constitutional symptoms, such as fever, chills, or malaise (**Fig. 7**). Physical examination usually

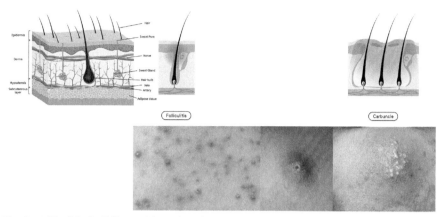

Fig. 6. Folliculitis, boil (furuncle), carbuncle (collection of boils) diagram and image. https://www.istockphoto.com/photo/skin-of-woman-with-big-and-painfull-furuncle-medicine-and-skincare-concept-gm1191905865-338457818?clarity=false. December 08, 2019. Accessed July 14, 2023. nymphoenix. Large abscess with pus under inflamed skin stock photoID 1338889918. https://www.istockphoto.com/photo/large-abscess-with-pus-under-inflamed-skin-gm1338889918-419353277?clarity=false. September 07, 2021. Accessed July 14, 2023. MicrovOne. Human skin. Layered epidermis with hair follicle, sweat and sebaceous glands. Healthy skin anatomy medical vector illustration stock illustration ID 1262260786. https://www.istockphoto.com/vector/human-skin-layered-epidermis-with-hair-follicle-sweat-and-sebaceous-glands-healthy-gm1262260786-369328776?clarity=false. :July 29, 2020. Accessed July 14, 2023. TAK. Image of skin problems, rough skin/acne, early to advanced folliculitis stock illustration ID 1411956564. https://www.istockphoto.com/vector/image-of-skin-problems-rough-skin-acne-early-to-advanced-folliculitis-gm1411956564-461587056?clarity=false. July 31, 2022. Accessed July 14, 2023. Created from: HengDao. Folliculitis stock photo ID 1332856446. https://www.istockphoto.com/photo/folliculitis-gm1332856446-415581289?phrase=pimples+folliculitis. August 07, 2021. Accessed July 14, 2023. Aleksej Sarifulin. Skin of woman with big and painfull furuncle. Medicine and skincare concept stock photo ID 1191905865.

shows erythema with advancing borders, tenderness, edema, increased warmth to touch, or fluctuance. Lymphangitis characterized by an erythematous linear streak that extends to a draining lymph node basin may be present. Perirectal abscesses have similar signs and symptoms but are located in the perineal area.

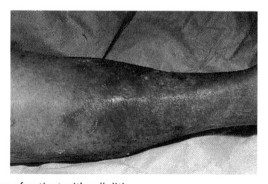

Fig. 7. Presentation of patient with cellulitis.

Microbiology

Most cellulitis in healthy adults is caused by a single aerobic pathogen, with the 2 most common organisms being *Streptococcus pyogenes* and *Staphylococcus aureus* (**Fig. 8**). *Streptococcus pneumoniae* is more common in patients with diabetes mellitus, alcoholism, systemic lupus erythematosus, and hematologic malignancies.[75] *Pseudomonas aeruginosa* is a particularly prevalent microorganism in diabetic infections and is discussed later in this article. Many diabetic infections can be polymicrobial, especially in the foot. Attempts to isolate a causative pathogen in general are usually unsuccessful, as needle aspiration and skin biopsy at an advancing margin of erythema are positive in only 15% and 40% of cases, respectively.

Treatment

Antibiotic therapy

Cellulitis can usually be treated with empirical antibiotic regimens that include medications effective against *S pyogenes* and *S aureus*. Methicillin-resistant *Staphylococcus aureus* (MRSA) can be present in up to 70% of all *S aureus* infections acquired in the community[76,77] and are more closely associated with diabetic patients. Bacteremia is uncommon, and only 2% to 4% of all patients with cellulitis will have positive blood cultures.[77,78] For otherwise healthy adults with a diagnosis of uncomplicated, early cellulitis without systemic manifestations, treatment can be provided with an oral antibiotic on an outpatient basis. The most empiric agents are the following: cephalexin, dicloxacillin, cefadroxil, erythromycin, or clindamycin. When MRSA is suspected, trimethoprim-sulfamethoxazole or clindamycin is often given. Appropriate analgesic agents should also be provided for pain control.

Patients that have diabetes mellitus or are immunocompromised, or who have systemic manifestations including high fever/chills or sepsis, rapidly expanding erythema, or cellulitis refractory to oral antibiotic treatment, should be admitted to the hospital for intravenous antibiotic therapy. For diabetic patients, ampicillin-sulbactam or piperacillin-tazobactam should be considered to cover gram-negative organisms. Vancomycin, linezolid, daptomycin, or tigecycline should be given to patients with high-risk or confirmed MRSA infections. Although not common, untreated or inadequately treated nonnecrotizing cellulitis can progress to necrotizing cellulitis. The diagnosis and management of NSTIs are discussed separately in this article.

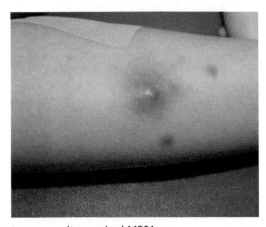

Fig. 8. Abscess due to community-acquired MRSA.

Surgical management
For fluctuant skin abscesses greater than 2 cm, treatment often consists of providing an antibiotic regimen and performing an incision and drainage procedure. A thorough search for loculated areas should be undertaken once the abscess cavity is unroofed to facilitate adequate drainage. The incision must be large enough to prevent premature closure and recurrence of the abscess. Culture of debrided material should be considered for patients with diabetic mellitus given higher presence of polymicrobial infection. For skin abscesses less than 2 cm that are spontaneously draining, close observation is an acceptable alternative. Although needle aspiration is less invasive, it is not recommended to perform needle aspiration of abscess contents unless the abscess is on the breast.[73,74]

NECROTIZING SOFT TISSUE INFECTIONS
Epidemiology

NSTIs are aggressive infections that can be difficult to recognize and diagnose but are rapidly progressive and are associated with high morbidity and mortality. These risks are drastically increased in patients who present in shock, are elderly, or are immunocompromised.[79,80] It is important for the evaluating physician to maintain a high index of suspicion for NSTIs, as early intervention with broad-spectrum antibiotics and surgical debridement has been consistently shown to improve survival.[81]

Pathophysiology

NSTIs are classified into 4 types, based on the pathogen of the underlying infection. Each has different features and predicted mortality. Type I NSTIs are the most common type of infection, are polymicrobial, and involve both aerobic and anaerobic bacteria.[79,80] Type II NSTIs are monomicrobial, with the most common pathogen being group A streptococcus. Less common are NSTIs caused by *Clostridium* and *Vibrio*, which fall under type III infections, and *Aeromonas* and fungi, which are found in type IV infections (**Table 4**).

Regardless of the pathogen causing the NSTI, the hallmark of these infections involves necrosis caused by bacterial toxins leading to cytokine activation, local thrombosis, and ischemia.[80] The resultant ischemia leads to further spread of the inciting pathogen, which leads to a cycle of further dissemination of infection with the potential for widespread disease (**Fig. 9**). It is the release of endotoxins and exotoxins by the causative pathogen that leads to the systemic illness often seen in NSTIs.

Clinical manifestation

The clinical presentation of NSTI can often be subtle and in approximately 50% of patients does not involve traumatic inoculation of the underlying bacteria.[82,83] Manifestations of NSTIs that are not associated with an open injury are often more subtle than those that are caused by traumatic inoculation. In the early stages of infection, patients present with pain and mild systemic symptoms. Cutaneous manifestations may include erythema (which can be mistaken for a simple cellulitis), bullae, skin necrosis, and/or local anesthesia[83,84] (**Figs. 10 and 11**).

Pain out of proportion to clinical findings, or pain extending beyond physical examination findings, should lead to a higher clinical suspicion for an underlying NSTI. It is very important to remember that even with more advanced disease, patients may present with varying severity of sepsis and without any notable physical examination findings.[84] In addition, lack of sensation can seem to be a reassuring symptom but may actually be a late finding when extensive necrosis destroys peripheral nerve fibers.

Table 4
Features of type I to IV necrotizing soft tissue infections

Types	Organisms	Population	Cause	Features	Mortality
Type I (70%–80%)	Polymicrobial	Multiple comorbidities	Polymicrobial, bowel flora	More indolent, better prognosis	Variable depending on comorbidities
Type II (20%–30%)	Group A strep (S aureus, MRSA)	Young, often healthy, intravenous drug user (IVDU)	Trauma, bites, IVDU	Aggressive, frequently missed, ± toxic shock syndrome	>30%
Type III (rare)	Monomicrobial (vibrio, clostridium)		Seafood ingestion, water contamination		30%–40%
Type IV (rare)	Fungal (Candida, Zygomycetes)	Immunocompromised	Trauma (wounds, bones)	Aggressive	>50%

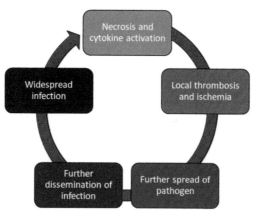

Fig. 9. Continuous dissemination cycle of NSTIs.

Diagnosis of NSTIs mostly relies on clinical findings. It is crucial for the provider to maintain a high index of suspicion when working up a patient for NSTI. When the diagnosis is unclear, the adjuncts listed in later discussion may help the physician make a diagnosis and initiate treatment. The authors want to emphasize that if there is any concern, prompt surgical intervention, which can include bedside cut-down, is warranted to rule out potentially rapidly progressing and life-threatening infection.

Laboratory workup
The Laboratory Risk Indicator for Necrotizing Fasciitis (LRINEC) score was initially created to allow physicians to detect NSTIs before the progression of the infection, as clinical signs are often subtle.[79] As noted above, physical examination findings may not correlate with severity of underlying infection. Therefore, the LRINEC score can be used to support clinical findings and aid in the diagnosis of an underlying NSTI[81] (**Table 5**). Importantly, the utility of the LRINEC score is supportive only because studies evaluating its sensitivity and specificity vary widely.[79] It is imperative that the physician not rely on a negative score to rule out NSTI, particularly if clinical suspicion remains high.[81,85] In particular, the LRINEC score's positive predictive value to diagnose NSTI is even less reliable in patients with diabetes, who already have a higher risk of morbidity and mortality with delayed treatment.[79]

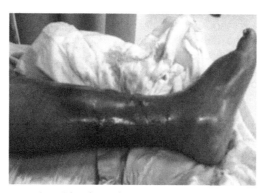

Fig. 10. Left lower extremity with edema, hemorrhagic bullae, and skin necrosis with foul-smelling discharge.

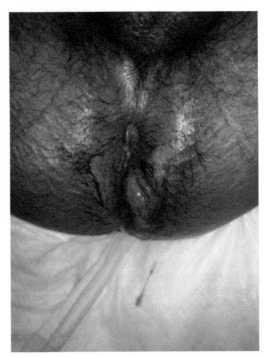

Fig. 11. Clinical presentation of perineal necrotizing soft tissue infection.

Radiography

Both plain film and axial imaging can be used in conjunction with physical examination findings to support the diagnosis of an NSTI. In the hemodynamically unstable patient, plain film imaging may be useful to quickly identify gas or edema within the soft tissue[8] **(Fig. 12)**. CT or MRI may show decreased enhancement, edema, or air along the fascial planes[80,83] but obtaining them may delay treatment. The absence of positive CT or MRI findings does not rule out a necrotizing infection and may delay initiation of treatment.[83]

Treatment

Once an NSTI is diagnosed, rapid initiation of treatment is crucial to successful management of NSTIs, as the rates of morbidity and mortality, intensive care unit, and hospital length of stays have been shown to decrease when surgical intervention is rapid.[81,86] The hallmarks of treatment for NSTIs involve both broad-spectrum antibiotic therapy and operative debridement.

Antibiotic therapy

Initial antibiotic therapy in patients in whom an NSTI is suspected should be broad to cover both aerobic and anaerobic activity, as well as MRSA, and can be narrowed based on cultures and sensitivities. Guidelines recommend empiric treatment with vancomycin, linezolid, or daptomycin, along with piperacillin-tazobactam, a carbapenem, or ceftriaxone with metronidazole, or a fluoroquinolone with metronidazole.[83] The addition of clindamycin also aids to suppress toxin-mediated cytokine production caused by group A streptococci.

Table 5
The laboratory risk indicator for necrotizing fasciitis

Variable	Score
C-reactive protein	
<15	0
≥15	4
Total WBC (1000 per mm³)	
<15	0
15–25	1
>25	2
Hemoglobin (g/dL)	
>13.5	0
11–13.5	1
<11	2
Sodium (mmol/L)	
≥135	0
<135	2
Creatinine (mg/dL)	
≤1.59	0
>1.59	2
Glucose (mg/dL)	
<180	0
≥180	1

Adapted from Wong CH, Khin LW, Heng KS, Tan KC, Low CO. The LRINEC (Laboratory Risk Indicator for Necrotizing Fasciitis) score: a tool for distinguishing necrotizing fasciitis from other soft tissue infections. Crit Care Med. 2004;32(7):1535-1541; with permission.

Surgical management

Although rapid initiation of antibiotic therapy is crucial, early surgical intervention and debridement of infected tissue is the key to successful management of the infection and improvement of survival.[82] Operative management is geared toward achieving source control by aggressive removal of infected and necrotic tissue (**Fig. 13**). Multiple debridements are often required to ensure true control of the infection, and progressive infection can often be seen during serial debridements[80] (**Fig. 14**). Once adequate control of the infection has been achieved, large disfiguring wounds can be managed using an interdisciplinary approach for appropriate tissue coverage.[80]

Perioperative care

Severe NSTIs often lead to severe systemic illness and multiorgan failure. The perioperative management in these patients is an important component of management. Close monitoring and management of a patient's hemodynamic status, frequent and careful serial examinations of wounds, strict glucose control and early nutritional support are all important adjuncts to management.[81] Rapid treatment of systemic disease, such as shock, respiratory or renal failure, is also key to survival.[84]

PSEUDOMONAS INFECTIONS
Epidemiology

P aeruginosa infections complicate DFIs. Although the presentation can vary, classic physical examination findings include a blue-green hue or the presence of Erythema

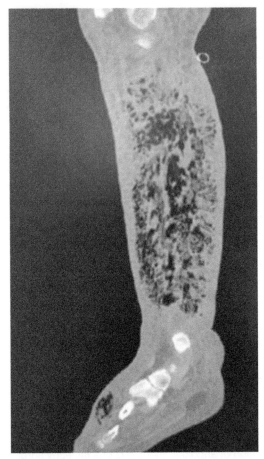

Fig. 12. Evidence of air tracking along the leg on coronal CT images of the right lower extremity.

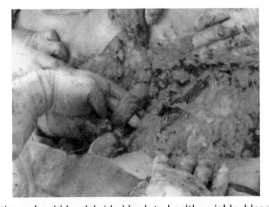

Fig. 13. Necrotic tissue should be debrided back to healthy, viable, bleeding tissue.

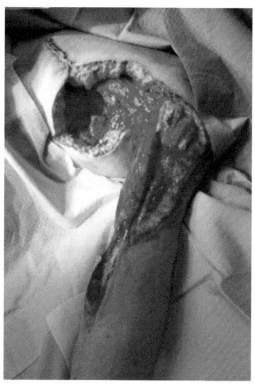

Fig. 14. Serial debridements occur until no infection remains and attention can be turned to closure of the defect.

Gangrenosum.[87] Diagnosis relies on blood and tissue cultures. Treatment largely depends on a multipronged antimicrobial approach given its high rate of drug resistance and tapering of antibiotics as soon as clinically possible.

   Pseudomonas remains a challenging diagnosis in the setting of diabetic infections. *Pseudomonas* is a gram-negative, flagellated, aerobic rod that is both catalase and oxidase positive.[88] It can grow in water and soil as well as on animals and plants. Although *Pseudomonas* strains are not the most common organism in DFIs, *P aeruginosa* specifically is the most common and virulent strain of *Pseudomonas* that occurs in DFIs. *Pseudomonas* most commonly occurs in the setting of polymicrobial infections and portends a poor prognosis as compared with DFIs without pseudomonal inoculation.[88,89] DFIs with *P aeruginosa* account for roughly 10% to 30% of all diabetic foot wounds[89,90] (**Fig. 15**).

   Risk factors for pseudomonal infections[88] include the following:
- Smoking
- Failure of outpatient antibiotic treatment for DFI within the past 90 days
- Advanced age
- Immunocompromised

Clinical Manifestation

The diagnosis of *Pseudomonal* infection in DFIs requires high clinical suspicion and an astute physical examination. Skin infection of *Pseudomonas* can occur owing to direct

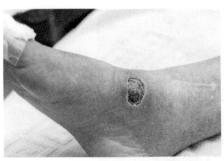 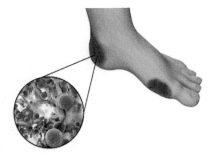

Fig. 15. Clinical examples of pseudomonal foot wounds. (*Left*) Nedomacki/iStock/Getty Images. (*Right*) Dr_Microbe/iStock/Getty Images.

organism inoculation in a wound or secondary seeding from a bacteremia.[89–91] *Pseudomonas* creates blue-green pigments owing to its creation of pyocyanin and pyoverdine.[92] Although wounds infected with *Pseudomonas* can have a blue-green hue or purulence, not all wounds infected with *Pseudomonas* will have this finding.[92]

Laboratory workup

An elevated ESR, as well as leukocytosis, more commonly occurs with pseudomonal DFIs, whereas ESR may not be elevated with other microbial infections.

Ecthyma Gangrenosum is a common manifestation of *Pseudomonas* infection and is characterized by erythematous nodules or hemorrhagic bullae that then progress into necrotic ulcers with eschar formation.[88,93] Interestingly, this can occur both with and without the presence of *Pseudomonas* bacteremia. If bacteremia is present, there are often multiple lesions in different locations that can be identified on physical examination. In the absence of bacteremia, there is typically one wound due to direct inoculation. Tissue culture, in addition to blood culture, is necessary to make this diagnosis. Histopathology of Ecthyma Gangrenosum reveals necrotic vasculitis with vascular thrombosis and may reveal gram-negative rods along the adventitia of the blood vessels[88] (**Fig. 16**).

Treatment

Antibiotic therapy

Treatment of pseudomonal DFIs is a challenging effort. The prevalence of multidrug-resistant *P aeruginosa* makes treatment increasingly difficult.[88] There are many

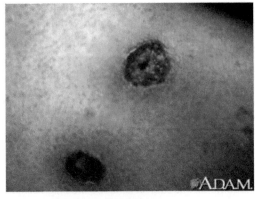

Fig. 16. Clinical appearance of Ecthyma Gangrenosum.

mechanisms identified in the cause of drug resistance. *P aeruginosa* is known to form early (<24 hour) biofilms more so than other bacterial species, especially in DFIs.[94–96] In addition, it has shown beta-lactamase and amp-C cephalosporinase activity against multiple generations of cephalosporins and carbapenems.[88,95] Many pseudomonal strains carry several aminoglycoside-modifying enzymes, acting on different aminoglycoside substituents, rendering them all ineffective.[88,94] Furthermore, *P aeruginosa* can secrete toxins, promote membrane impermeability and porin alteration, and perform quorum sensing, all of which contribute to drug resistance. These mechanisms allow *Pseudomonas* to evade the immune system and antimicrobials.[88,92]

Mainstays of antipseudomonal antibiotic therapy are combination therapy with an antipseudomonal beta-lactam, carbapenem, and fluoroquinolone, such as piperacillin/tazobactam, ceftazidime/avibactam, cefepime, or meropenem.[88,95] Ceftolozane/tazobactam can be used in extreme drug-resistant *Pseudomonas* infection.[97] As always, narrowing antibiotics based on culture susceptibility as soon as possible is of the utmost importance given the high rates of antibiotic resistance by this organism in particular. Antibiotic duration is typically 10 to 14 days.[97] If deep space infection is suspected, or an underlying abscess is formed, surgical debridement may be necessary. Rarely will *Pseudomonas* cause a necrotizing infection.

COMPLICATIONS OF PUNCTURE WOUNDS
Epidemiology

Puncture wounds are common injuries with self-limiting symptoms in many cases. Many individuals never seek care following puncture wounds, so the true incidence of puncture wounds is unknown.[98] These wounds may occur in any location, but the plantar surface of the feet, the palmar surface of the hands, and the fingertips are most commonly affected (**Fig. 17**). Nails are the most common source of puncture injuries, but glass, wood, and other metal objects can frequently cause these wounds.[98–100] Although their course can be relatively benign most of the time, the sequelae of puncture wounds can also include serious complications with the potential for limb loss and death. Cellulitis, foreign body granuloma, abscess, osteomyelitis, septic arthritis, NSTIs, tenosynovitis, and sepsis are a few of the serious morbidities that can result from puncture wounds.

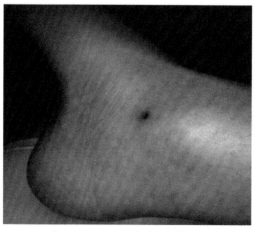

Fig. 17. Clinical appearance of puncture wound. Jim Still-Pepper/iStock/Getty Images.

Pathophysiology

Microbiology

The most common gram-positive organisms isolated from puncture wounds are *S aureus*, *Staphylococcus epidermidis*, and alpha-hemolytic streptococci. Gram-negative organisms include *P aeruginosa*, *Escherichia coli*, *Proteus*, and *Klebsiella*.[101,102] Diabetic patients generally develop polymicrobial infections.[101] Extensive variability exists based on the setting where the injury occurs. Water, soil, and farm exposures add a significant number of possible infecting organisms. Fungal and mycobacterial infections following puncture wound injury have also been reported.[102,103]

Pseudomonal infections are of particular importance in plantar puncture wounds. *Pseudomonas* is the most common organism causing osteomyelitis after puncture wounds.[99,104,105] Several investigators have hypothesized that this occurs when a puncture wound occurs through shoes harboring *Pseudomonas*. This hypothesis is supported by positive pseudomonal cultures taken from patients' shoes following punctures that progress to osteomyelitis.[96,101,106–110]

Clinical Manifestation

The clinical course of puncture wounds depends on multiple factors, including patient comorbidities, immunosuppression, depth of injury, type and degree of contamination, presence of a retained foreign body, and time to presentation. The authors do not know the exact impact each of these factors has, largely because so many patients do not seek medical care following injury. Not surprisingly, diabetic patients have more complications and more serious morbidity following puncture wounds. Truong and colleagues[104,105] evaluated 114 consecutive patients with a foot infection following puncture wounds and found that greater than 70% of the patients presenting with infections following puncture wounds were diabetic. In looking at the hospital course for these 114 patients, they found that diabetic patients had a higher surgery rate, had more surgeries, were 14 times more likely to undergo amputation, and were 9 times more likely to develop osteomyelitis compared with nondiabetic patients. Numerous studies have shown that there is an association between a higher infection rate and delayed presentation greater than 24 hours from the time of injury.[111,101] This is confounded by the fact that a patient not immediately seeking care may only present once signs of infections develop. Despite this possible confounding factor, later presentation is still a predictor for a worse outcome.

Treatment

Antibiotic therapy

For puncture wounds that do not appear infected, it is important to confirm the patient's tetanus immunization status and administer tetanus vaccine or booster as indicated.[112] Irrigation and local wound care may be performed without prophylactic antibiotics for these wounds. Infected puncture wounds should be treated swiftly with appropriate laboratory studies, imaging, antibiotic therapy, and surgical source control as indicated by the specific characteristics of the wound and patient comorbidities. All patients presenting with puncture wounds should be evaluated for the presence of a foreign body at the site of injury. Foreign bodies should be removed, as they confer higher risk of complications. The specifics of the object, puncture location, and depth should dictate whether this is performed in the operating room or at the bedside.

CLINICS CARE POINTS

- Because diabetes is a risk factor for the development of many soft tissue infections, a high index of suspicion should be maintained when evaluating these patients, and prompt surgical treatment is needed for more severe wounds.
- Necrotizing soft tissue infections can be life-threatening infections that progress rapidly especially in diabetic patients. Workup should not precede operative intervention when clinical suspicion is high.

DISCLOSURE

The authors have nothing to disclose.

REFERENCES

1. Llorente L, De La Fuente H, Richaud-Patin Y, et al. Innate immune response mechanisms in non-insulin dependent diabetes mellitus patients assessed by flow cytoenzymology. Immunol Lett 2000;74(3):239–44.
2. Delamaire M, Maugendre D, Moreno M, et al. Impaired leucocyte functions in diabetic patients. Diabet Med 1997;14(1):29–34.
3. Zykova SN, Jenssen TG, Berdal M, et al. Altered cytokine and nitric oxide secretion in vitro by macrophages from diabetic type II-like db/db mice. Diabetes 2000;49(9):1451–8.
4. Amano H, Yamamoto H, Senba M, et al. Impairment of endotoxin-induced macrophage inflammatory protein 2 gene expression in alveolar macrophages in streptozotocin-induced diabetes in mice. Infect Immun 2000;68(5):2925–9.
5. Mazade MA, Edwards MS. Impairment of type III group B Streptococcus-stimulated superoxide production and opsonophagocytosis by neutrophils in diabetes. Mol Genet Metab 2001;73:259.
6. Al-Mashat HA, Kandru S, Liu R, et al. Diabetes enhances mRNA levels of proapoptotic genes and caspase activity, which contribute to impaired healing. Diabetes 2006;55:487.
7. Price CL, Hassi HO, English NR, et al. Methylglyoxal modulates immune responses: relevance to diabetes. J Cell Mol Med 2010;14:1806.
8. Ilyas R, Wallis R, Soilleux EJ, et al. High glucose disrupts oligosaccharide recognition function via competitive inhibition: a potential mechanism for immune dysregulation in diabetes mellitus. Immunobiology 2011;216:126.
9. Graham PL 3rd, Lin SX, Larson EL. A U.S. population-based survey of Staphylococcus aureus colonization. Ann Intern Med 2006;144(5):318–25.
10. de Leon EM, Jacober SJ, Sobel JD, et al. Prevalence and risk factors for vaginal Candida colonization in women with type 1 and type 2 diabetes. BMC Infect Dis 2002;2:1.
11. Hostetter MK. Handicaps to host defense. Effects of hyperglycemia on C3 and Candida albicans. Diabetes 1990;39:271.
12. Ferguson BJ. Mucormycosis of the nose and paranasal sinuses. Otolaryngol Clin North Am 2000;33:349.
13. Martin ET, Kaye KS, Knott C, et al. Diabetes and Risk of Surgical Site Infection: A Systematic Review and Meta-analysis. Infect Control Hosp Epidemiol 2016; 37(1):88–99.

14. Golden SH, Peart-Vigilance C, Kao WH, et al. Perioperative glycemic control and the risk of infectious complications in a cohort of adults with diabetes. Diabetes Care 1999;22(9):1408–14.

15. Brem H, Tomic-Canic M. Cellular and molecular basis of wound healing in diabetes. J Clin Invest 2007;117(5):1219–22.

16. Ata A, Lee J, Bestle SL, et al. Postoperative hyperglycemia and surgical site infection in general surgery patients. Arch Surg 2010;145(9):858–64.

17. Latham R, Lancaster AD, Covington JF, et al. The association of diabetes and glucose control with surgical-site infections among cardiothoracic surgery patients. Infect Control Hosp Epidemiol 2001;22(10):607–12.

18. Furnary AP, Zerr KJ, Grunkemeier GL, et al. Continuous intravenous insulin infusion reduces the incidence of deep sternal wound infection in diabetic patients after cardiac surgical procedures. Ann Thorac Surg 1999;67(2):352–62.

19. Boreland L, Scott-Hudson M, Hetherington K, et al. The effectiveness of tight glycemic control on decreasing surgical site infections and readmission rates in adult patients with diabetes undergoing cardiac surgery: A systematic review. Heart Lung 2015;44(5):430–40.

20. International Diabetes Federation. IDF Diabetes Atlas, 10th edn. Brussels, Belgium: 2021. Available at: https://www.diabetesatlas.org. Accessed February 26, 2023.

21. Singh N, Armstrong DG, Lipsky BA. Preventing foot ulcers in patients with diabetes. JAMA 2005;293(2):217–28.

22. McInnes AD. Diabetic foot disease in the United Kingdom: about time to put feet first. J Foot Ankle Res 2012;5(1):26.

23. Walsh JW, Hoffstad OJ, Sullivan MO, et al. Association of diabetic foot ulcer and death in a population-based cohort from the United Kingdom. Diabet Med 2016; 33(11):1493–8.

24. Harding JL, Andes LJ, Rolka DB, et al. National and State-Level Trends in Nontraumatic Lower-Extremity Amputation Among U.S. Medicare Beneficiaries With Diabetes, 2000-2017. Diabetes Care 2020;43(10):2453–9.

25. Reiber GE, Ledoux WR. Epidemiology of diabetic foot ulcers and amputations: Evidence for prevention. In: Williams R, Herman W, Kinmonth AL, et al, editors. The evidence base for diabetes care. Chichester; Hoboken (NJ): John Wiley & Sons, Ltd; 2003. p. 641–65. https://doi.org/10.1002/0470846585.ch28.

26. Pendsey SP. Understanding diabetic foot. Int J Diabetes Dev Ctries 2010; 30(2):75–9.

27. Bowering CK. Diabetic foot ulcers. Pathophysiology, assessment, and therapy. Can Fam Physician 2001;47:1007–16.

28. Rubitschung K, Sherwood A, Crisologo AP, et al. Pathophysiology and Molecular Imaging of Diabetic Foot Infections. Int J Mol Sci 2021;22(21):11552.

29. Ababneh A, Bakri FG, Khader Y, et al. Prevalence and Associates of Foot Deformities among Patients with Diabetes in Jordan. Curr Diabetes Rev 2020;16(5): 471–82.

30. Cancelliere P. A review of the pathophysiology and clinical sequelae of diabetic polyneuropathy in the feet. Journal of Diabetes, Metabolic Disorders & Control 2016;3(2). https://doi.org/10.15406/jdmdc.2016.03.00062.

31. Bandyk DF. The diabetic foot: Pathophysiology, evaluation, and treatment. Semin Vasc Surg 2018;31(2–4):43–8.

32. Boulton AJ. Diabetic neuropathy and foot complications. Handb Clin Neurol 2014;126:97–107.

33. Kolluru GK, Bir SC, Kevil CG. Endothelial dysfunction and diabetes: effects on angiogenesis, vascular remodeling, and wound healing. Int J Vasc Med 2012; 2012:918267.
34. Moura J, Rodrigues J, Gonçalves M, et al. Impaired T-cell differentiation in diabetic foot ulceration. Cell Mol Immunol 2017;14(9):758–69.
35. Daryabor G, Atashzar MR, Kabelitz D, et al. The Effects of Type 2 Diabetes Mellitus on Organ Metabolism and the Immune System. Front Immunol 2020;11:1582.
36. Oliver T.I., Mutluoglu M., Diabetic Foot Ulcer. [Updated 2022 Aug 8]. In: StatPearls [Internet]. Treasure Island (FL): StatPearls Publishing; 2023. Available at: https://www.ncbi.nlm.nih.gov/books/NBK537328/. Accessed February 17, 2023.
37. Alexiadou K, Doupis J. Management of Diabetic Foot Ulcers. Diabetes Ther 2012;3:4.
38. Armstrong DG, Lavery LA. Diabetic foot ulcers: prevention, diagnosis and classification. Am Fam Physician 1998;57(6):1325–38.
39. Williams DT, Price P, Harding KG. Amputation and mortality in new-onset diabetic foot ulcers stratified by etiology: response to Moulik, Mtonga, and Gill. Diabetes Care 2003;26(11):3199–200.
40. American Diabetes Association. Consensus Development Conference on Diabetic Foot Wound Care: 7-8 April 1999, Boston, Massachusetts. American Diabetes Association. Diabetes Care 1999;22(8):1354–60.
41. Forsythe RO, Hinchliffe RJ. Assessment of foot perfusion in patients with a diabetic foot ulcer. Diabetes Metab Res Rev 2016;32(Suppl 1):232–8.
42. Boulton AJ, Armstrong DG, Albert SF, et al. Comprehensive foot examination and risk assessment: a report of the task force of the foot care interest group of the American Diabetes Association, with endorsement by the American Association of Clinical Endocrinologists. Diabetes Care 2008;31(8):1679–85.
43. Mayfield JA, Reiber GE, Sanders LJ, et al. Preventive foot care in people with diabetes. Diabetes Care 1998;21(12):2161–77.
44. Mayfield JA, Reiber GE, Sanders LJ, et al, American Diabetes Association. Preventive foot care in people with diabetes. Diabetes Care 2003;26(Suppl 1):S78–9.
45. Abbott CA, Carrington AL, Ashe H, et al. The North-West Diabetes Foot Care Study: incidence of, and risk factors for, new diabetic foot ulceration in a community-based patient cohort. Diabet Med 2002;19(5):377–84.
46. Reiber GE, Vileikyte L, Boyko EJ, et al. Causal pathways for incident lower-extremity ulcers in patients with diabetes from two settings. Diabetes Care 1999; 22(1):157–62.
47. Boulton AJ, Kirsner RS, Vileikyte L. Clinical practice. Neuropathic diabetic foot ulcers. N Engl J Med 2004;351(1):48–55.
48. Boulton AJ, Malik RA, Arezzo JC, et al. Diabetic somatic neuropathies. Diabetes Care 2004;27(6):1458–86.
49. Frykberg RG, Zgonis T, Armstrong DG, et al. Diabetic foot disorders. A clinical practice guideline (2006 revision). J Foot Ankle Surg 2006;45(5 Suppl):S1–66. https://doi.org/10.1016/S1067-2516(07)60001-5.
50. Armstrong DG, Boulton AJM, Bus SA. Diabetic Foot Ulcers and Their Recurrence. N Engl J Med 2017;376(24):2367–75.
51. Senneville É, Lipsky BA, Abbas ZG, et al. Diagnosis of infection in the foot in diabetes: a systematic review. Diabetes Metab Res Rev 2020;36(Suppl 1):e3281.
52. Bader MS. Diabetic foot infection. Am Fam Physician 2008;78(1):71–9.
53. Punchard NA, Whelan CJ, Adcock I. The Journal of Inflammation. J Inflamm 2004;1(1):1.

54. Armstrong DG, Lavery LA, Sariaya M, et al. Leukocytosis is a poor indicator of acute osteomyelitis of the foot in diabetes mellitus. J Foot Ankle Surg 1996; 35(4):280–3.

55. Eneroth M, Apelqvist J, Stenström A. Clinical characteristics and outcome in 223 diabetic patients with deep foot infections. Foot Ankle Int 1997;18(11):716–22.

56. Iyengar KP, Jain VK, Awadalla Mohamed MK, et al. Update on functional imaging in the evaluation of diabetic foot infection. J Clin Orthop Trauma 2021;16: 119–24.

57. Ibrahim A, Berkache M, Morency-Potvin P, et al. Diabetic foot infections: how to investigate more efficiently? A retrospective study in a quaternary university center. Insights Imaging 2022;13(1):88.

58. Malhotra R, Chan CS, Nather A. Osteomyelitis in the diabetic foot. Diabet Foot Ankle 2014;5. https://doi.org/10.3402/dfa.v5.24445.

59. Everett E, Mathioudakis N. Update on management of diabetic foot ulcers. Ann N Y Acad Sci 2018;1411(1):153–65.

60. Lipsky BA, Berendt AR, Cornia PB, et al. 2012 Infectious Diseases Society of America clinical practice guideline for the diagnosis and treatment of diabetic foot infections. Clin Infect Dis 2012;54(12):e132–73.

61. Schaper NC, van Netten JJ, Apelqvist J, et al. Practical Guidelines on the prevention and management of diabetic foot disease (IWGDF 2019 update). Diabetes Metab Res Rev 2020;36(Suppl 1):e3266.

62. Lipsky BA, Pecoraro RE, Larson SA, et al. Outpatient management of uncomplicated lower-extremity infections in diabetic patients. Arch Intern Med 1990; 150(4):790–7.

63. Santema TB, Lenselink EA, Balm R, et al. Comparing the Meggitt-Wagner and the University of Texas wound classification systems for diabetic foot ulcers: inter-observer analyses. Int Wound J 2016;13(6):1137–41.

64. Oyibo SO, Jude EB, Tarawneh I, et al. A comparison of two diabetic foot ulcer classification systems: the Wagner and the University of Texas wound classification systems. Diabetes Care 2001;24(1):84–8.

65. Pemayun TG, Naibaho RM, Novitasari D, et al. Risk factors for lower extremity amputation in patients with diabetic foot ulcers: a hospital-based case-control study. Diabet Foot Ankle 2015;6:29629.

66. Tan JS, Friedman NM, Hazelton-Miller C, et al. Can aggressive treatment of diabetic foot infections reduce the need for above-ankle amputation? Clin Infect Dis 1996;23(2):286–91.

67. Singh S, Jajoo S, Shukla S, et al. Educating patients of diabetes mellitus for diabetic foot care. J Family Med Prim Care 2020;9(1):367–73.

68. Krishnan S, Nash F, Baker N, et al. Reduction in diabetic amputations over 11 years in a defined U.K. population: benefits of multidisciplinary team work and continuous prospective audit. Diabetes Care 2008;31(1):99–101.

69. Jørgensen ME, Almdal TP, Faerch K. Reduced incidence of lower-extremity amputations in a Danish diabetes population from 2000 to 2011. Diabet Med 2014; 31(4):443–7.

70. Wang C, Mai L, Yang C, et al. Reducing major lower extremity amputations after the introduction of a multidisciplinary team in patient with diabetes foot ulcer. BMC Endocr Disord 2016;16(1):38.

71. Swartz MN. Cellulitis. N Engl J Med 2004;350:904.

72. Quirke M, Ayoub F, McCabe A, et al. Risk factors for nonpurulent leg cellulitis: a systematic review and meta-analysis. Br J Dermatol 2017 Aug;177(2):382–94.

73. Stulberg DL, Penrod MA, Blatny RA. Common bacterial skin infections. Am Fam Phys 2002;66:119.
74. Sadick NS. Current aspects of bacterial infections of the skin. Dermatol Clin 1997;15:341.
75. Parada JP, Maslow JN. Clinical syndromes associated with adult pneumococcal cellulitis. Scand J Infect Dis 2000;32:133.
76. King MD, Humphrey BJ, Yang YF, et al. Emergence of community-acquired methicillin-resistant Staphylococcus aureus. USA 300 clone as the predominant cause of skin and soft tissue infections. Ann Intern Med 2006;144:309–17.
77. Moran GJ, Krishnadasan A, Gorwitz RJ, et al. Methicillin-resistant S. aureus infections among patients in the emergency department. N Engl J Med 2006;355: 666–74.
78. Perl B, Gottehrer NP, Ravek D, et al. Cost-effectiveness of blood cultures for adult patients with cellulitis. Clin Infect Dis 1999;29:1483.
79. Johnson LJ, Crisologo PA, Sivaganesan S, et al. Evaluation of the laboratory risk indicator for necrotizing fasciitis (LRINEC) score for detecting necrotizing soft tissue infections in patients with diabetes and lower extremity infection. Diabetes Res Clin Pract 2021;171:108520.
80. Bonne SL, Kadri SS. Evaluation and management of necrotizing soft tissue infections. Infect Dis Clin 2017;31(3):497–511.
81. Anaya DA, Dellinger EP. Necrotizing soft-tissue infection: Diagnosis and management. Clin Infect Dis 2007;44(5):705–10.
82. Stevens DL, Bryant AE, Goldstein EJC. Necrotizing soft tissue infections. Infect Dis Clin 2021;35(1):135–55.
83. Stevens DL, Bisno AL, Chambers HF, et al. Practice guidelines for the diagnosis and management of skin and soft tissue infections: 2014 update by the Infectious Diseases Society of America. Clin Infect Dis 2014;59(2). https://doi.org/10.1093/cid/ciu296.
84. Elliott DC, Kufera JA, Myers RA. Necrotizing soft tissue infections. Ann Surg 1996;224(5):672–83.
85. Fernando SM, Tran A, Cheng W, et al. Necrotizing soft tissue infection: Diagnostic accuracy of physical examination, imaging, and LRINEC score. Ann Surg 2019;269(1):58–65.
86. Hadeed GJ, Smith J, O'Keeffe T, et al. Early Surgical Intervention and its impact on patients presenting with necrotizing soft tissue infections: A single academic center experience. J Emergencies, Trauma, Shock 2016;9(1):22–7.
87. Korte AKM, Vos JM. Ecthyma Gangrenosum. N Engl J Med 2017;377(23):e32.
88. Reynolds D, Kollef M. The Epidemiology and Pathogenesis and Treatment of Pseudomonas aeruginosa Infections: An Update. Drugs 2021;81(18):2117–31.
89. Veve MP, Mercuro NJ, Sangiovanni RJ, et al. Prevalence and Predictors of Pseudomonas aeruginosa Among Hospitalized Patients With Diabetic Foot Infections. Open Forum Infect Dis 2022;9(7):ofac297.
90. Spernovasilis N, Psichogiou M, Poulakou G. Skin manifestations of Pseudomonas aeruginosa infections. Curr Opin Infect Dis 2021;34(2):72–9.
91. Sivanmaliappan TS, Sevanan M. Antimicrobial Susceptibility Patterns of Pseudomonas aeruginosa from Diabetes Patients with Foot Ulcers. Int J Microbiol 2011;2011:605195.
92. Surme S, Saltoglu N, Kurt AF, et al. Changing Bacterial Etiology and Antimicrobial Resistance Profiles as Prognostic Determinants of Diabetic Foot Infections: A Ten-Year Retrospective Cohort Study. Surg Infect 2022;23(7):667–74.

93. Vaiman M, Lazarovitch T, Heller L, et al. Ecthyma gangrenosum and ecthyma-like lesions: review article. Eur J Clin Microbiol Infect Dis 2015;34(4):633–9.
94. Mottola C, Mendes JJ, Cristino JM, et al. Polymicrobial biofilms by diabetic foot clinical isolates. Folia Microbiol (Praha) 2016;61(1):35–43.
95. Bassetti M, Vena A, Croxatto A, et al. How to manage Pseudomonas aeruginosa infections. Drugs Context 2018;7:212527.
96. Amin AN, Cerceo EA, Deitelzweig SB, et al. Hospitalist perspective on the treatment of skin and soft tissue infections. Mayo Clin Proc 2014;89(10):1436–51.
97. Escolà-Vergé L, Pigrau C, Los-Arcos I, et al. Ceftolozane/tazobactam for the treatment of XDR Pseudomonas aeruginosa infections. Infection 2018;46(4):461–8.
98. Chisholm CD, Schlesser JF. Plantar puncture wounds: controversies and treatment recommendations. Ann Emerg Med 1989;18(12):1352–7.
99. Haverstock BD. Puncture wounds of the foot. Clin Podiatr Med Surg 2012;29(2): 311–22, ix.
100. Fitzgerald RH, Cowan JD. Puncture wounds of the foot. Orthop Clin North Am 1975;6(4):965–72.
101. Laughlin TJ, Armstrong DG, Caporusso J, et al. Soft tissue and bone infections from puncture wounds in children. West J Med 1997;166(2):126–8.
102. Lavery LA, Harkless LB, Felder-Johnson K, et al. Bacterial pathogens in infected puncture wounds in adults with diabetes. J Foot Ankle Surg 1994;33(1):91–7.
103. Lavery LA, Walker SC, Harkless LB, et al. Infected puncture wounds in diabetic and nondiabetic adults. Diabetes Care 1995;18(12):1588–91.
104. Truong DH, Johnson MJ, Crisologo PA, et al. Outcomes of Foot Infections Secondary to Puncture Injuries in Patients With and Without Diabetes. J Foot Ankle Surg 2019;58(6):1064–6.
105. Truong DH, La Fontaine J, Malone M, et al. A Comparison of Pathogens in Skin and Soft Tissue Infections and Pedal Osteomyelitis in Puncture Wound Injuries Affecting the Foot. J Am Podiatr Med Assoc 2020. https://doi.org/10.7547/20-206.
106. Palmore TN, Shea YR, Childs RW, et al. Fusarium proliferatum soft tissue infection at the site of a puncture by a plant: recovery, isolation, and direct molecular identification. J Clin Microbiol 2010;48(1):338–42.
107. Cruz AT, Antekeier SB. Chronic multifocal Mycobacterium fortuitum osteomyelitis following penetrating plantar trauma. Am J Orthop (Belle Mead NJ) 2012; 41(8):E109–11.
108. Laughlin RT, Reeve F, Wright DG, et al. Calcaneal osteomyelitis caused by nail puncture wounds. Foot Ankle Int 1997;18(9):575–7.
109. Fisher MC, Goldsmith JF, Gilligan PH. Sneakers as a source of Pseudomonas aeruginosa in children with osteomyelitis following puncture wounds. J Pediatr 1985;106(4):607–9.
110. Graham BS, Gregory DW. Pseudomonas aeruginosa causing osteomyelitis after puncture wounds of the foot. South Med J 1984;77(10):1228–30.
111. Patzakis MJ, Wilkins J, Brien WW, et al. Wound site as a predictor of complications following deep nail punctures to the foot. West J Med. May 1989;150(5): 545–7.
112. HOUSTON AN, ROY WA, FAUST RA, et al. Tetanus prophylaxis in the treatment of puncture wounds of patients in the deep South. J Trauma 1962;2:439–50.

General Surgery During Pregnancy and Gynecologic Emergencies

Raymond Traweek, MD, Vivy Phan, MD, Chad Griesbach, MD, Chad Hall, MD*

KEYWORDS

- Emergency general surgery • Pregnancy • Obstetrical emergencies

KEY POINTS

- Evaluation of the pregnant patient with abdominal pain.
- Perioperative care of pregnant patients.
- Management of general surgery and obstetrical emergencies that occur in pregnancy.

INTRODUCTION

Nonobstetrical surgical emergencies can occur throughout gestation and may present unique challenges for the surgical team. Current recommendations from the American College of Obstetricians and Gynecologists state that medically necessary surgery should not be denied or delayed, regardless of trimester, due to increased risk to the mother and fetus.[1] Fortunately, nonobstetric surgery in pregnancy is relatively rare, with estimates of incidence ranging from 0.5% to 2% of pregnant patients.[2] Acute appendicitis is the most common indication for nonobstetric surgery, followed by acute cholecystitis, adnexal surgery, and surgery for trauma.[3,4] Analysis of the American College of Surgeons National Surgical Quality and Improvement Program database demonstrated a major postoperative complication rate of 5.8% among pregnant patients undergoing nonobstetric antenatal surgery.[4] As such, surgeons must thoughtfully consider the perioperative care of pregnant patients to ensure the safety of both the patient and the fetus.

EVALUATION OF ACUTE ABDOMINAL PAIN DURING PREGNANCY

The evaluation of acute abdominal pain in a pregnant patient is complex and requires the medical provider to maintain a broad understanding of possible obstetrical and

The authors have no financial interests to disclose.
Baylor Scott & White Medical Center, 2401 South 31st Street, Temple, TX 76508, USA
* Corresponding author.
E-mail address: Chad.hall@bswhealth.org

nonobstetrical causes. Patients should be carefully screened for history of trauma and undergo a trauma evaluation, if appropriate. Obstetrical causes of abdominal pain must be quickly evaluated because they are potentially life threatening to mother and fetus. Although not always present, vaginal bleeding and hypertension in the setting of acute abdominal pain are ominous signs of an obstetrical emergency. Nonobstetrical surgical diagnoses should be considered once obstetrical causes have been ruled out. This requires insight into the physiologic changes of pregnancy and knowledge of alternative diagnostic studies for thorough investigation of the patient's pain.

Physiology Changes During Pregnancy

Nearly every organ system is affected by predictable physiologic changes that will affect the vital signs, physical examination, and laboratory abnormalities of a pregnant patient with acute abdominal pain. A summary of physiologic changes by organ system is shown in **Table 1**.[5] Plasma volume increases throughout a normal pregnancy, resulting in a relative anemia because the expansion in plasma volume exceeds the increase in red blood cell mass. Oxygen demand is significantly increased in pregnancy, due to changes in metabolic rate and oxygen consumption. Increased minute ventilation and a mild compensated respiratory alkalosis, pH 7.40 to 7.47, is considered normal in pregnancy.

Changes in Vital Signs and Physical Examination

Blood pressure is known to decrease during the first trimester, reaching a nadir by 22 to 24 weeks gestation. Blood pressure will then slowly increase throughout the remainder of pregnancy to normal values by 36 weeks. The upper limit of normal heart rate increases with gestational age, with 115 beats per minute as an appropriate upper limit in the third trimester of pregnancy.[6]

The abdominal physical examination of a pregnant patient requires consideration of the gravid uterus and its effect on intra-abdominal structures, limitation to your examination, and pathologic condition specific to pregnant patients. The fundus of the

Table 1 Physiologic changes during pregnancy by organ system	
System	**Expected Change**
Cardiovascular	50% increase in plasma volume Physiologic anemia from hemodilution Increased baseline heart rate Increased cardiac output
Pulmonary	Decreased functional residual capacity Increased minute ventilation Mild respiratory alkalosis
Gastrointestinal	Delayed gastric emptying Decreased resting pressure of lower esophageal sphincter Increased gastrointestinal transit time
Renal	Increased glomerular filtration rate Increased renal mass Decreased serum creatinine
Endocrine	Increased thyroid hormone production Increased plasma free cortisol
Hematologic	Increased RBC mass Increased production of coagulation factors

uterus will be located at the pubic symphysis at 12 weeks' gestation, at the umbilicus at 20 weeks' gestation, and the xiphoid at approximately 36 weeks' gestation. Between 20 and 36 weeks, the fundus can be expected to reach 1 cm cephalad to the umbilicus for each week gestation over 20 weeks. The uterus can displace intra-abdominal structures and may reduce the diagnostic accuracy of abdominal palpation. Patient positioning for an examination may need to be modified. In the first and second trimesters, supine position with mild elevation of the head of the bed is appropriate. However, in the third trimester, a left lateral position is appropriate in order to reduce the compression of the uterus on the inferior vena cava (IVC).

Abdominal Imaging Modalities in Pregnancy

Imaging studies are a pertinent adjunct to the clinical examination for the evaluation of acute abdominal pain but must be chosen wisely in pregnant patients. Ultrasound (US) and MRI are preferred imaging modalities because they do not use radiation and are not associated with risk to the fetus.[7] Computerized tomography (CT), x-rays, nuclear scanning, and PET all involve exposure of mother and fetus to ionizing radiation. Estimated threshold dose and effect on the fetus will vary during gestation.[7] As a general rule, there is a negligible risk to the fetus for radiation doses less than 50 mGy. A CT of the abdomen and pelvis provides a fetal dose of 10 to 50 mGy. This suggests that a single CT of the abdomen and pelvis poses minimal risk to the fetus; however, studies are additive and can exceed that threshold of 50 mGy if multiple ionizing studies are necessary. If ionizing imaging modalities are required to make a diagnosis, great care should be taken to shield the fetus and limit radiation doses when able. Importantly, the selection of the imaging modality should be discussed and made as an informed decision with the patient.

PERIOPERATIVE CONSIDERATIONS DURING PREGNANCY

The perioperative management of pregnant patients begins with the identification of risk factors that may contribute to anesthetic complications. In addition to a physical assessment, a thorough history must be obtained to delineate a personal or family history of bleeding disorders, coagulopathies, or severe complications resulting from anesthetic agents such as malignant hyperthermia.[8]

Pregnant patients undergo physiologic changes of the airway that include swelling and increased friability of the oropharyngeal tissue, both of which contribute to a reduced size of the glottic opening. These changes are more pronounced near the end of pregnancy but may be encountered in the second trimester.[9] As a result, pregnant patients may be more difficult to bag-mask ventilate or endotracheally intubate, particularly when unconscious.[10] A higher Mallampati score, a tool that assesses the size and shape of the tongue and esophageal airway to predict difficulty of endotracheal intubation, has been suggested to be more predictive of a difficult intubation in pregnant patients when compared with nonpregnant patients.[11] How significantly these physiologic changes contribute to failed endotracheal intubation is controversial; however, loss of maternal airway is the most common cause of anesthesia-related maternal mortality.[12–14] As such, steps that must be taken to reduce the risk of maternal airway loss include the utilization of regional anesthesia when possible, well-rehearsed emergency airway algorithms, ready availability of advanced airway devices, and the involvement of experienced anesthesia personnel.[15]

There has been no clear evidence suggesting teratogenicity of commonly used anesthetic agents. A large meta-analysis did not demonstrate an increased risk of major birth defects associated with nonobstetric surgery.[16] Historically, there has been concern that benzodiazepine administration is associated with an increased incidence of cleft palate and cardiac anomalies; however, multiple recent studies have refuted these data.[17,18] Additionally, preclinical mouse models have demonstrated increased neuronal apoptosis following volatile anesthetic administration, resulting in abnormal behavior patterns in adult rodents.[19] However, retrospective cohort studies have yielded no evidence associating antenatal anesthetic administration with postpartum cognitive or behavioral disturbances in children.[20,21] Ultimately, the administration of commonly used anesthetic agents such as propofol, barbiturates, and neuromuscular blocking agents seems safe for fetal development.

Regional anesthesia is preferred when appropriate for the clinical context because it eliminates maternal airway manipulation and abrogates the risk of fetal hypoxia as well as placental transfer of general anesthetic. Although short, transient periods of mild fetal hypoxemia are well tolerated, prolonged reductions in uteroplacental perfusion because of anesthetic-induced hypotension significantly increase the risk of hypoxemia, acidosis, and fetal demise.[22,23] Almost all anesthetic agents have been observed to transfer across the placenta, with the exception of neuromuscular blockading agents.[24] However, the exact effects of these drugs on overall fetal well-being remain poorly understood. Retrospective studies examining fetal outcomes in pregnant women requiring surgery have observed an increased risk of spontaneous abortion and low birth weight; however, these may be due to the underlying maternal pathophysiology rather than anesthetic exposure.[25] As such, regional anesthetic has become increasingly used in pregnant patients to the reduce risk of anesthesia-related maternal and fetal mortality.[26]

Postoperatively, The American College of Obstetricians and Gynecologists (ACOG) recommends consideration of corticosteroid administration for patients with viable fetuses of premature gestational ages due to the risk of preterm delivery following surgery.[1] Additionally, pregnant patients are 5 times more likely to develop deep vein thromboses compared with nonpregnant women.[27] Increased age, body mass index, and periods of immobility, such as surgery, increase this risk. As such, ACOG guidelines recommend close monitoring for venous thromboembolic events following surgery and pregnant patients should receive the appropriate chemoprophylaxis and mechanical prophylaxis perioperatively.[1]

RECOMMENDATIONS FOR FETAL MONITORING DURING SURGERY

Data supporting specific recommendations regarding intraoperative fetal heart rate (FHR) monitoring in nonobstetric surgery are limited. As such, recommendations proposed by ACOG have been formulated by expert opinion.[1] Broadly, FHR monitoring is recommended for all pregnant patients undergoing surgery, with the choice of monitoring technique dependent on the stage of pregnancy. For pregnancies that are considered previable (<22 weeks), ACOG states that obtaining FHR by Doppler before and after surgery is generally sufficient.

For pregnancies that are considered viable (≥22 weeks), intraoperative electronic FHR and contraction monitoring is recommended because FHR variability can be more readily observed.[1,28] Loss of FHR variability intraoperatively may not represent fetal distress but may instead be an expected physiologic reaction in response to the effects of general anesthetic on the fetal autonomic nervous system. However, fetal bradycardia intraoperatively is more concerning, because this may represent prolonged fetal hypoxemia and developing acidosis, and may require intervention.[29]

Uterine contractions can be monitored using an external or internal tocodynamometer; there have been no differences in maternal or fetal outcomes observed between the 2 modalities.[30] If premature labor occurs, tocolytic therapy will be necessary to preserve the pregnancy. If tocolytics are not immediately available, adjunctive measures to achieve uterine relaxation are required. Volatile anesthetics have been observed to be potent uterine relaxants; however, proper dosing requires administration of high concentrations.[31,32] Additionally, intravenous nitroglycerin has been observed to produce profound uterine relaxation. Fetal effects seem mild due to the large degree of placental metabolization, although its effects are short-acting and may require redosing.[33]

PATIENT POSITIONING AND ANATOMIC CONSIDERATIONS

Optimal patient position is largely determined by the gravid uterus and its effects on surrounding organs, most notably the IVC. These effects become more pronounced as pregnancy progresses, and surgical providers must be aware of these changes to best manage acute surgical pathology in the pregnant patient.

During the first trimester of pregnancy, the uterus does not seem to affect maternal physiology with changes in positioning. Although there are a paucity of data examining aortocaval compression in early pregnancy, Spiropoulos and colleagues examined changes in arterial oxygen tension (PaO_2) and arterial carbon dioxide tension ($PaCO_2$) in pregnant patients while sitting and supine throughout pregnancy. The authors observed no significant difference in mean PaO_2 or $PaCO_2$ in first trimester patients that were supine when compared with those that were sitting.[34] However, significant reductions in PaO_2 occurred when supine when compared with sitting as pregnancy progressed, with the most pronounced difference occurring late in the third trimester. Considered together, these data suggest that the supine position is likely safe for patients in early-pregnancy, and adequate patient positioning may be determined at the discretion of surgical providers.

By 20 weeks gestation, the gravid uterus has sufficient volume such that posterior displacement may compress the IVC. Caval compression has been observed to reduce venous return by up to 30%, with notable decreases in maternal cardiac output; as a result, supine positioning should be avoided to reduce the risk of placental hypoperfusion.[35] Left lateral decubitus position is often recommended to minimize caval compression; however, the decubitus position may not be necessary because only slight left-sided elevation may be sufficient to relieve IVC compression. Higuchi and colleagues conducted a single-institution retrospective review of third trimester patients undergoing MRI and measured caval compression with respect to degrees of left lateral elevation. The authors observed that maximum caval decompression occurred with 30° left-sided elevation, suggesting that a bump may be sufficient to alleviate caval compression and restore maternal physiology intraoperatively.[36]

So long as adequate measures are taken to accommodate the gravid uterus, the prone position is safe in all stages of pregnancy. A large meta-analysis by Cavalcante and colleagues[37] examined reported maternal and fetal outcomes for patients requiring prone positioning for acute respiratory distress syndrome or surgery. Based on these data, the authors concluded that prone positioning is safe in patients undergoing surgery; however, the authors do note that adequate support of the hips and chest must be implemented to reduce abdominal pressure.

ROLE OF LAPAROSCOPY IN PREGNANCY

Minimally invasive surgery is safe in pregnancy and is the surgical approach of choice when clinically appropriate. Multiple meta-analyses have demonstrated that minimally invasive surgery, both laparoscopic and robotic-assisted, has been associated with an improved postoperative control, shorter length of stay, and earlier return to activity across a multitude of pathologic conditions when compared with an open approach.[38–40] Historic concerns regarding the implementation of minimally invasive surgery in pregnancy have revolved around possible injury to or manipulation of the gravid uterus, decreased uterine or placental blood flow from abdominal insufflation, and the possibility of fetal hypercarbia secondary to maternal and fetal absorption of carbon dioxide. Although prospective data are limited, clinical experience and retrospective studies suggest that minimally invasive surgery is safe in pregnant patients when performed by an experienced surgeon.[41]

Early studies examining the use of laparoscopic surgery in pregnancy have demonstrated no apparent association between injury to the gravid uterus and trocar or Veress needle insertion. In a small series, Lemaire and Erp did not observe any iatrogenic injury or pregnancy-related complications following successful laparoscopic surgery for acute appendicitis and acute cholecystitis.[42] The choice of approach for initial abdominal insufflation, however, remains somewhat controversial. Early studies have suggested that an open approach was best used in the later stages of pregnancy, particularly the second and third trimesters.[43] However, subsequent studies have found no differences in rates of iatrogenic injury when using a Veress needle compared with the Hasson technique.[44,45]

The risk of uteroplacental insufficiency from abdominal insufflation and subsequent compression of the uterine vessels seems minimal. Candiani and colleagues performed a single-institution case series in which uteroplacental perfusion was measured among a small number of pregnant patients undergoing laparoscopic pelvic surgery. Using noninvasive ultrasonography, the authors observed no significant differences in mean uterine resistance index or umbilical artery pulsatility index following abdominal insufflation.[46] The authors additionally noted that both of these parameters, as well as FHR, remained stable throughout surgery, suggesting no evidence of fetal hypoxemia because of insufflation.

Despite these data, there remain concerns that transient disruptions of uteroplacental vasculature may affect birth outcomes, particularly birth weight. A large retrospective study examining birth outcomes of pregnant patients in Korea who underwent both laparoscopic and open pelvic surgery identified a significantly increased risk of low birth weight in both the minimally invasive and open surgery patients.[47] Notably, although a laparoscopic approach had a significantly lower risk of low birth weight when compared with an open approach, laparoscopic surgery was itself significantly associated with low birth weight when compared with nonsurgical controls. However, there are data suggesting that severe intra-abdominal pathologic condition, particularly acute appendicitis, is associated with low birth weight and spontaneous abortion.[48,49] Therefore, it remains difficult to determine if reductions in birth weight are a result of surgery or the underlying abdominal pathologic condition.

Considered together, these data suggest that laparoscopic surgery is both safe and feasible in pregnancy. As such, the Society of American Gastrointestinal and Endoscopic Surgeons (SAGES) recommend the implementation of laparoscopy when clinically indicated based on moderate-quality and high-quality evidence.[50] According to the SAGES clinical practice guidelines regarding the use of laparoscopic surgery in pregnancy, laparoscopy offers similar benefits in pregnant patients as nonpregnant patients when compared with laparotomy and can be safely used in all trimesters of pregnancy.[51] Specifically, laparoscopy confers superior postoperative pain control and lowered narcotic requirement, resulting in a decreased fetal respiratory depression and maternal hypoventilation.[52] Laparoscopic surgery may additionally reduce the risk of uterine irritability by reducing the need manual manipulation of the gravid uterus.[53]

As surgical technology continues to advance, robotic-assisted laparoscopic surgery (RALS) has become increasingly common in the treatment of acute surgical pathologic condition. Due to its recent and ongoing implementation, there are little data exploring the use of robotic surgery in pregnancy. Clinical experience and case-reports have proposed that robotic surgery is safe and efficacious in the treatment of various nonobstetric conditions in pregnant patients, including benign adnexal masses, urologic dysfunction, and colon cancer.[54–56] The decision to perform RALS is therefore at the discretion of the operating surgeon and should be made in the context of the patient's clinical presentation and the health-care team's experience with robotic surgery.

Emergency General Surgery During Pregnancy

Acute appendicitis

Acute appendicitis is the most common cause of acute abdomen in pregnancy.[57] The prevalence of appendicitis is similar in pregnant women to nonpregnant women; however, the reported risk of perforation, is higher in the obstetric population.[58] This is thought to be due to the often-delayed diagnosis of appendicitis in pregnant patients due to overlap in symptoms with pregnancy. Presentation of appendicitis in pregnant patients is often misdiagnosed as indigestion, urinary infection, and impending labor.[57]

Similar to nonpregnant patients, patients most commonly present with periumbilical pain that migrated to the right lower quadrant, often associated with fever, nausea, and vomiting. However, due to displacement of the appendix by the uterus, the pain may present atypically as well. During pregnancy, the appendix shifts from its normal position in the iliac fossa upward and outward above the iliac crest as pregnancy progresses. This displacement starts approximately around the third month of pregnancy. Tenderness can be found in the right upper quadrant and right costal margin in the later months of pregnancy.[59] Additionally, given altered anatomy, guarding and rebound tenderness due to peritoneal irritation may not be as pronounced. Leukocytosis can be physiologic in pregnancy, thus may be nonspecific concerning appendicitis. However, a left shift and band formation may be more indicative of inflammation and infection.

US is the first-line diagnostic modality for appendicitis in pregnancy. US has a sensitivity of 67% to 100% and specificity of 83% to 96% for appendicitis in pregnancy and is typically favored over CT due to the risk of radiation exposure.[60] If US is inconclusive, American College of Radiology recommends MRI next for suspicion of appendicitis given high sensitivity and specificity for appendicitis and minimizing risk of radiation.[61]

Delay in diagnosis and treatment of acute appendicitis can often lead to adverse maternal and fetal outcomes.[62] In uncomplicated appendicitis, fetal loss rate has been reported to be 3% to 5% with insignificant effects on maternal mortality, whereas in cases of perforated appendicitis, fetal loss rates increase to 20% to 25% and maternal mortality rates are about 4%.[63] A high suspicion for acute appendicitis can expedite operative management and decrease postoperative maternal and fetal complications.

Given the high fetal mortality rates and preterm delivery rates associated with perforation, the early operative management of acute appendicitis is the gold standard. The treatment is similar for complicated appendicitis as well. Studies have shown that failed nonoperative management of complicated appendicitis increased chances of amniotic infection and sepsis compared with immediate operation. Additionally, failed nonoperative management of complicated appendicitis with delayed operation increased chances of preterm delivery, preterm labor, and abortion compared with immediate operation.[64]

Acute cholecystitis

Acute cholecystitis is the second most common cause of nonobstetric acute abdominal pain in pregnant patients. During pregnancy, estrogen increases cholesterol secretion and progesterone reduces bile acid secretion and decreases gallbladder motility, predisposing patients to the formation of gallstones. Even with hormone changes causing increased gallstones in pregnancy, the incidence of acute cholecystitis does not seem to increase with pregnancy.[65]

Presentation of pregnant patients with cholecystitis is similar to that of nonpregnant patients: right upper quadrant pain, fever, nausea, and vomiting. Murphy sign can be variable depending on patient's body habitus and gestational age of the fetus. Right upper quadrant US is the diagnostic study of choice with sensitivity greater than 95%. Findings indicative of cholecystitis are similar to nonpregnant patients: gallstones, gallbladder wall thickening, pericholecystic fluid, and dilated biliary ducts in cases of biliary obstruction.[66] Leukocytosis can be physiologic in pregnancy, thus again may be nonspecific concerning cholecystitis but a left shift and presence of bands may point toward cholecystitis. Comprehensive metabolic panel and lipase to assess for biliary obstruction is also crucial for accurate diagnosis.

Traditionally, pregnant patients were admitted and treated with antibiotics, resuscitation, and analgesics. Studies have shown, however, that there is a higher risk of fetal death among patients treated nonoperatively to those who were treated with laparoscopic cholecystectomy, so there is a push toward operative treatment given the risk to the fetus in the setting of acute infection.[67] In addition, nonoperative approaches still had a high relapse rate of 40% to 70%.[68]

Earlier surgical intervention has shown a lower rate of preterm delivery in surgical patients, less medication usage, shorter hospital stays, and lower rates of complications from cholecystitis.[68] There has also been reported success with percutaneous cholecystostomy tube treatment without neonatal complications; however, there are not enough data to offer this as an alternative to cholecystectomy.[69]

In patients with biliary obstruction such as cholangitis, choledocholithiasis, or gallstone pancreatitis, studies have shown that endoscopic retrograde cholangiopancreatography with sphincterotomy and stone extraction to relieve obstruction is safe in pregnancy with minimal risk of radiation exposure to the fetus.[70] Cholecystectomy in these instances can be deferred until postpartum.

Small bowel obstruction

Small bowel obstruction (SBO) is a rare, yet adverse cause of acute abdominal pain in pregnant patients. The rate of fetal loss in setting of SBO can be as high as 17% and maternal mortality rate up to 2%.[71] Similar to nonpregnant patients, they are most commonly due to adhesions. The incidence of mechanical SBO increases throughout gestation, with more occurring in the second and third trimesters.[72] Symptoms are similar to nonpregnant patients with nausea, vomiting, abdominal pain, and obstipation. Diagnosis can be made with plain films and MRI. If a patient does not respond well to conservative management, MRI may help delineate further cause of obstruction without ionizing radiation to the fetus.[73] Initial treatment is similar to nonpregnant patients: bowel rest, resuscitation, and nasogastric decompression. Surgical intervention should be considered in the setting of peritonitis, threatened or ischemic bowel, and for patients who fail conservative management. Close monitoring of patient and fetus is critical because urgent surgical management may be necessary should the fetus begin to show signs of stress. An additional consideration is management of bowel obstruction conservatively to allow fetus to grow to a later gestational age to allow greater chances of survival should the fetus not tolerate surgery.[71]

Gynecologic emergencies

There are several gynecological emergencies that should be considered as a source of acute abdominal pain in pregnancy. Adnexal torsion can be seen in pregnancy, with increased incidence in patients undergoing in vitro fertilization, likely due to hyperstimulation of ovarian follicles.[74] Displacement of the ovary by an enlarging uterus may also cause torsion as well.[75] Patients will present with acute onset, unilateral pain that may be intermittent and associated with nausea and vomiting. On examination, there is tenderness unilaterally in the lower abdomen. Diagnosis is made with pelvic US, which can evaluate blood flow to the ovary.[76] The treatment of ovarian torsion is surgical detorsion. Salpingo-oophorectomy of the affected side should only be considered if the perfusion is severely compromised.[77] Surgical detorsion has no increased risk to mother or fetus.[78]

Ectopic pregnancy

Although ectopic pregnancies are rare, with an incidence of 1% to 2% of all pregnancies, ruptured ectopic pregnancies are the cause of 6% of maternal deaths.[79] Patients present with abdominal pain, vaginal bleeding, amenorrhea, lightheadedness, and general pregnancy symptoms. On physical examination, they may have abdominal tenderness, adnexal tenderness, peritonitis, rebound, or guarding, depending on the progression of the ectopic pregnancy to rupture. Diagnosis is based on transvaginal US and laboratory tests such as complete blood count (CBC) and beta-human chorionic gonadotropin (HCG). It is important to obtain a blood type in order to assess the need for prophylactic Rhogam. If the ectopic pregnancy has not ruptured and the patient is stable, the patient may be treated conservatively with methotrexate or with surgery. If the ectopic pregnancy has ruptured and the patient is unstable, the patient will need to go to the operating room for an emergent salpingectomy.[75]

Severe vaginal bleeding

Severe vaginal bleeding in a pregnant patient can be life threatening. It may be due to a wide variety of causes from placenta abruption to trauma to ruptured ectopic pregnancy, as previously discussed. Treatment of these patients is similar to the approach to a trauma patient, starting with the assessment of airway, breathing, and circulation. Obtaining large bore intravenous access and appropriate activation of massive transfusion protocol is critical in the unstable patient. If the patient continues to be unstable, emergent delivery of the fetus may be necessary. After delivery, oxytocin and other uterotonics should be used initially to treat hemorrhage in conjunction with uterine massage. Should initial measures not stop bleeding, tranexamic acid and intrauterine balloon tamponade are next-line conservative measures to control hemorrhage. If hemorrhage is not controlled with conservative treatment, uterine artery embolization, or hysterectomy may be necessary to control life-threatening bleeding.[80]

SUMMARY

Nonobstetrical and obstetrical surgical emergencies occur throughout pregnancy and must be approached with a thorough understanding of the physiologic changes and perioperative nuances of pregnant patients. In the setting of a surgical emergency, care of a pregnant patient should not be withheld because this may be detrimental to the mother and fetus. The management of these surgical emergencies may be performed using standard surgical techniques, including minimally invasive surgery.

CLINICS CARE POINTS

- The evaluation and management of acute abdominal pain in a pregnant patient requires an understanding of key physiologic changes that occur during pregnancy.
- General anesthesia and minimally invasive surgical techniques are safe for pregnant patients in any trimester; however, options for patient positioning and fetal monitoring should be discussed among treatment team.
- Obstetrical and nonobstetrical surgical emergencies often have similar signs and symptoms that can delay definitive treatment. Surgeons must maintain a thorough understanding of these conditions to minimize risk to the patient and fetus.

REFERENCES

1. ACOG Committee Opinion No. 775 summary: nonobstetric surgery during pregnancy. Obstet Gynecol 2019;133(4):844–5.
2. Reitman E, Flood P. Anaesthetic considerations for non-obstetric surgery during pregnancy. Br J Anaesth 2011;107(Suppl 1):i72–8.
3. Gilo NB, Amini D, Landy HJ. Appendicitis and cholecystitis in pregnancy. Clin Obstet Gynecol 2009;52(4):586–96.
4. Erekson EA, Brousseau E, Dick-Biascoechea M, et al. Maternal postoperative complications after nonobstetric antenatal surgery. J Matern Fetal Neonatal Med 2012;25(12):2639–44.
5. Kepley JM, Bates K, Mohiuddin SS. Physiology, maternal changes. StatPearls [Internet]. Treasure Island (FL): StatPearls Publishing; 2022. Available at: https://www.ncbi.nlm.nih.gov/books/NBK539766/.
6. Green L, Mackillop L, Salvi D, et al. Gestation-specific vital sign reference ranges in pregnancy. Obstet Gynecol 2020;135(3):653–64.
7. ACOG Committee Opinion No 723. Guidelines for diagnostic imaging during pregnancy and lactation. Obstet Gynecol 2017;130(4):e210–6.
8. Ravindra GL, Madamangalam AS, Seetharamaiah S. Anaesthesia for non-obstetric surgery in obstetric patients. Indian J Anaesth 2018;62(9):710–6.
9. Kodali BS, Chandrasekhar S, Bulich L, et al. Airway changes during labor and delivery. Anesthesiology 2008;108(3):357–62.
10. Pilkington S, Carli F, Dakin MJ, et al. Increase in Mallampati score during pregnancy. Br J Anaesth 1995;74(6):638–42.
11. Rocke D, Murray WB, Rout CC, et al. Relative risk analysis of factors associated with difficult intubation in obstetric anesthesia. Anesthesiology 1992;77(1):67–73.
12. Rahman K, Jenkins JG. Failed tracheal intubation in obstetrics: no more frequent but still managed badly. Anaesthesia 2005;60(2):168–71.
13. Djabatey E, Barclay P. Difficult and failed intubation in 3430 obstetric general anaesthetics. Anaesthesia 2009;64(11):1168–71.
14. Hawkins JL, Chang J, Palmer SK, et al. Anesthesia-related maternal mortality in the United States: 1979-2002. Obstet Gynecol 2011;117(1):69–74.
15. Cheek TG, Baird E. Anesthesia for nonobstetric surgery: maternal and fetal considerations. Clin Obstet Gynecol 2009;52(4):535–45.
16. Cohen-Kerem R, Railton C, Oren D, et al. Pregnancy outcome following non-obstetric surgical intervention. Am J Surg 2005;190(3):467–73.
17. McElhatton PR. The effects of benzodiazepine use during pregnancy and lactation. Reprod Toxicol 1994;8(6):461–75.

18. Shiono P, Mills J. Oral clefts and diazepam use during pregnancy. N Engl J Med 1984;311(14):919–20.
19. Palanisamy A, Baxter MG, Keel PK, et al. Rats exposed to isoflurane in utero during early gestation are behaviorally abnormal as adults. Anesthesiology 2011; 114(3):521–8.
20. Bartels M, Althoff RR, Boomsma DI. Anesthesia and cognitive performance in children: no evidence for a causal relationship. Twin Res Hum Genet 2009; 12(3):246–53.
21. DiMaggio C, Sun LS, Kakavouli A, et al. A retrospective cohort study of the association of anesthesia and hernia repair surgery with behavioral and developmental disorders in young children. J Neurosurg Anesthesiol 2009;21(4):286–91.
22. Itskovitz J, LaGamma EF, Rudolph AM. The effect of reducing umbilical blood flow on fetal oxygenation. Am J Obstet Gynecol 1983;145(7):813–8.
23. Dilts PV Jr, Brinkman CR, Kirschbaum TH, et al. Uterine and systemic hemodynamic interrelationships and their response to hypoxia. Am J Obstet Gynecol 1969;103(1):138–57.
24. Pacifici GM, Nottoli R. Placental transfer of drugs administered to the mother. Clin Pharmacokinet 1995;28(3):235–69.
25. Allaert SE, Carlier SP, Weyne LP, et al. First trimester anesthesia exposure and fetal outcome. A review. Acta Anaesthesiol Belg 2007;58(2):119–23.
26. Eltzschig HK, Lieberman ES, Camann WR. Regional anesthesia and analgesia for labor and delivery. N Engl J Med 2003;348(4):319–32.
27. Devis P, Knuttinen MG. Deep venous thrombosis in pregnancy: incidence, pathogenesis and endovascular management. Cardiovasc Diagn Ther 2017;7: S309–19.
28. ACOG Practice Bulletin No. 106: Intrapartum fetal heart rate monitoring: nomenclature, interpretation, and general management principles. Obstet Gynecol 2009;114(1):192–202.
29. Kuczkowski KM. Nonobstetric surgery during pregnancy: what are the risks of anesthesia? Obstet Gynecol Surv 2004;59(1):52–6.
30. Bakker JJ, Janssen PF, van Halem K, et al. Internal versus external tocodynamometry during induced or augmented labour. Cochrane Database Syst Rev 2012 Dec 12;12:CD006947.
31. Myers LB, Cohen D, Galinkin J, et al. Anaesthesia for fetal surgery. Paediatr Anaesth 2002;12(7):569–78.
32. Okutomi T, Saito M, Kuczkowski KM. The use of potent inhalational agents for the ex- utero intrapartum treatment (exit) procedures: what concentrations? Acta Anaesthesiol Belg 2007;58(2):97–9.
33. Smith GN, Brien JF. Use of nitroglycerin for uterine relaxation. Obstet Gynecol Surv 1998;53(9):559–65.
34. Spiropoulos K, Prodromaki E, Tsapanos V. Effect of body position on PaO2 and PaCO2 during pregnancy. Gynecol Obstet Invest 2004;58(1):22–5.
35. Lees MM, Scott DB, Kerr MG, et al. The circulatory effects of recumbent postural change in late pregnancy. Clin Sci 1967;32(3):453–65.
36. Higuchi H, Takagi S, Zhang K, et al. Effect of lateral tilt angle on the volume of the abdominal aorta and inferior vena cava in pregnant and nonpregnant women determined by magnetic resonance imaging. Anesthesiology 2015;122(2): 286–93.
37. Cavalcante FML, Fernandes CDS, Rocha LDS, et al. Use of the prone position in pregnant women with COVID-19 or other health conditions. Rev Lat Am Enfermagem 2021;29:e3494.

38. Coccolini F, Catena F, Pisano M, et al. Open versus laparoscopic cholecystectomy in acute cholecystitis. Systematic review and meta-analysis. Int J Surg 2015;18:196–204.

39. Martínez-Pérez A, de'Angelis N, Brunetti F, et al. Laparoscopic vs. open surgery for the treatment of iatrogenic colonoscopic perforations: a systematic review and meta-analysis. World J Emerg Surg 2017;12:8.

40. Quah GS, Eslick GD, Cox MR. Laparoscopic appendicectomy is superior to open surgery for complicated appendicitis. Surg Endosc 2019;33(7):2072–82.

41. Fatum M, Rojansky N. Laparoscopic surgery during pregnancy. Obstet Gynecol Surv 2001;56(1):50–9.

42. Lemaire BM, van Erp WF. Laparoscopic surgery during pregnancy. Surg Endosc 1997;11(1):15–8.

43. Al-Fozan H, Tulandi T. Safety and risks of laparoscopy in pregnancy. Curr Opin Obstet Gynecol 2002;14(4):375–9.

44. Guterman S, Mandelbrot L, Keita H, et al. Laparoscopy in the second and third trimesters of pregnancy for abdominal surgical emergencies. J Gynecol Obstet Hum Reprod 2017;46(5):417–22.

45. Upadhyay A, Stanten S, Kazantsev G, et al. Laparoscopic management of a nonobstetric emergency in the third trimester of pregnancy. Surg Endosc 2007;21(8): 1344–8.

46. Candiani M, Maddalena S, Barbieri M, et al. Adnexal masses in pregnancy: fetomaternal blood flow indices during laparoscopic surgery. J Minim Invasive Gynecol 2012;19(4):443–7.

47. Cho HW, Cho GJ, Noh E, et al. Pregnancy outcomes following laparoscopic and open surgery in pelvis during pregnancy: a nationwide population-based study in Korea. J Korean Med Sci 2021;36(29):e192.

48. Wei PL, Keller JJ, Liang HH, et al. Acute appendicitis and adverse pregnancy outcomes: a nationwide population-based study. J Gastrointest Surg 2012; 16(6):1204–11.

49. Theilen LH, Mellnick VM, Shanks AL, et al. Acute appendicitis in pregnancy: predictive clinical factors and pregnancy outcomes. Am J Perinatol 2017;34(6): 523–8.

50. Pearl JP, Price RR, Tonkin AE, et al. SAGES guidelines for the use of laparoscopy during pregnancy. Surg Endosc 2017;31(10):3767–82.

51. Oelsner G, Stockheim D, Soriano D, et al. Pregnancy outcome after laparoscopy or laparotomy in pregnancy. J Am Assoc Gynecol Laparosc 2003;10(2):200–4.

52. Curet MJ, Allen D, Josloff RK, et al. Laparoscopy during pregnancy. Arch Surg 1996;131(5):546–50 [discussion: 550-1].

53. Soriano D, Yefet Y, Seidman DS, et al. Laparoscopy versus laparotomy in the management of adnexal masses during pregnancy. Fertil Steril 1999;71(5): 955–60.

54. Capella CE, Godovchik J, Chandrasekar T, et al. Nonobstetrical robotic-assisted laparoscopic surgery in pregnancy: a systematic literature review. Urology 2021; 151:58–66.

55. Hagen ER, Gerson L, Rashidi L, et al. Robotic surgical management of sigmoid colon cancer in pregnancy: a case series. Am J Surg 2021;221(6):1291–2.

56. Baldwin LA, Podzielinski I, Goodrich ST, et al. Robotic surgery for adnexal masses in pregnancy. J Robot Surg 2011;5(3):231–3.

57. Horowitz MD, Gomez GA, Santiesteban R, et al. Acute appendicitis during pregnancy. Diagnosis and management. Arch Surg 1985;120(12):1362–7.

58. Mourad J, Elliott J, Erickson L, et al. Appendicitis in pregnancy: new information that contradicts long-held clinicalbeliefs. Am J Obstet Gynecol 2000;182:1027–9.
59. Baer JL, Reis RA, Arens RA. Appendicitis in pregnancy: with changes in position and axis of the normal appendix in pregnancy. JAMA 1932;98(16):1359–64.
60. Williams R, Shaw J. Ultrasound scanning in the diagnosis of acute appendicitis in pregnancy. Emerg Med J 2007;24(5):359–60.
61. Rosen MP, Ding A, Blake MA, et al. ACR Appropriateness Criteria right lower quadrant pain – suspected appendicitis. J Am Coll Radiol 2011;8(11):749–55.
62. Chwat C, Terres M, Duarte MR, et al. Laparoscopic treatment for appendicitis during pregnancy: retrospective cohort study. Ann Med Surg (Lond) 2021;68: 102668.
63. Doberneck RC. Appendectomy during pregnancy. Am Surg 1985;51(5):265–8.
64. Ashbrook M, Cheng V, Sandhu K, et al. Management of complicated appendicitis during pregnancy in the US. JAMA Netw Open 2022;5(4):e227555.
65. Dietrich CS, Hill CC, Hueman M. Surgi-cal diseases presenting in pregnancy. Surg Clin North Am 2008;88:408–19.
66. Borzellino G, Massimiliano Motton AP, Minniti F, et al. Sonographic diagnosis of acute cholecystitis in patients with symptomatic gallstones. J Clin Ultrasound 2016;44(3):152–8.
67. Jelin EB, Smink DS, Vernon AH, et al. Management of biliary tract disease during pregnancy: a decision analysis. Surg Endosc 2008;22(1):54–60.
68. Swisher SG, Schmit PJ, Hunt KK, et al. Biliary disease during preg-nancy. Am J Surg 1994;168(6):576–81.
69. Caliskan K. The use of percutaneous cholecystostomy in the treatment of acute cholecystitis during pregnancy. Clin Exp Obstet Gynecol 2017;44(1):11–3.
70. Tham TC, Vandervoort J, Wong RC, et al. Safety of ERCP during pregnancy. Am J Gastroenterol 2003;98(2):308–11, 40.
71. Webster PJ, Bailey MA, Wilson J, et al. Small bowel obstruction in pregnancy is a complex surgical problem with a high risk of fetal loss. Ann R Coll Surg Engl 2015; 97(5):339–44.
72. Augustin G, Majerovic M. Non-obstetrical acute abdomen during pregnancy. Eur J Obstet Gynecol Reprod Biol 2007;131(1):4–12.
73. McKenna DA, Meehan CP, Alhajeri AN, et al. The use of MRI to demonstrate small bowel obstruction during pregnancy. Br J Radiol 2007;80:e11–4.
74. Robson S, Kerin JF. Acute adnexal torsion before oocyte retrieval in an in vitro fertilization cycle. Fertil Steril 2000;73:650–1.
75. McWilliams GDE, Hill MJ, Dietrich CS. Gynecologic emergencies. Surg Clin 2008; 88(2):265–83.
76. Albayam F, Hamper UM. Ovarian and adnexal torsion: spectrum of sonographic findings with pathologic correlation. J Ultrasound Med 2001;20:1083–9.
77. Zweizig S, Perron J, Grubb D, et al. Conservative management of adnexal torsion. Am J Obstet Gynecol 1993;168:1791–5.
78. Daykan Y, Bogin R, Sharvit M, et al. Adnexal torsion during preg-nancy: pregnancy outcomes after surgical intervention – a retrospective case–control study. J Minim Invasive Gynecol 2019;26(1):117–21.
79. Berg CJ, Callaghan WM, Syverson C, et al. Pregnancy-related mortality in the United States, 1998 to 2005. Obstet Gynecol 2010;116(6):1302–9.
80. WHO recommendations for the prevention and treatment of postpartum haemor-rhage. Geneva (Switzerland): World Health Organization; 2012. p. 3. Results.

Surgical Emergencies in Patients with Significant Comorbid Diseases

Jacqueline Blank, MD[a], Adam M. Shiroff, MD[a,b], Lewis J. Kaplan, MD, FCCP, FCCM[a,b],*

KEYWORDS

- Surgical emergency • Critical care • Frailty • Comorbidities • Chronic critical illness
- Organ failure

KEY POINTS

- Emergency surgical care in patients with significant comorbidities offers little time to pre-operatively improve physiology, especially for time-sensitive conditions.
- Deciding whether to offer surgical intervention in this unique but growing patient population is essential and often requires rapidly engaging family members or other surrogates.
- Intra-operative interventions should leverage a damage control approach.
- Postoperative interventions are numerous, reflect standard critical care, but should ensure goal-concordant care.
- Outcomes vary widely based on age and comorbidities and are adversely impacted by the development of chronic critical illness.

INTRODUCTION

Unlike elective procedures, surgical urgencies and emergencies often do not provide opportunity for preop interventions that improve operation or anesthesia tolerance. In this way, surgical emergency patients share broad overlap with those who present with hemorrhagic shock after injury, procedural intervention, or gastrointestinal hemorrhage. The lack of opportunity to address underlying physiologic derangements related to comorbid conditions is complicated by population aging as well as

[a] Department of Surgery, Division of Trauma, Surgical Critical Care, and Emergency Surgery, Perelman School of Medicine, University of Pennsylvania, 51 North 39th Street, MOB 1, Suite 120, Philadelphia, PA 19104, USA; [b] Surgical Services, Section of Surgical Critical Care and Emergency General Surgery, Corporal Michael J. Crescenz VA Medical Center, 3900 Woodland Avenue, Philadelphia, PA 19104, USA
* Corresponding author. Department of Surgery, Division of Trauma, Surgical Critical Care, and Emergency Surgery, Perelman School of Medicine, University of Pennsylvania, 51 North 39th Street, MOB 1, Suite 120, Philadelphia, PA 19104.
E-mail address: Lewis.Kaplan@pennmedicine.upenn.edu

Surg Clin N Am 103 (2023) 1231–1251
https://doi.org/10.1016/j.suc.2023.06.003
0039-6109/23/Published by Elsevier Inc.
surgical.theclinics.com

concomitant frailty.[1] Patient care is also adversely impacted by concurrent therapeutic agents and complex medication regimens.[2,3] Outcomes after emergency intervention are derailed by preoperative cognitive impairment, reduced health literacy and limited access to care that may deprive patients of optimal health maintenance.[1] Therefore, surgeons at institutions spanning critical access hospitals to quaternary care centers need to be prepared to manage emergency surgery patients with substantial single or multiple comorbidities immediately prior to surgical rescue, within the OR, as well as through the postoperative period into convalescence. Accordingly, this chapter will primarily focus on emergency general surgery (EGS) but will articulate lessons and guidance that are applicable to a broad range of surgical specialties.

PREVALENCE

Emergency operative care occurs with great frequency across US acute care facilities.[4] However, those cases include low risk ones such as acute non-perforated appendicitis in a healthy 24 year-old to a necrotizing soft tissue infection of the perineum and buttocks in a 76 year-old individual with diabetes, COPD, and coronary artery disease with a transplanted kidney on immune suppression. Up to 40% of patients who undergo an EGS procedure require postoperative critical care.[5,6] It is this group of patients – those with an accelerated mortality risk based upon disease process and comorbidities – that is part of the focus of the now well-established discipline of Acute Care Surgery.[7] Moreover, this group of patients demonstrates an asymmetric proportion of the elderly (aged > 65 years). Indeed, the elderly commonly evidence substantial comorbidities that influence care as well as outcome (**Fig. 1**). Responding to either the need for more complex surgical or postoperative care, or concomitant comorbidities, patients are commonly transferred into a tertiary or quaternary care facility in need of both EGS intervention as well as ICU management.[8,9] An ACS service at a complex care facility can serve as a rescue service for inpatients as well as the portal of entry for the region. Such services provide operative intervention in 33% of patients for whom they are unanticipatedly engaged within their home facility.[10] Increasingly, health systems are articulating critical care networks and organizations that span all of the facilities within the system.[11] These networks may also funnel complex patients into the "hub" facility from their feeder "spoke" sites to align patient needs with existing resources – including those relevant for the OR and the ICU.

PATIENT EVALUATION OVERVIEW

Once it has been determined that the patient has a condition that may be addressed with an urgent or emergent surgical intervention, the surgeon has only limited time to address imperatives that improve outcome. Complex evaluations and diagnostic or provocative testing that assesses cardiovascular or pulmonary fitness for anesthesia and surgical intervention are precluded by the time sensitive nature of the patient's condition. Therefore, in general, the surgeon needs to decide on a course of therapy without being able to modify comorbidity-related risk factors for morbidity or mortality. Certain conditions such as hypovolemia, acute anemia, hyperglycemia, and hypoxia, hypercarbia, hypo- or hyperthermia, as well as life-threatening metabolic acidosis may be addressed while preparing the patient for the OR – if the surgeon agrees to offer operation including palliative operation.[12–14] In other circumstances, the surgeon may choose to pursue non-operative management, and for those with a variety of conditions that render operative care inadvisable, only comfort care (**Fig. 2**). Some patients may be unable to help the surgeon understand their goals and preferences due to underlying cognitive failure, dementia, shock, or acute organ failure.

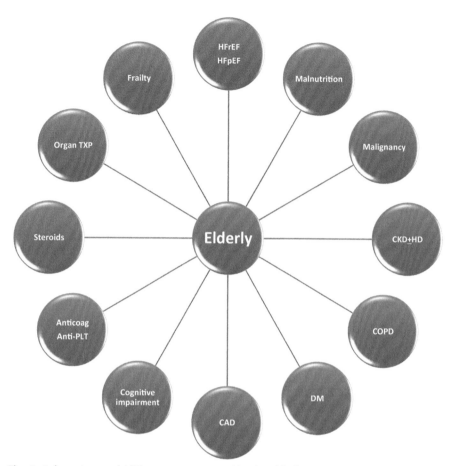

Fig. 1. Relevant comorbidities overrepresented in the elderly.

Instead, a surrogate, including a legally authorized representative (LAR), is essential in understanding what the patient would have likely thought about their current condition, and not what the surrogate thinks about the current condition and potential care. This point is critical especially when there is an abrupt change in physiology or life circumstance and the surrogate has not had a conversation with the patient about their goals, values, and preferences in that kind of situation. When such conversations have not occurred, engaging with a Palliative Care Medicine (PCM) clinician is often helpful.[15] The surrogate gains a clinician who is there for them, as opposed to the surgeon, who may be viewed as being engaged on behalf of the patient – despite the surgeon delivering patient and family-centered care. PCM clinicians may be particularly helpful when there is family conflict and discord around end-of-life issues as they are specifically trained in communication and conflict management.[16,17]

Reasonable indications for acute PCM consultation are presented in **Fig. 3**. At times, the surgeon will encounter conditions that are so time sensitive that prolonged discussion is unable to occur.

Key time-sensitive conditions relevant for the emergency surgeon – as opposed to the trauma surgeon – include necrotizing soft tissue infection, acute intestinal ischemia, and massive gastrointestinal hemorrhage.[18] Each of these are linked by demonstrating

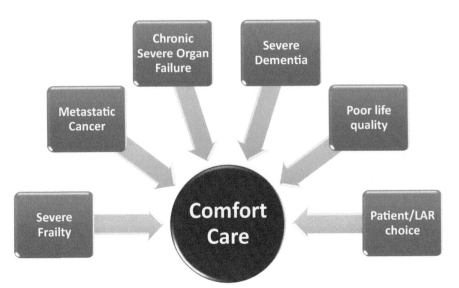

Fig. 2. Key conditions that often drive comfort care discussions.

a high degree of lethality, and by not benefitting from a period of preoperative resuscitation to achieve stabilization prior to acute operation. Other conditions including intestinal perforation demonstrate improved outcomes as a result of resuscitation ahead of general anesthesia and acute operation. Accordingly, for those with time-sensitive conditions, acute intervention may be viewed as acute rescue to allow time for family to gather, evaluate their loved one's response to an attempt at initial intervention, and

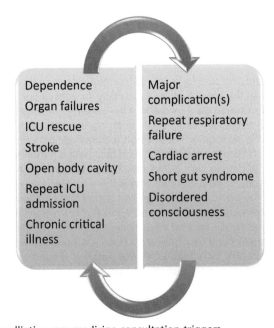

Fig. 3. Common palliative care medicine consultation triggers.

then reach consensus about how the patient would likely perceive their current condition and care trajectory. This kind of approach may be selected by family members despite the patient suffering from chronic serious illness. It is important to recognize that acute operation may be viewed as the family portion of patient and family-centered care, especially if the patient has not otherwise stated their desires with regard to intervention in case of life-threatening illness. Nonetheless, the surgeon must be facile with preoperative assessment tools that may also help inform patients or their surrogates or family members regarding likely outcomes including morbidity and mortality.

TREATMENT OPTIONS
Preoperative Assessment Scoring Tools

Clearly, certain comorbidities confer an increased risk for survival failure as well as an increased likelihood of per-operative morbidity.[19,20] Many of those are identified in **Fig. 1**. Unsurprisingly, there are a variety of calculators that one may use to forecast postoperative risks.[21–23] Examples include the National Surgery Quality Improvement Program (NSQIP) calculator as well as the related Veterans Affairs SQIP (VASQIP) calculator. Others exist including but not limited to POSSUM, the Preoperative Mortality Predictor Score (PMP), the Society of Thoracic Surgeons Risk Calculator, Revised Cardiac Risk Index, the Gupta Perioperative Risk for Myocardial Infarction/Cardiac Arrest calculator, the Surgical Outcome Risk Tool (SORT), the Emergency Surgery Score (ESS), the American Society of Anesthesiologists (ASA) score, as well as the Predictive OpTimal Trees in Emergency Surgery Risk (POTTER) tool. All of these tools incorporate fixed elements such as age with measures of comorbidity, measures of function and some also include vital signs and acute laboratory elements. Some include the urgency of surgery, or the potential for non-operative therapies, while others include features that are only known once surgery has begun such as the presence of peritoneal soiling, or after surgery has been completed such as estimated blood loss. Given the plethora of scoring systems, it is not clear that one is superior. Some like the RCRI and the Gupta score are more specifically focused.

In general, the above scoring systems treat scoring elements as unique factors whose impact on outcome is treated in a binary (present vs absent) and additive fashion devoid of comorbid condition interaction. For example, heart failure with an ejection fraction of 45% is quite different from that with an EF of 15% and each of those will interface differently with concomitant cirrhosis. Scoring systems often do not account for degrees of organ failure, and typically do not adjust predicted outcomes based upon comorbid condition interactions. Furthermore, tools vary in complexity and greatly differ in their ability to be used at the bedside ahead of a decision to proceed with surgery. More recent ones such as the POTTER tool leverage machine learning/artificial intelligence to forecast outcomes rendering it less suitable for rapid bedside analysis and may be unable to be applied in resource-limited settings.[21] Finally, most of the tools are derived from outcome data related to elective procedures and may not be as precise as desired when applied to emergency ones, even after "correcting" for the urgency of the intended procedure. Regardless of predicted outcome for those who are appropriate for, and are willing to undergo, an emergency procedure, there are a limited number of preoperative interventions that are of acute value that help with intra- as well as post-operative management.

Preoperative Interventions of Value

It is assumed that the diagnostic interventions that engaged the surgeon and established the admitting diagnosis have already occurred, and that the surgeon and the patient or their surrogate have embraced a surgical solution. Once that has occurred, the surgeon may pursue a limited number of interventions ahead of urgent or emergent surgery (**Fig. 4**). Point-Of-Care-UltraSound (POCUS) helps identify the presence of hypovolemia versus hypovolemia and hyperdynamic cardiac function as opposed to biventricular or univentricular decreased contractility.[24] This examination is not intended to serve as a precision diagnostic interrogation (like a typical Echocardiogram), but is instead focused on determining the advisability of acute interventions. On occasion, left or right ventricular function will be severely compromised by a extrinsic process (ie, non-cardiac) such as septic shock. In the uncommon patient, unilateral or bilateral ventricular support is appropriate.[24] In general, that kind of support should drive reevaluation of the appropriateness of surgical intervention, and engender a surrogate or family discussion regarding goals of care.

Since most who need acute surgical rescue have a fluid deficit, plasma volume expansion (PVE) is commonplace and is central to the bundled management approach for those with sepsis or septic shock from the Surviving Sepsis Campaign.[12,25,26] Having a starting point helps one evaluate the impact of PVE on contractility as well as chamber volume and inferior vena cava volume. Patients with concomitant heart failure or hepatic failure may not demonstrate a plasma volume deficit, and may instead be better managed with a vasopressor to address hypotension. Of course, timely administration – within 1 hour of identifying sepsis or septic shock – of empiric antibiotics is

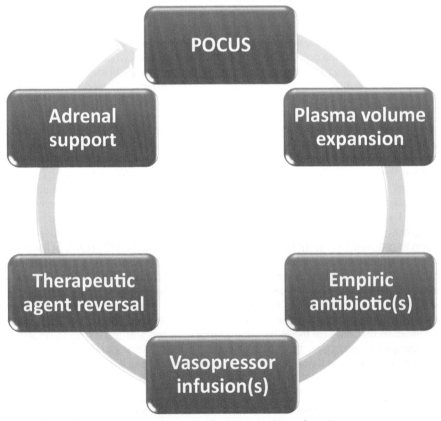

Fig. 4. Urgent/emergent surgery preoperative interventions of merit.

optimal and also conforms to the Hour-1 bundle of the 2016 and 2021 SSC guidelines.[25,27]

Moreover, the reversal of therapeutic agents that impede coagulation is imperative for operations that are likely to have high blood loss, substantial dissection, or those that would have substantial consequences even with small-volume bleeding. The range of reversal agents spans Vitamin K, fresh frozen plasma (FFP), 4-factor pro-thrombin complex concentrate (4F-PCC), as well as agents that specifically reverse direct acting oral anticoagulants.[28,29] Patients on dabigatran may be treated with idar-ucizumab while all others may receive either 4F-PCC or andexanet-alpha.[28,29] DOAC reversal may be accompanied by an increased risk of thromboembolism but is gener-ally perceived as a lesser risk compared to DOAC-related hemorrhage in the postop-erative patient.[28] A variety of guiding documents are available and are often translated into local algorithms in conjunction with Hematology as well as Pharmacy. None of these interventions should impede rapid transit to the OR for source or bleeding con-trol. Finally, preoperative preparation with either stress dose steroids (100 mg hydro-cortisone, initially, and 300 mg in divided doses over 24 hours) or critical illness-related corticoadrenal insufficiency (CIRCI) steroids (50 mg hydrocortisone initially, and 200 mg in divided doses over 24 hours) benefit those with either moderate or greater home steroid dosing, or those with pressor-resistant septic shock.[30] Low-intensity steroid therapy does not, in general, require adrenal support.[31,32]

Intra-operative Interventions of Value

Intra-operative interventions that enhance outcome occur in three major domains: monitoring hemodynamics, improving perfusion, and utilizing a damage control approach (**Fig. 5**). The specific method of hemodynamic monitoring is less important than that there is a monitoring approach. Both invasive and non-invasive approaches may be successful.[33] The principal goals are the restoration of euvolemia and support of biventricular function. With regard to the latter, both vasopressors and inotropic agents may be utilized and are augmented by calcium supplementation especially in the setting of large volume packed red blood cell transfusion.[34–36] Citrate-associated calcium chelation may lead to clinically-relevant hypocalcemia and should be specifically assessed. The efficacy of support may be assessed using extremity temperature monitoring as well as plasma lactate dynamics. Confounders of the latter approaches are severe peripheral arterial disease and pulmonary lactate release or hepatic lactate clearance failure as well as hyperlactatemia unassociated with anaer-obic metabolism respectively.

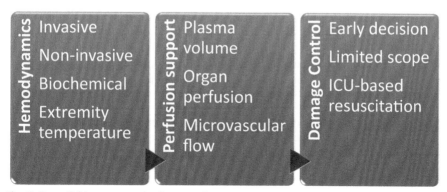

Fig. 5. Essential intra-operative interventions.

Improving bulk systemic flow does not always also enhance microvascular flow, especially in the presence of acidosis and after correction of severe hypovolemia. Reduced pH is associated with RBC volume swelling by approximately 7%, an increase that can impede cell wall deformation that is required for capillary traversal; this may be identified as the "no reflow" phenomenon in unanticipatedly obstructed capillary beds.[37,38] Thus, abrogating severe acidosis as part of an approach to perfusion management is reasonable. Since most resuscitation fluids that are used to correct hypoperfusion are relatively hyperchloremic compared to plasma, hyperchloremic metabolic acidosis (HCMA) is a common consequence of their infusion.[39] Accordingly, specific attention should be paid to avoiding or correcting dyschloremia. To the extent possible, 0.9% NSS should be avoided, and balanced crystalloid solutions such as Normosol or Plasmalyte may be prioritized.[39,40] Lactated Ringer's solution is less abnormal than is 0.9% NSS, but is less ideal than solutions that nearly approximate plasma electrolytes. For those with established HCMA, a solution with markedly reduced chloride can correct the imbalance. A maintenance type of fluid such as D_5W+75 mEq $NaHCO_3/L$, or a resuscitation and bolus-suitable fluid such as ½NSS+75 mEq $NaHCO_3/L$ may be utilized to great effect. Enhanced microvascular flow is designed to help support organ recovery, reduce the extent of organ injury, and therefore, potentially reduce the need for specific organ support such as intermittent or continuous hemodialysis techniques.

An early decision to pursue a damage control approach to operative management is essential, even if the operation is designed to be palliative.[41,42] This allows the OR team and the ICU team to anticipate timing and prepare for rapid transfer between care zones. A truncated operation reduces evaporative loss, exposure to anesthetics that are vasodilators and negative inotropes, and more swiftly delivers the patient to the ICU for ongoing metabolic resuscitation. An open body cavity that is commonly managed using negative pressure wound therapy facilitates managing pressure-volume relationships in the immediate postoperative period where ascites, organ edema, and less commonly hemorrhage may induce intraabdominal hypertension (IAH) or abdominal compartment syndrome (ACS).[42,43] Intestinal discontinuity is common, and intraperitoneal packing may be required. Patients are routinely left with an indwelling oral endotracheal tube for invasive mechanical ventilation, and undergo gastric and bladder decompression; multiple venous and arterial access and monitoring lines are typical and should be shared with family members ahead of operation. Relatedly, the need for a second, and perhaps a third or more returns to the OR should also be shared. Routinely monitoring for IAH and the ACS throughout the postoperative period supports early recognition of pressure-volume dysregulation and drives therapy (see below).[43]

Intra-operative temperature regulation may prove problematic, especially in those with concomitant infection as thermal dysregulation is common. The goal is to maintain euthermia and is easier to address in those with hyperthermia as cooler fluids may be infused, the open body cavity or tissue space during operation increases heat loss, and device-integrated heaters (ventilator, fluid infusion pump) may be deactivated. Patients who demonstrate hypothermia benefit from a warmer room temperature, warmed fluid(s) and inhaled gas, but also external active convective warming; active internal warming using an extracorporeal device is uncommon in this setting.

Microvascular bleeding is commonly encountered during emergency operation and is linked with concomitant hypothermia. Since standard coagulation measures generally require an hour to return after being collected, an alternative approach has been leveraged. Thromboelastography (TEG) and related methods including rotational thromboelastomometry (ROTEM) provides rapid assessment of all elements of the coagulation cascade and does so within approximately 20 minutes of sample acquisition.[44] Both approaches provide a graphic and numeric analysis of the interlinked elements of the coagulation system. While TEG and ROTEM are not universally available, they are particularly helpful in assessing unexplained bleeding, especially during ongoing component transfusion that is expected to lead to normal coagulation.[45]

A related element of utilizing a damage control approach occurs outside of the OR, and involves the care transition between the OR and the ICU. A routine, systematic, and clearly structured handoff optimally involves members from every team (Anesthesia, Surgery, Critical Care Nursing, Respiratory Therapy, Pharmacy, and Critical Care) (physician and/or APP) at the bedside at the same time to support information transfer fidelity. This has been explored using an approach known as HATRICC (Handoffs And Transitions In Critical Care) and is associated with reduced communication-related errors.[46] Postoperative interventions – directed toward critical care issues and family engagement - that may impact outcome are more plentiful than those that may be readily deployed in the preoperative or intra-operative time frames for those requiring urgent or emergent surgical rescue.

Postoperative Interventions of Value

Patients with critical illness benefit from management using a team-based approach including critical care directed by a specifically trained intensivist.[47,48] At present, only half of all of US acute care facilities are staffed by an intensivist.[49] Therefore, when patient care needs outstrip the ability of the facility's clinicians to render required care, transfer is ideal. Preexisting transfer agreements may facilitate both transfer and repatriation. Other health care systems have developed critical care organizations that align care needs with facility resources, including clinicians and specialized equipment such as extracorporeal membrane oxygenation (ECMO).[50]

Critical care management routinely includes actions that prevent complications such as venous thromboembolism, pressure ulceration, and iatrogenic infections related to invasive devices (intravenous or intra-arterial catheters, nasoenteric tube, oral endotracheal tube, tracheostomy tube, chest tube).[51–54] In light of the opioid epidemic, a multimodal approach to analgesia and sedation is increasingly leveraged to include non-pharmacologic methods (ice, heat, environmental cues), routine Tylenol, non-opioid analgesics (NSAIDs, gabapentin), local or regional anesthetics, patient-controlled epidural analgesia (PCEA), and patient-controlled analgesia (PCA).[55,56] Sedation is minimized in this approach and prioritizes typical or atypical antipsychotic agents as opposed to benzodiazepines as they seem to be more deliriogenic, especially in the elderly. Newer approaches such as cryoablation are more common in those with rib fractures or in those who need a sternotomy.[57] Regardless, reduced opioid analgesia often allows the patient to be more interactive and engaged in their postoperative health care, even if they were unable to participate in shared preoperative decision making.

Since many patients with critical illness require invasive mechanical ventilation, an approach to liberating patients from mechanical ventilation that addresses penumbra concerns is essential to deploy in the ICU. Such an approach was initially known as the A-through-F approach, but has been renamed the ICU Liberation Bundle (**Fig. 6**).[58–60] The elements Assess and address pain, spontaneous awakening and Breathing, Choice of sedation and analgesia, Delirium recognition, prevention and management, Early mobilization and exercise, and Family engagement and empowerment. Bundle utilization improves survival, reduces delirium and coma, but does so at the expense of patients being more awake and therefore reporting more pain – a quite acceptable trade-off – that reinforces the importance of adequate pain control.[60] Decreased ICU

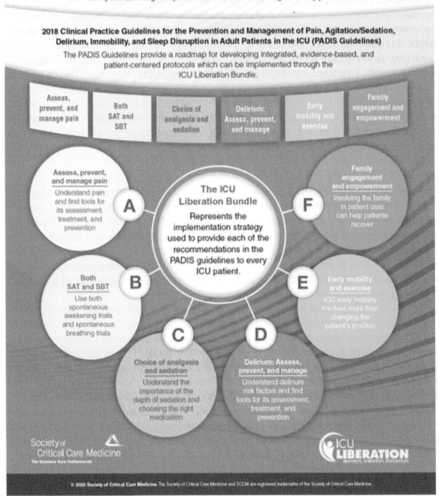

Fig. 6. ICU liberation bundle.

time and decreased delirium also helps mitigate against the development of the post-intensive care syndrome (PICS).[61] The "F" portion of the bundle also helps to reduce how PICS impacts families as well (PICS-F).[62] Synergistic approaches also include the use of an ICU diary, and ICU support group and perhaps most importantly, a post-ICU clinic.[63,64] A post-ICU clinic also has a variety of benefits for the ICU and related clinicians that span improved morale, the creation of new survivor roles, improved understanding of the patient experience, and the development of additional post-ICU programs.[63] All of this supports patient and family centered care as does including family members on rounds.

Fluid management is intertwined with the development of organ edema that influences intra-abdominal pressure, IAH and the ACS as noted above. There is a rubric for fluid management named "ROSE" which stands for resuscitation, optimization, stabilization, and evacuation and reflects the 4 phases of acute patient care with regard to salt and water balance (**Fig. 7**).[65] The importance of this approach is that the different phases are coupled with clinical interventions. Avoiding salt and water excess – and the undesirable acid-base imbalances that occur – are vital aspects of the postoperative critical care of patients with surgical emergencies and serious comorbidities. These interfaces are most readily apparent as one assesses acute kidney injury (AKI) and the work of breathing associated with the minute ventilation (VE; respiratory rate x tidal volume) required to achieve a target carbon dioxide (CO_2) clearance during invasive mechanical ventilation.

Acidosis decreases renal blood flow by afferent arteriolar vasoconstriction and can contribute to AKI development or worsening.[66,67] Septic AKI comprises approximately 50% of the AKI identified in ICU patients in developed nations, but is exacerbated by flow derangements as well as exposure to nephrotoxic agents including certain antibiotics.[68] For healthy individuals, requiring a higher VE to offset metabolic acidosis with respiratory alkalosis is generally well tolerated. In those with serious comorbidities, the increased work of breathing may preclude liberation from invasive mechanical ventilation, increases metabolic demand, and may lead to diaphragm fatigue during spontaneous breathing trials. Therefore, normalizing acid-base balance as rapidly as possible – or preventing it from becoming deranged to the greatest extent possible – is advantageous for those with serious comorbidities who require urgent or emergent surgical rescue.

Coupled with fluid therapy is planned monitoring for IAH and the ACS in those who require emergency laparotomy, but is especially important for those with serious comorbidities. IAH without the ACS will decrease venous return and therefore cardiac output, but also increases renal, splanchnic, and hepatic venous hypertension leading to intra-organ hypertension and organ edema. These untoward consequences in turn increase pressure-volume derangements within the closed or temporarily closed peritoneal space. Thus, regular monitoring is required to detect IAH and respond to it before the ACS ensues.[43] The World Society of the Abdominal Compartment Syndrome (WSACS; now known as the Abdominal Compartment Society; www.wsacs.org) has articulated and revised guidelines on IAH and ACS management that are relevant for bedside decision-making and intervention.[69] Unsurprisingly, the WSACS guideline dovetails with actions encoded in the ROSE approach. It is essential to recognize that utilizing an open abdomen approach does not preclude developing IAH or the ACS. Bedside re-exploration may be required for ACS management if the

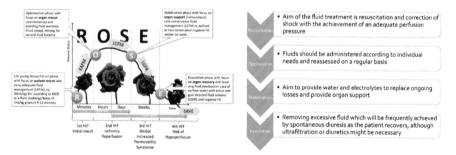

Fig. 7. The ROSE approach to fluid management.

patient is hemodynamically unstable, unsuitable for transport due to care devices, or an OR is unavailable.[70,71]

The clinical condition that drives surgical rescue – as well as operative intervention – may worsen preexisting chronic organ failure, or induce new organ failure. Clinicians should assess organ failure(s) on a daily basis to assess patient trajectory, decide on newly required interventions, and to help family members or surrogates understand the evolving clinical course. Three broad approaches are utilized: Acute Physiology and Chronic Health Evaluation (APACHE) scoring, Sequential Organ Failure Assessment (SOFA) scoring, and a numeric tally of organs demonstrating failure; other scoring systems exist but offer no specific advantage.[72–75] Each of these may be useful and often reflect an institutional approach to acuity assessment. However, APACHE (multiple iterations exist) is difficult for non-clinicians to understand and use in their assessment of how the patient would think about their condition, and SOFA does not include an assessment of gastrointestinal failure. Therefore, perhaps the most simple, and most readily understood by all, is the numeric tally of failing organs. As organ failures increase, so too does mortality with 5 or more organ failures reflecting a mortality in excess of 90%.[76] Organ failure is often managed using invasive devices such acute dialysis or invasive mechanical ventilation; increased use of ECMO for rescue has defined the last 5 years in particular. In particular, the new need for hemodialysis that is anticipated to persist into the postdischarge period is highly associated with an accelerated 1-year mortality when it occurs in the aged, and in those with increased numbers of comorbidities.[77] These sobering observations should be shared with family members or surrogates when assessing patient trajectory to enable accurate shared decision-making.

While nutritional support is an important part of postoperative care, those with serious comorbidities represent a vulnerable group. In comparison to the healthy acutely injured patient, this group often demonstrates preexisting moderate to severe protein-calorie malnutrition.[78–80] Therefore, the common practice of waiting up to 7 days prior to pursuing nutritional support while awaiting return of bowel motility is inappropriate for this group. Instead, early enteral access and luminal nutritional support is preferred, and often requires an elemental diet for success. After 3 days of a lack of oral intake, the luminal brush border enzyme system that is required to complex nutrient processing has degraded.[81] Therefore, an elemental diet (single and double amino acids, simple sugars, and medium chain triglycerides) is ideal as the components may be directly absorbed and do not require luminal processing. After a 72-h period of rebuilding of the brush border enzyme system, non-elemental formulae may be utilized without risking formula-associated diarrhea due to processing failure and subsequent malabsorption. Importantly, luminal nutritional support also helps cells migrate form the villus crypt to the tip and elaborate the mucosal barrier that helps protect against bacteria and bacterial product translocation.[82] Furthermore, luminal nutrition helps support a normal microbiome instead of allowing a destructive pathobiome to flourish.[82,83] The latter is highly associated with anastomotic failure and should inform nutrition support decision-making.

Finally, the resumption of preadmission medications may be quite relevant, especially when there is a withdrawal syndrome associated with therapeutic agent cessation. Key medications in this grouping include beta-blockers, anticonvulsant agents, pulmonary vasodilators, antiarrhythmic agents, steroids, and organ transplant-related immune suppressant agents. Often intravenous equivalents are required due to intestinal discontinuity or ongoing resuscitation and high dose pressor infusions. For some, therapeutic agent concentration monitoring is essential and a PharmD is a key team member that enables safe care.[84] When patients are not native to the health care system in which they are receiving care, medication reconciliation is essential; a PharmD can often aid in this activity and commonly interfaces with family members, other clinicians, and pharmacies to ensure accuracy.

Communication is a foundational action in the postoperative care of the complex postoperative patient with serious comorbidities. One approach that also supports patient and family centered care is to include family members or the patient's surrogate on daily bedside rounds.[58,85] Doing so helps to ensure that every aspect of care is clearly shared with the patient (if they are awake and can process information appropriately), and their loved ones or decision-maker. When evaluated, this approach reduces the number of after-rounds family meetings, improves knowledge of the daily plan, and affords ample opportunity for questions to be raised.[85,86] Depending on Attending and family member comfort, goals of care may also be explored on rounds. This allows diverse team members, many of whom are excluded from the after-rounds meetings due to workhours restrictions or competing duties, to participate and share key perspectives with the patient's decision-maker. The recent SARS-CoV-2 pandemic excluded family members from the acute care facility in large part. Accordingly, much of the family communication occurred across digital platforms with great success.[87,88] Such platforms may also be key in linking families whose loved ones may have been transferred from an outlying facility, or if family members cannot reasonably regularly get to the hospital to participate in daily discussions. Relatedly, as patients awaken, being able to see and hear familiar faces and voices may strongly support both orientation and comfort. Nonetheless, and especially when end-of-life decisions are being discussed, there may be conflict between the family or surrogate and the care team, between different family members, or within the care team.[89]

Often, PCM clinicians are able to help successfully resolve conflict.[16] Despite their efficacy in that role, it would be better to utilize an approach that identifies the potential for conflict, and addresses those drivers ahead of conflict eruption. When that is unsuccessful, or incapable of occurring due to established conflict, de-escalation techniques that the entire clinical team can use may be invaluable. These techniques are collectively known as Conflict Management Training and help clinicians understand the root causes of conflict and offers several paths to successful conflict resolution.[90] Urgent or emergent surgical rescue in those with serious preexisting comorbidities is often freighted with outcome bias by families, especially when the rescue occurs at a complex care facility known for care excellence. This aspect is often magnified when the patient and their family arrive as a result of transfer from a less complex facility where successful transfer is often linked with life-saving intervention expectation. If the expectation and the ability to render successful care are not aligned, conflict may ensue. Conflict Management techniques are generally well suited to this kind of conflict. However, when this approach fails, a related one is needed – Conflict Mediation.[91] Conflict Mediation is a longer process that leverages a neutral mediator to help parties find a successful resolution; the mediator is not invested in a specific resolution, only in finding a resolution that is acceptable for all. Conflict mediators may be clinicians but may also flow from other specialties including law enforcement, the legal system, and administrators. It is imperative to not have a clinician on the care team serve in this role as the mediator must be perceived as neutral and unaligned with either party.

EVALUATION OF OUTCOMES/LONG-TERM RECOMMENDATIONS

Engagement with the acute health care system is common with the 6 months prior to death. Often, surgical care is rendered within the month prior to death. When evaluated among Medicare and Medicaid recipients, acute operation occurred in 20% of patients within the year prior to their demise.[92] These data underpin the importance of ensuring that offered surgical care can reasonably achieve an outcome that is aligned with the patient's goals, values, and preferences. Readmission following surgical rescue in those with serious comorbidities is common and is often related to a surgical complication or an infection, especially those related to the pulmonary system or an indwelling care device.[93] Given the complexity of their preoperative medical care, postdischarge destinations are more often to another care site such as a Long-Term Acute Care Hospital (LTACH), Rehabilitation facility, Skilled Nursing Facility (SNF) or Nursing Home (NH).[94,95] Transfer to a facility such as an NH is not an acceptable outcome and is unlikely to support a desired quality of life. Therefore, it is imperative to understand what constitutes an acceptable outcome ahead of providing surgical rescue to the greatest extent possible. Sometimes, the patient's trajectory is unable to be forecast with any degree of reliability until after operation and initial care has occurred.

Ongoing ICU care that persists for 2 weeks or more, that is characterized by repeated infections, and non-resolving organ dysfunction defines chronic critical illness.[96] Outcomes for such patients, examined quite thoroughly in surgical patients, are quite poor with high mortality and loss of independence in those who survive but who do not rapidly recover. It is in this setting – chronic ICU care – that trajectories such as NH placement may be better defined for patients and family members or surrogates. If such a destination is unacceptable, Comfort Care offers a path that honors the patient's values and preferences. Routine PCM consultation for such patients, a feature that often characterizes Geriatric Centers of Excellence is invaluable for the patient and the family.[97] PCM consultation is also ideal for those who survive their critical illness and have a destination other than a NH. Such patients often have a substantial change in life circumstance (new colostomy, stroke, etc.) and may have symptoms that will benefit from ongoing management (pain, nausea, anxiety, etc.) especially when the operation was palliative in nature that are not typically undertaken by the surgeon. PCM clinicians excel in this role and remain engaged well beyond the acute care hospitalization.[98,99]

Another key element of Geriatric Centers of Excellence that is increasingly adopted at other care facilities is the High-Risk Surgery Committee.[100] This committee is designed to be multi-professional and establish an inclusive approach to the advisability of offering surgical care to those with comorbidities that render the patient high risk for serios complication including mortality. Many, but not necessarily all, committee members can be rapidly assembled in an impromptu fashion to help assess and guide decision-making for those who need surgical rescue in the setting of serious comorbidities. This approach provides multiple perspectives and may be especially valuable when the surgeon does not believe that offering surgical care can meet the patients stated goals.

Facilities should ideally establish and maintain a database of patients and their outcomes to identify successes as well as opportunities for improvement. The American College of Surgeons has recently launched a program to this effect that includes an EGS-specific morbidity and mortality conference.[101] The patients who have been explored above will comprise a substantial proportion of such discussions and their outcome evaluation will benefit from team-based discourse, just as does their acute care.

SUMMARY

Caring for patients with significant comorbid diseases who present with urgent or emergent surgical conditions is complex and is supported by utilizing a phase-based structured approach to decision-making and intervention. While operation is appropriate for many, goal-concordant care may be better realized using non-operative management, including Comfort Care. Partners in this process may be the patient, their family members, a legally authorized representative, or consultants such as Palliative Care Medicine clinicians. Since many conditions are time-sensitive, rapid decision-making is necessary and resuscitation and operation may occur simultaneously. Certain preoperative interventions enhance outcome but are outnumbered by those that are useful intra-operatively as well as postoperatively. Utilizing a damage control approach to operation helps prioritize addressing life-threatening conditions and rapidly delivers the patient to the ICU for ongoing resuscitation. A team-based approach during ICU care is ideal. Goals of care are imperative to reassess in the ICU to help align care with the anticipated trajectory to assure that interventions are targeted to an acceptable outcome. Those discussions may be informed by the course of organ failure and the development of chronic critical illness to guide shared decision-making.

CLINICS CARE POINTS

- Surgical emergencies in patients with significant comorbidities is common
- Surgeons must rapidly decide if surgical therapy can meet the patient's goals, and if not, help patient pursue non-operative management that may include Comfort Care
- Be aware of family or surrogate-based optimism bias, especially for critically ill patients transferred from a less complex facility
- Preoperative interventions to improve physiology and outcome are few, especially for those with time-sensitive conditions
- Intra-operative interventions should leverage a damage control approach to limit OR time and prioritize ICU-based resuscitation
- Postoperative management reflects critical care interventions and should track progress, organ failure(s), while surveilling for the development of chronic critical illness
- Goals of care reevaluation is essential for those who do not demonstrate rapid recovery
- Palliative Care Medicine consultation is appropriate for this patient population who demonstrates comorbidities that influence outcome
- A facility-based database addressing outcomes of patients who require emergency surgery facilitate performance improvement
- Conflict regarding care, especially end-of-life care, is common and benefits from a team-based approach to detection, mitigation, and management

DISCLOSURE

No author has any relevant financial disclosures. Dr L.J. Kaplan is a past-president of the Society of Critical Care Medicine (2020–2021). Dr A.M. Shiroff is a past-president of the Chest Wall Injury Society (2019–2020). Drs L.J. Kaplan and A.M. Shiroff are employed in part by the Veterans Health Administration (VHA). The views, opinions, and thoughts expressed in this article are independent and are do not represent an official position of the VHA or the federal government.

REFERENCES

1. Hanna K, Ditillo M, Joseph B. The role of frailty and prehabilitation in surgery. Curr Opin Crit Care 2019;25(6):717–22.

2. Xue L, Boudreau RM, Donohue JM, et al. Persistent polypharmacy and fall injury risk: the Health, Aging and Body Composition Study. BMC Geriatr 2021; 21(1):710.
3. Fried TR, Tinetti ME, Iannone L. Primary care clinicians' experiences with treatment decision making for older persons with multiple conditions. Arch Intern Med 2011;171(1):75–80.
4. To KB, Kamdar NS, Patil P, et al. Acute Care Surgery Model and Outcomes in Emergency General Surgery. J Am Coll Surg 2019;228(1):21–8.e7.
5. Fakhry SM, Martin B, Al Harakeh H, et al. Proportional costs in trauma and acute care surgery patients: dominant role of intensive care unit costs. J Am Coll Surg 2013;216(4):607–14.
6. Thevathasan T, Copeland CC, Long DR, et al. The Impact of Postoperative Intensive Care Unit Admission on Postoperative Hospital Length of Stay and Costs: A Prespecified Propensity-Matched Cohort Study. Anesth Analg 2019; 129(3):753–61.
7. Hamidi M, Zeeshan M, Leon-Risemberg V, et al. Frailty as a prognostic factor for the critically ill older adult trauma patients. Am J Surg 2019;218(3):484–9.
8. Yelverton S, Rozario N, Matthews BD, et al. Interhospital transfer for emergency general surgery: an independent predictor of mortality. Am J Surg 2018;216(4): 787–92.
9. Iwashyna TJ, Christie JD, Moody J, et al. The structure of critical care transfer networks. Medical Care 2009;47(7):787.
10. Reinke CE, Thomason M, Paton L, et al. Emergency general surgery transfers in the United States: a 10-year analysis. J Surg Res 2017;219:128–35.
11. Pastores SM, Halpern NA, Oropello JM, et al. Critical care organizations in academic medical centers in North America: A descriptive report. Crit Care Med 2015;43(10):2239–44.
12. Eissa D, Carton EG, Buggy DJ. Anaesthetic management of patients with severe sepsis. Br J Anaesth 2010;105(6):734–43.
13. Chreiman KM, Kim PK, Garbovsky LA, et al. Blueprint for Implementing New Processes in Acute Care: Rescuing Adult Patients With Intraosseous Access. J Trauma Nur 2015;22(5):266–73.
14. Dorken Gallastegi A, Mikdad S, Kapoen C, et al. Intraoperative Deaths: Who, Why, and Can We Prevent Them? J Surg Res 2022;274:185–95.
15. Bleicher J, McGuire LE, Robbins RB, et al. Preoperative Advance Care Planning for Older Adults Undergoing Major Abdominal Surgery. Am J Hosp Palliat Care 2022;39(4):406–12.
16. Chiarchiaro J, White DB, Ernecoff NC, et al. Conflict Management Strategies in the ICU Differ Between Palliative Care Specialists and Intensivists. Crit Care Med 2016;44(5):934–42.
17. Schram AW, Hougham GW, Meltzer DO, et al. Palliative Care in Critical Care Settings: A Systematic Review of Communication-Based Competencies Essential for Patient and Family Satisfaction. Am J Hosp Palliat Care 2017;34(9):887–95.
18. Daniel VT, Rushing AP, Ingraham AM, et al. Association between operating room access and mortality for life-threatening general surgery emergencies. J Trauma Acute Care Surg 2019;87(1):35–42.
19. Rosen CB, Roberts SE, Wirtalla CJ, et al. Analyzing Impact of Multimorbidity on Long-Term Outcomes after Emergency General Surgery: A Retrospective Observational Cohort Study. J Am Coll Surg 2022;235(5):724–35.

20. Ho VP, Bensken WP, Warner DF, et al. Association of Complex Multimorbidity and Long-term Survival After Emergency General Surgery in Older Patients With Medicare. JAMA Surg 2022;157(6):499–506.
21. El Hechi MW, Maurer LR, Levine J, et al. Validation of the Artificial Intelligence-Based Predictive Optimal Trees in Emergency Surgery Risk (POTTER) Calculator in Emergency General Surgery and Emergency Laparotomy Patients. J Am Coll Surg 2021;232(6):912–9.e1.
22. Mitka M. Data-based risk calculators becoming more sophisticated–and more popular. JAMA 2009;302(7):730–1.
23. Long AM, Hildreth AN, Davis PT, et al. Evaluation of the Performance of ACS NSQIP Surgical Risk Calculator in Emergency General Surgery Patients. Am Sur 2020;86(2):83–9.
24. Bughrara N, Diaz-Gomez JL, Pustavoitau A. Perioperative Management of Patients with Sepsis and Septic Shock, Part II: Ultrasound Support for Resuscitation. Anesthesiol Clin 2020;38(1):123–34.
25. Rhodes A, Evans LE, Alhazzani W, et al. Surviving Sepsis Campaign: International Guidelines for Management of Sepsis and Septic Shock: 2016. Intensive Care Med 2017;43(3):304–77.
26. Font MD, Thyagarajan B, Khanna AK. Sepsis and Septic Shock - Basics of diagnosis, pathophysiology and clinical decision making. Med Clin North Am 2020; 104(4):573–85.
27. Evans L, Rhodes A, Alhazzani W, et al. Surviving sepsis campaign: international guidelines for management of sepsis and septic shock 2021. Intensive Care Med 2021;47(11):1181–247.
28. Cuker A, Burnett A, Triller D, et al. Reversal of direct oral anticoagulants: Guidance from the Anticoagulation Forum. Am J Hematol 2019;94(6):697–709.
29. Dhakal P, Rayamajhi S, Verma V, et al. Reversal of Anticoagulation and Management of Bleeding in Patients on Anticoagulants. Clin Appl Thromb Hemost 2017; 23(5):410–5.
30. Annane D, Pastores SM, Rochwerg B, et al. Guidelines for the diagnosis and management of critical illness-related corticosteroid insufficiency (CIRCI) in critically ill patients (Part I): Society of Critical Care Medicine (SCCM) and European Society of Intensive Care Medicine (ESICM) 2017. Intensive Care Med 2017; 43(12):1751–63.
31. Allen JM, Feild C, Shoulders BR, et al. Recent Updates in the Pharmacological Management of Sepsis and Septic Shock: A Systematic Review Focused on Fluid Resuscitation, Vasopressors, and Corticosteroids. Ann Pharmacother 2019;53(4):385–95.
32. MacKenzie CR, Goodman SM. Stress Dose Steroids: Myths and Perioperative Medicine. Curr Rheumatol Rep 2016;18(7):47.
33. Bartels K, Esper SA, Thiele RH. Blood Pressure Monitoring for the Anesthesiologist: A Practical Review. Anesth Analg 2016;122(6):1866–79.
34. Vasudeva M, Mathew JK, Groombridge C, et al. Hypocalcemia in trauma patients: A systematic review. J Trauma Acute Care Surg 2021;90(2):396–402.
35. Chanthima P, Yuwapattanawong K, Thamjamrassri T, et al. Association Between Ionized Calcium Concentrations During Hemostatic Transfusion and Calcium Treatment With Mortality in Major Trauma. Anesth Analg 2021;132(6):1684–91.
36. Byerly S, Inaba K, Biswas S, et al. Transfusion-Related Hypocalcemia After Trauma. World J Surg 2020;44(11):3743–50.
37. Kloner RA, King KS, Harrington MG. No-reflow phenomenon in the heart and brain. Am J Physiol Heart Circ Physiol 2018;315(3):H550–62.

38. Kloner RA. No-reflow phenomenon: maintaining vascular integrity. J Cardiovasc Pharmacol Ther 2011;16(3–4):244–50.

39. Astapenko D, Navratil P, Pouska J, et al. Clinical physiology aspects of chloremia in fluid therapy: a systematic review. Periop Med 2020;9(1):1–8.

40. Piper GL, Kaplan LJ. Fluid and electrolyte management for the surgical patient. Surgical Clinics 2012 Apr 1;92(2):189–205.

41. Tolstrup MB, Jensen TK, Gögenur I. Intraoperative surgical strategy in abdominal emergency surgery. World J Surg 2023;47(1):162–70.

42. Stawicki SP, Brooks A, Bilski T, et al. The concept of damage control: extending the paradigm to emergency general surgery. Injury 2008;39(1):93–101.

43. Coccolini F, Roberts D, Ansaloni L, et al. The open abdomen in trauma and non-trauma patients: WSES guidelines. World J Emerg Surg 2018;13:7.

44. Subramanian M, Kaplan LJ, Cannon JW. Thromboelastography-Guided Resuscitation of the Trauma Patient. JAMA Surg 2019;154(12):1152–3.

45. Da Luz LT, Nascimento B, Shankarakutty AK, et al. Effect of thromboelastography (TEG®) and rotational thromboelastometry (ROTEM®) on diagnosis of coagulopathy, transfusion guidance and mortality in trauma: descriptive systematic review. Crit Care 2014;18(5):518.

46. Lane-Fall MB, Beidas RS, Pascual JL, et al. Handoffs and transitions in critical care (HATRICC): protocol for a mixed methods study of operating room to intensive care unit handoffs. BMC Surg 2014;14:96.

47. Napolitano LM, Fulda GJ, Davis KA, et al. Challenging issues in surgical critical care, trauma, and acute care surgery: a report from the Critical Care Committee of the American Association for the Surgery of Trauma. J Trauma 2010;69(6):1619–33.

48. Wilcox ME, Chong CA, Niven DJ, et al. Do intensivist staffing patterns influence hospital mortality following ICU admission? A systematic review and meta-analyses. Crit Care Med 2013;41(10):2253–74.

49. Halpern NA, Tan KS, DeWitt M, et al. Intensivists in United States acute care hospitals. Crit Care Med 2019 Apr;47(4):517.

50. Combes A, Hajage D, Capellier G, et al. Extracorporeal Membrane Oxygenation for Severe Acute Respiratory Distress Syndrome. N Engl J Med 2018;378(21):1965–75.

51. Buesing KL, Mullapudi B, Flowers KA. Deep venous thrombosis and venous thromboembolism prophylaxis. Surg Clin North Am 2015;95(2):285–300.

52. Moore Z, Patton D, Avsar P, et al. Prevention of pressure ulcers among individuals cared for in the prone position: lessons for the COVID-19 emergency. J Wound Care 2020;29(6):312–20.

53. Boev C, Kiss E. Hospital-Acquired Infections: Current Trends and Prevention. Crit Care Nurs Clin North Am 2017;29(1):51–65.

54. Montpetit AJ, Sessler CN. Optimizing safe, comfortable ICU care through multi-professional quality improvement: just DO it. Crit Care 2013;17(2):1–2.

55. Wick EC, Grant MC, Wu CL. Postoperative Multimodal Analgesia Pain Management With Nonopioid Analgesics and Techniques: A Review. JAMA Surg 2017;152(7):691–7.

56. Keating J, Kane-Gill SL, Kaplan LJ. Interaction of Opioids with Sedative Practices in the ICU. In: Pascual JL, Gaulton TG, editors. Opioid use in critical care. Cham: Springer; 2021. p. 147–64.

57. Bauman ZM, Loftus J, Raposo-Hadley A, et al. Surgical stabilization of rib fractures combined with intercostal nerve cryoablation proves to be more cost

effective by reducing hospital length of stay and narcotics. Injury 2021;52(5): 1128–32.

58. Stollings JL, Devlin JW, Lin JC, et al. Best Practices for Conducting Interprofessional Team Rounds to Facilitate Performance of the ICU Liberation (ABCDEF) Bundle. Crit Care Med 2020;48(4):562–70.

59. Devlin JW, Skrobik Y, Gélinas C, et al. Clinical practice guidelines for the prevention and management of pain, agitation/sedation, delirium, immobility, and sleep disruption in adult patients in the ICU. Crit Care Med 2018;46:e825–73.

60. Pun BT, Balas MC, Barnes-Daly MA, et al. Caring for critically ill patients with the ABCDEF bundle: results of the ICU liberation collaborative in over 15,000 adults. Crit Care Med 2019;47(1):3.

61. Voiriot G, Oualha M, Pierre A, et al. Chronic critical illness and post-intensive care syndrome: from pathophysiology to clinical challenges. Ann Intensive Care 2022;12(1):58.

62. Lobato CT, Camões J, Carvalho D, et al. Risk factors associated with post-intensive care syndrome in family members (PICS-F): A prospective observational study. J Intensive Care Soc 2022. https://doi.org/10.1177/17511437221108904.

63. Haines KJ, Sevin CM, Hibbert E, et al. Key mechanisms by which post-ICU activities can improve in-ICU care: results of the international THRIVE collaboratives. Intensive Care Med 2019;45(7):939–47.

64. Misak C, Herridge M, Ely EW, et al. Patient and family engagement in critical illness. Crit Care Med 2021;49(9):1389–401.

65. Malbrain MLNG, Langer T, Annane D, et al. Intravenous fluid therapy in the perioperative and critical care setting: Executive summary of the International Fluid Academy (IFA). Ann Intensive Care 2020;10(1):64.

66. Raghunathan K, Shaw A, Nathanson B, et al. Association between the choice of IV crystalloid and in-hospital mortality among critically ill adults with sepsis. Crit Care Med 2014;42(7):1585–91.

67. Chowdhury AH, Cox EF, Francis ST, et al. A randomized, controlled, double-blind crossover study on the effects of 2-L infusions of 0.9% saline and plasma-lyte® 148 on renal blood flow velocity and renal cortical tissue perfusion in healthy volunteers. Ann Surg 2012;256(1):18–24.

68. Chua HR, Wong WK, Ong VH, et al. Extended Mortality and Chronic Kidney Disease After Septic Acute Kidney Injury. J Intensive Care Med 2020;35(6):527–35.

69. Kirkpatrick AW, Roberts DJ, De Waele J, et al. Intra-abdominal hypertension and the abdominal compartment syndrome: updated consensus definitions and clinical practice guidelines from the World Society of the Abdominal Compartment Syndrome. Intensive Care Med 2013;39(7):1190–206.

70. Schreiber J, Nierhaus A, Vettorazzi E, et al. Rescue bedside laparotomy in the intensive care unit in patients too unstable for transport to the operating room. Crit Care 2014;18(3):R123.

71. Piper GL, Maerz LL, Schuster KM, et al. When the ICU is the operating room. J Trauma Acute Care Surg 2013;74(3):871–5.

72. Knaus WA, Draper EA, Wagner DP, et al. APACHE II: a severity of disease classification system. Crit Care Med 1985;13(10):818–29.

73. Capuzzo M, Valpondi V, Sgarbi A, et al. Validation of severity scoring systems SAPS II and APACHE II in a single-center population. Intensive Care Med 2000;26(12):1779–85.

74. Vincent JL, Moreno R, Takala J, et al. The SOFA (Sepsis-related Organ Failure Assessment) score to describe organ dysfunction/failure. On behalf of the

Working Group on Sepsis-Related Problems of the European Society of Intensive Care Medicine. Intensive Care Med 1996;22(7):707–10.

75. Cárdenas-Turanzas M, Ensor J, Wakefield C, et al. Cross-validation of a Sequential Organ Failure Assessment score-based model to predict mortality in patients with cancer admitted to the intensive care unit. J Crit Care 2012;27(6): 673–80.

76. Barie PS, Hydo LJ, Fischer E. A prospective comparison of two multiple organ dysfunction/failure scoring systems for prediction of mortality in critical surgical illness. J Trauma 1994;37(4):660–6.

77. Shah S, Leonard AC, Harrison K, et al. Mortality and Recovery Associated with Kidney Failure due to Acute Kidney Injury. Clin J Am Soc Nephrol 2020;15(7): 995–1006.

78. Barazzoni R, Gortan Cappellari G. Double burden of malnutrition in persons with obesity. Rev Endocr Metab Disord 2020;21(3):307–13.

79. Sze S, Pellicori P, Zhang J, et al. The impact of malnutrition on short-term morbidity and mortality in ambulatory patients with heart failure. Am J Clin Nutr 2021;113(3):695–705.

80. Gupta A, Gupta E, Hilsden R, et al. Preoperative malnutrition in patients with colorectal cancer. Can J Surgery 2021;64(6):E621.

81. Kelly P. Starvation and Its Effects on the Gut. Adv Nutr 2021;12(3):897–903.

82. Oami T, Chihade DB, Coopersmith CM. The microbiome and nutrition in critical illness. Curr Opin Crit Care 2019;25(2):145–9.

83. Alverdy JC, Luo JN. The influence of host stress on the mechanism of infection: lost microbiomes, emergent pathobiomes, and the role of interkingdom signaling. Front Microbiol 2017;8:322.

84. Lee H, Ryu K, Sohn Y, et al. Impact on Patient Outcomes of Pharmacist Participation in Multidisciplinary Critical Care Teams: A Systematic Review and Meta-Analysis. Crit Care Med 2019;47(9):1243–50.

85. Allen SR, Pascual J, Martin N, et al. A novel method of optimizing patient-and family-centered care in the ICU. J Trauma Acute Care Surg 2017;82(3):582–6.

86. Donovan AL, Aldrich JM, Gross AK, et al. Interprofessional Care and Teamwork in the ICU. Crit Care Med 2018;46(6):980–90.

87. Kennedy NR, Steinberg A, Arnold RM, et al. Perspectives on Telephone and Video Communication in the Intensive Care Unit during COVID-19. Ann Am Thorac Soc 2022;18(5):838–47.

88. Hollander JE, Carr BG. Virtually Perfect? Telemedicine for Covid-19. N Engl J Med 2020;382(18):1679–81.

89. Rose L, Cook A, Onwumere J, et al. Psychological distress and morbidity of family members experiencing virtual visiting in intensive care during COVID-19: an observational cohort study. Intensive Care Med 2022;48(9):1156–64.

90. Bajwa NM, Bochatay N, Muller-Juge V, et al. Intra versus interprofessional conflicts: implications for conflict management training. J Interprofessional Care 2020;34(2):259–68.

91. Kayser JB, Kaplan LJ. Conflict Management in the ICU. Crit Care Med 2020; 48(9):1349–57.

92. Yefimova M, Aslakson RA, Yang L, et al. Palliative Care and End-of-Life Outcomes Following High-risk Surgery. JAMA Surg 2020;155(2):138–46.

93. Rossi IR, Ross SW, May AK, et al. Readmission After Emergency General Surgery: NSQIP Review of Risk, Cause and Ideal Follow-Up. J Surg Res 2021; 260:359–68.

94. Hyder JA, Wakeam E, Habermann EB, et al. Derivation and validation of a simple calculator to predict home discharge after surgery. J Am Coll Surg 2014; 218(2):226–36.

95. AlSowaiegh R, Naar L, Mokhtari A, et al. Does the Emergency Surgery Score predict failure to discharge the patient home? A nationwide analysis. J Trauma Acute Care Surg 2021;90(3):471–6.

96. Carmichael ED, Apple CG, Kannan KB, et al. Chronic Critical Illness in Patients With Sepsis is Associated With Persistent Anemia, Inflammation, and Impaired Functional Outcomes. Am Surg 2022. https://doi.org/10.1177/00031348221104252.

97. Reuben DB, Kaplan DB, van der Willik O, et al. Hartford Foundation Centers of Excellence Program: History, Impact, and Legacy. J Am Geriatr Soc 2017;65(7): 1396–400.

98. Aslakson RA, Curtis JR, Nelson JE. The changing role of palliative care in the ICU. Crit Care Med 2014;42(11):2418–28.

99. Henson LA, Maddocks M, Evans C, et al. Palliative care and the management of common distressing symptoms in advanced cancer: pain, breathlessness, nausea and vomiting, and fatigue. J Clin Oncol 2020;38(9):905.

100. McDonald SR, Heflin MT, Whitson HE, et al. Association of Integrated Care Coordination With Postsurgical Outcomes in High-Risk Older Adults: The Perioperative Optimization of Senior Health (POSH) Initiative. JAMA Surg 2018;153(5): 454–62.

101. American College of Surgeons Emergency General Surgery Verification Program. Available at: https://www.facs.org/quality-programs/accreditation-and-verification/emergency-general-surgery/; Accessed January 21. 2023.

Optimization of Care for the Elderly Surgical Emergency Patient

Rachel Lynne Warner, DO[a], Nadia Iwanyshyn, PharmD, BCPS[b],
Donald Johnson, PharmD, BCPS, BCCP[b], David J. Skarupa, MD, FCCM[a],*

KEYWORDS

- Emergency general surgery • Geriatric • Frailty • EGS outcomes

KEY POINTS

- Emergency general surgery (EGS) patients aged older than 65 years are at increased risk of morbidity and mortality.
- Multidisciplinary care including comprehensive geriatric assessment can improve outcomes in geriatric EGS patients.
- Cognitive impairment and delirium play a role in complications and discharge disposition in the elderly emergency surgical patient.
- Frailty is a driving factor of postoperative outcomes in the geriatric population.
- High-volume EGS centers and geriatric verification programs improve the quality of care for older adults with surgical emergencies.

BACKGROUND

In 2012 the American Association for the Surgery of Trauma defined emergency general surgery (EGS) as "any patient (inpatient or emergency department) requiring an emergency surgical evaluation (operative or nonoperative) for diseases within the realm of general surgery as defined by the American Board of Surgery."[1] The scope of practice is large and includes diagnosis and management of surgical emergencies in various body regions including thoracic, abdominal, vascular, and soft tissue pathologic conditions. EGS patients comprise more than 3 million hospital visits annually, a number that outstrips that of new diabetes and heart failure admissions, and this number is only expected to increase particularly as the population ages.[2] These patients with surgical emergencies have a higher burden of comorbidities and increased

[a] University of Florida College of Medicine -Jacksonville, 655 West 8th Street, Jacksonville, FL 32209, USA; [b] University of Florida College of Pharmacy -Jacksonville, 655 West 8th Street, Jacksonville, FL 32209, USA
* Corresponding author.
E-mail address: David.Skarupa@Jax.ufl.edu

Surg Clin N Am 103 (2023) 1253–1267
https://doi.org/10.1016/j.suc.2023.05.017
0039-6109/23/© 2023 Elsevier Inc. All rights reserved.

mortality when compared with the elective general surgery patients.[2–4] In fact, when compared with non-EGS patients, EGS is independently associated with an increased risk of death and major complications.[5] Given their higher burden of comorbidities and generally lower physiologic reserve, elderly patients are especially at risk for worse outcomes after EGS.

The population is rapidly aging, currently in the United States alone, persons aged older than 65 years make up approximately 17% of the population with 52 million people.[6] This number is expected to increase to 92 million and 23% of the population by the year 2060.[6] Adults are living longer and working longer leading to increased healthcare usage by this population. Nearly 35% of EGS patients are aged older than 70 years, and most of these patients have at least one comorbidity.[2]

The definition of "elderly" or "geriatric" varies depending on the source thus, multiple age cutoffs have been used to define and study this population in literature. From an anthropological viewpoint, "aging" is a social construct that is continually disputed and not necessarily based on chronologic age but rather a combination of social, cultural, and medical parameters.[7,8] However, as this concept is difficult to define, literature uses chronologic age to classify the elderly population. Conventionally a person aged 65 years is considered elderly; however, several organizations as well as various studies on the aging population have considered people aged as young as 45 years as "elderly" or "geriatric." Currently, the United Nations and Center for Disease Control define persons aged older than 60 years as elderly.[9,10] The World Health Organization has previously defined patients aged greater than 65 years as elderly, yet several reports adjust this age to 60 years and even as low as 50 years in developing nations.[11] Traditionally, 65 years is the age of retirement and the age of Medicare eligibility, which leads to an assumption that this is considered "elderly." Those aged 65 to 74 years are considered "early elderly" while patients aged greater than 75 year old are often considered "late elderly."[7] However, these classifications have become a moving target given the increased life expectancy of the aging population in which octogenarians will account for 400 million people by the year 2050.[12] There is great variation in overall health and health-care utilization among those defined as "geriatric." Although chronic disease has become more prevalent in younger populations, when comparing octogenarians to those aged 65 to 79 years, patients aged older than 80 years have higher prescription drug usage, are twice as likely to be hospitalized and are more likely to be discharged to long-term care facilities.[12] Thus, there is certainly a distinction between age cohorts even within the overall population considered "elderly." Recent studies published regarding geriatric patients in EGS use the age cutoff of 65 years or older, and this tends to be the most accepted definition. However, with more research, it is clear that age is in fact just a number rather it is physical fitness and frailty that is an important driver in outcomes and management of the geriatric patient.

Currently, 30% of EGS operations are performed on elderly patients and the number of older persons being admitted to the hospital with EGS diagnosis has been steadily increasing.[13,14] Given the increasing number of older EGS patients, it is pertinent to focus on the challenges that this population presents including polypharmacy, physiologic changes, multiple comorbidities, and baseline frailty, all of which lead to worse outcomes in these patients. Despite increased admission rates, overall EGS inpatient mortality and length of stay has decreased overtime, nevertheless, older EGS patients have a 2-fold to 5-fold increased odds of postoperative complications and mortality when compared with younger patients.[15] With increasing numbers of older individuals presenting with a need for EGS services, it is important to understand how to optimize these patients and provide care to reduce complications and mortality wherever possible.

DISCUSSION
Multidisciplinary Approach to Care

A multidisciplinary approach to the elderly patient with a surgical emergency is essential. Comanagement of the geriatric surgical patient results in trends toward improved function, survival, and length of stay.[16] Each member of the health-care team has a role in the optimization of these patients. Due to the acute nature of emergency surgical diagnosis, there is often little time for preoperative optimization without leading to a potentially harmful delay in surgical care. At the onset of diagnosis, communication from the surgeon to the patient and family is of utmost importance. Given the known increased perioperative complications of older individuals, a direct goal concordant care conversation should take place during the consultation and surgical consent process. Where possible minimally invasive or local techniques should be considered because they place less physiologic demand on an elderly patient. A frame work that uses discussing the acute problem in the setting of the patients chronic illness and age, formulating a prognosis, describing both surgical and palliative options, eliciting the patients goals and priorities, formulating a treatment plan, and assuring ongoing support for the patient and family has been suggested to assist in discussions with high-risk patients.[17] It is also helpful to frame possible outcomes in a best case/worst case scenario for both patient and families to better grasp the possible outcomes. In particular, the surgeon should also discuss with the patient and family perioperative do not resuscitate orders and wishes where possible.

The anesthesia provider plays an important role and faces unique challenges when caring for the geriatric EGS patient. With little time for preparation to undergo general anesthesia, acute optimization must be done without delaying urgent surgical care. Intraoperatively, the avoidance of hypotension can reduce risk of myocardial infarction, stroke, and acute kidney injury.[16] Thus, the goal should be to maintain mean arterial pressure greater than 65 mmHg or within 10% of baseline where possible.[16] In addition, goal-directed fluid therapy intraoperatively has been shown to reduce morbidity and length of stay.[16] In terms of type of anesthetic, there is mixed evidence on the effect of types of anesthetic and their effects on cognitive recovery for elderly individuals. Although some studies suggest propofol or IV-based anesthetic leads to lower postoperative delirium when compared with volatile inhaled gases, others found no differences in delirium rates or mortality.[16,18,19] Immediately postoperatively it is important to consider appropriate disposition and level of care considering frailty, preexisting comorbids, and acute physiology.

The geriatric medicine specialist has proven to be an integral part of the team to improve outcomes when caring for the older EGS patient. Geriatrician consultants provide assessments and patient-centered interventions. Most commonly they manage polypharmacy, provide targeted efforts for delirium prevention and treatment, risk stratification, assist in appropriate discharge disposition, and assist in end-of-life conversations.[20–23] Involvement of a trained geriatrician has even been shown to reduce hospital length of stay for elderly EGS patients. Finally, it is important to address the importance of the palliative care team in the perioperative care of the geriatric EGS patient. The appropriate time for in-depth palliative and goals of care conversations is unclear. Although preoperative determination of overall goals and perioperative code status is important in shared decision-making, a prolonged palliative discussion likely cannot take place due to the acute nature of surgical emergencies. The timing for these discussions is left up to the care team, patient, and family. Nearly 70% of older inpatient EGS patients have palliative care needs; however, only 5% of these patients receive specialized palliative medicine consultations.[23] Palliative care consultation for EGS patients results in reduced inpatient mortality and increased referral to Hospice care.[24] In particular, in older patients, undergoing emergency abdominal surgery admission from a skilled nursing facility is an independent predictor of death and one-third of these patients will die within 30 days, thus these patients should receive early palliative care consultations.[25,26] The involvement of trained palliative care physicians is underutilized in EGS patients.[23] Given the high burden of mortality and complications especially among the elderly EGS patient, early involvement of both a geriatrician and palliative medicine physician is suggested to optimize the care of elderly EGS patients.

Physiologic Changes in the Elderly Adult

Aging is associated with progressive changes in organ systems, mobility, and cognitive function. These changes can lead to increased perioperative mortality and in hospital complications. With decreased physiologic reserve, older individuals are less equipped to deal with the stress of acute illness and the demands of surgical intervention. Multiple organ systems are affected by aging. From a cardiovascular standpoint, as patients age, blood vessels increase in intimal thickness, cardiac ventricles and atria enlarge and become stiffer, and this leads to decreased regulation of vascular tone. In addition, cardiac reserve and ability to regulate heart rate and contractility is decreased.[25] Nearly 80% of patients aged older than 80 years have identifiable cardiac disease.[25] Pulmonary compliance is decreased in older individuals. With decreased chest wall compliance and elastic recoil of the lungs coupled with decrease strength of the respiratory muscles, the ability for an elderly patient to regulate and respond to hypoxia and/or hypercarbia is reduced.[25] Renal reserve and function also diminishes over time. Creatinine clearance and glomerular filtration rate decrease over time, which leads to compromised sodium homeostasis, renal drug tolerance, and autoregulation.[25] The physiologic changes of organ systems in older adults lead to special considerations in care perioperatively, in particular in safe medication use and management.

Considerations: Safe Medication Use in the Elderly

Medication management in older adults can be a complex process. There are several factors that contribute to increased complications, including adverse drug events, in older adults including polypharmacy due to higher prevalence of multiple comorbidities, increased medication sensitivity, increased frailty, and altered pharmacokinetics (altered metabolism and clearance of medications).[27] Prescribers should regularly review medication list to determine whether dose adjustments are necessary or if a medication can be discontinued to decrease the risk of complications and reduce the risk of drug interactions.

Another reason for older adults being at an increased risk for adverse effects to medications is the physiochemical properties of the medication itself and alterations in pharmacokinetic and pharmacodynamic seen with the aging population. The most common identified pharmacokinetic change with aging is a decrease in the excretory capacity of the kidneys versus the decline of hepatic drug metabolism. Evidence shows that pharmacodynamic alterations are commonly associated with being more sensitive to drugs.[28–30] This is most apparent with medications associated with the cardiovascular and central nervous system. There are described side effects of orthostatic hypotension and increased central nervous system depression with opioids, benzodiazepines, and psychotropic medications. It is important for the providers to consider that most medications that are being prescribed to our elderly patients will have impaired renal clearance and increase sensitivity to the effects of medications.

Therefore, the importance to follow the best practice in our elderly patients to "start low and go slow" especially if drug therapy is considered beneficial or absolutely necessary for them (**Boxes 1–3**).[28]

There are several tools available to help identify potentially inappropriate medications for use in older adults, including the Beer's criteria and the STOPP/START criteria.[31–33] These tools have been validated and are supported by evidence; however, prescribers need to use clinical judgment when caring for this population because strict adherence to these guidelines may not always be possible. The table below shows commonly used medications in Emergency General Surgery in Older Adults (**Tables 1–4**).

Considerations: Delirium

Baseline cognitive impairment is common in geriatric patients. As the brain ages, it undergoes physiologic changes that include decreased synapses, dendritic branching and changes in oxidative metabolism.[25] This leads to increased baseline impairment and higher risk for acute delirium in this population. One out of 5 EGS patients aged older than 65 years has cognitive impairment.[34] These patients have a higher rate of postoperative complications, in particular, respiratory and infectious complications.[34] In addition, elderly EGS patients with baseline cognitive impairment have higher readmission rates, less favorable discharge dispositions and higher mortality when compared with their cognitive intact counterparts.[34] Recognizing baseline cognitive impairment and its sequela can allow for preoperative and postoperative targeted strategies to mitigate worsening of baseline cognitive issues and development of acute delirium.

Delirium is classified as transient cognitive impairment with features of fluctuating levels of consciousness, disturbed sleep–wake cycles, and altered psychomotor function.[35] Postoperative delirium often develops 24 to 28 hours after surgery and can worsen based on time of day and is more common in elderly individuals.[35] Postoperative delirium is present in 26% of geriatric patients who undergo EGS. Many factors predispose to the development of delirium including baseline cognitive impairment, polypharmacy, multimorbid state, and overall frailty. The mainstay of treatment of delirium is aimed at preventative measures.[36] Prevention strategies that include multiple components are often the most effective. Pain at rest is a risk factor for acute delirium, given this it is important to appropriately treat postoperative pain without oversedating and keeping in mind that polypharmacy also contributes to confusion.[36–38] Multimodal pain control while minimizing narcotics is often the best route. Other important prevention strategies include daily orientation, enhanced sleep–wake cycles, sensory protocols, which include hearing/visual aids as the patient needs and minimizing lines/tubes where possible.[37,38] Acute delirium diagnosis leads to a more complicated postoperative period for the geriatric EGS patient. It is

---

Box 1
Because drug distribution, metabolism, and elimination vary widely among older patients, the following should be done

- Drug doses should be carefully titrated
- Creatinine clearance for renally excreted drugs should be calculated when doses are adjusted
- Serum drug levels should be measured
- Patient responses should be observed

Box 2
General principles in medication management in elderly

- Avoid inappropriate medications
- Ensure appropriate use of indicated medications
- Appropriately determine therapeutic endpoints—that is, blood pressure and Hgb A1c goals
- Monitor for side effects and drug levels
- Avoid drug–drug interactions
- Involve the patient, recognizing patient values
- Assess the timing of medications administered

---

associated with longer hospital stays, increased costs and discharge to a nursing facility. Directed prevention and management should take place for all geriatric EGS patients.[34–36] Comprehensive geriatric assessment by a trained geriatrician not only aids in the diagnosis and management of delirium but is associated with decreased incidence.[21,38]

Considerations: Frailty

Frailty is defined as "recognizable state of increased vulnerability resulting from aging-associated decline in reserve and function across multiple physiologic systems such that the ability to cope with everyday stress or acute stressors is compromised."[39] Much like the anthropological definition of elderly, frailty considers physiologic, cognitive, and social aspects of age rather than chronicity alone. Recent literature has demonstrated the importance of the frailty syndrome when it comes to predicting outcomes in the geriatric surgery population. In fact, the frailty index (FI) independently predicts postoperative complications and hospital stay in the older EGS patient.[40] Frail patients have higher rates of infectious complications, are more likely to be admitted to the ICU postoperatively, have longer hospital stays and are more likely to be discharged to a rehab or nursing facility.[40,41] When it comes to mortality, frailty is associated with 30-day mortality in geriatric patients undergoing both high-risk and low-risk procedures.[41–43] Failure to rescue (FTR) or morbidity after in-patient complications depends not only on system factors but also on patient level factors. Frailty status is associated with increased odds of FTR in geriatric EGS patients.[44–46] Identifying frail patients who are at high risk for FTR can allow for early mobilization of resources and directed efforts to reduce this risk.

Box 3
According to the American College of Surgeons NSQIP/AGS best practices guideline—optimal perioperative management of the geriatric surgical patient

- Obtain a complete medication list when able (including Over the Counter [OTC], supplements, vitamins, herbal)
- Discontinue nonessential medications—considering potential for withdrawal, progression of disease, progression without medication, and potential for interactions with anesthetic agents
- Resumption of all baseline outpatient medications in postoperative period with consideration for minimizing polypharmacy risk

---

Table 1
Pain medications

- Multimodal in nature and should be appropriately titrated for the increased sensitivity and altered physiology of older adult
- Include prophylactic pharmacologic bowel regimen and stimulant laxative when appropriate
- Avoid mineral oil[5]
- Avoid the concurrent use of opioids with either benzodiazepines, barbiturates, or gabapentinoids, due to the increased risk of overdose and severe sedation-related adverse events such as respiratory depression and death[5]
- Avoid potentially inappropriate medications determined by Beers Criteria
- Use opioid sparing techniques
- Use regional techniques if able to improve pain control, avoid opioids, and improve satisfaction/outcomes

Medication	Recommendation	Rationale
Skeletal muscle relaxants: Carisoprodol Cyclobenzaprine Methocarbamol	Avoid	Poorly tolerated due to anticholinergic adverse effects, sedation, increased risk of fractures
Nonselective cox inhibitor nonsteroidal anti-inflammatory drugs (NSAIDs): Aspirin > 325 mg/d Diclofenac Etodolac Ibuprofen Meloxicam Naproxen	Avoid chronic use, unless other alternatives are not effective and patient can take gastroprotective agent	Increased risk of gastrointestinal bleeding or peptic ulcer disease in high-risk groups, including those >75 y or taking oral or parenteral corticosteroids, anticoagulants, or antiplatelet agents
Indomethacin Ketorolac (including parenteral)	Avoid	• Increased risk of gastrointestinal bleeding/peptic ulcer disease and acute kidney injury in older adults • Indomethacin is more likely than other NSAIDs to have adverse CNS effects
Gabapentin Pregabalin[7]	Use with caution	• Consider its use for peripheral neuropathy and postherpetic neuralgia • Initiate at low dose and frequencies • Less or no benefit in the preoperative and postoperative settings • Monitor for mental status change, drowsiness, dry mouth, and renal function

Table 2
Sedation medications

- Older adults are more sensitive to the drug properties of benzodiazepines and barbiturates
- Drug clearance may be altered with declining renal function
- Risk of physical dependence
- Withdrawal may occur with abrupt cessation
- Extreme caution should be considered with combinations of sedatives, opiates, and other central nervous system medications
- If necessary, start at the lowest dose possible and titrate to effect
- Monitor for cognitive impairment, delirium and falls
- In the intensive care unit—Use a nonsedative approach or titrate to low level of sedation—RASS −1 to 0.[12]

Barbiturates: Butalbital Pentobarbital Phenobarbital	Avoid	• High rate of physical dependence, tolerance to sleep benefits, greater risk of overdose at low dosages • May be appropriate for ethanol withdrawal
Benzos: Alprazolam Lorazepam Temazepam Chlordiazepoxide Clonazepam Diazepam	Avoid	• Increased risk of cognitive impairment, delirium, falls, fractures, and motor vehicle crashes in older adults • May be appropriate for seizure disorders, rapid eye movement sleep behavior disorder, benzodiazepine withdrawal, ethanol withdrawal, severe generalized anxiety disorder, and periprocedural anesthesia
Nonbenzodiazepine, benzodiazepine receptor agonist hypnotics: Eszopiclone Zaleplon Zolpidem	Avoid	• Increased risk of delirium, falls, fractures • Increased emergency room visits/ hospitalizations; motor vehicle crashes; minimal improvement in sleep latency and duration

Preoperative frailty evaluation can predict postoperative complications and is associated with FTR. Given this, it is important to screen geriatric EGS patients for frailty. Multiple scoring systems have been used in an attempt to properly identify the "frail" patient. Many of these scoring models including the Edmonton and Robinson frailty scales have been used and validated in the elective surgical patient and have been shown to predict complications in these patients.[47–49] These frailty scales can be done at the bedside preoperatively and often incorporate multiple domains including cognition, social support, functional status, medication use, and other variables evaluable by practitioners.[47–49] Not all of these indices have been validated specifically in the EGS population in which patients undergo operations in a more acute manner when compared with elective surgical patients. The Rockwood FI, which uses social, physiologic, and cognitive factors to determine frailty and has been shown to be an independent predictor of major postoperative complications in older EGS patients even more so than age or American Society of Anesthesiologists (ASA) classification.[40] Given that EGS in itself carries higher morbidity and mortality in the general population when compared with elective surgery, further defining and recognizing frailty in geriatric EGS patients is of the utmost importance. The EGS specific frailty index (EGSFI) was developed and verified to predict postoperative outcomes for elderly patients undergoing EGS.[40] EGSFI is composed a 15-variable questionnaire that covers patient factors of activities of daily living, comorbidities, nutritional status, and health attitude. Geriatric

Table 3 Gastrointestinal (GI) medications		
Metoclopramide	Avoid	• If using for gastroparesis, do not exceed 12 wk • Monitor renal function • Associated with extrapyramidal effects
Proton pump inhibitors (PPI)	Avoid	• Caution use >8 wk unless for high-risk patients (eg, oral corticosteroids or chronic NSAID use), erosive esophagitis, Barrett esophagitis, or demonstrated need for maintenance treatment • Avoid due to risk of *Clostridium difficile* infection and bone loss and fractures
H2-receptor antagonists	Avoid	May cause delirium but may be used in patients with dementia
5-HT3 receptor antagonists (ondansetron)	Use with caution	Monitor for serotonin syndrome and QT prolongation
Corticosteroids (for postoperative nausea/vomiting prophylaxis)	Avoid	May worsen or induce delirium
Scopolamine	Avoid	• Highly anticholinergic • Increased risk for delirium/ cognitive impairment • Can worsen constipation
Promethazine Prochlorperazine	Avoid	• Anticholinergic • Increased risk for delirium/ cognitive impairment • Can worsen constipation
Mineral oil (given orally)	Avoid	Potential for aspiration and adverse effects

EGS patients who are deemed frail by the EGSFI have higher complication rates, mortality rates, and longer hospital stays compared with those who are nonfrail.[40] The EGSFI simplifies frailty scoring is efficient and reliable in the EGS population.

Once a patient is identified as frail, it is clear they are at higher risk for complications as well as FTR. Implementing a targeted frailty pathway with multidisciplinary input including a comprehensive geriatric medicine assessment and palliative care consults where needed and order sets aimed at appropriate medication use, nursing care, and delirium prevention decreases length of stay and readmission rates for frail EGS patients.[50]

Considerations: Risk Assessment and Consent

With higher morbidity and mortality among the elderly EGS patient, risk assessment preoperatively is imperative. Geriatric EGS patients are at high risk for morbidity and mortality after both traditionally high-risk and low-risk procedures.[42] Multiple risk assessment tools exist, and it is unclear which tool is the best for risk stratification. Since its development, the American College of Surgeons (ACS) National Surgical Quality Improvement Program (NSQIP) risk calculator has been used as a tool to aid in informed consent before surgical procedures and has been shown to be reliable; however, this tool was created based on elective procedures, and although there is an option to "risk adjust," it may not accurately reflect risk for EGS patients.[51,52] Several

Table 4
Central nervous system/antipsychotic agents

First-generation antihistamines: Diphenhydramine Hydroxyzine Meclizine Promethazine	Avoid	• Highly anticholinergic • Risk of confusion, dry mouth, and constipation • Acute treatment for severe allergic reaction may be appropriate
Antipsychotics: First and second generation	Avoid	• Increased risk of stroke and greater rate of cognitive decline and mortality in persons with dementia except in schizophrenia or bipolar disorder • May need to be used for short-term use as antiemetic during chemotherapy

EGS-specific risk assessment tools have been developed. The POTTER tool is an artificial intelligence-based calculator specific to EGS that has been shown to reliably predict 30-day outcomes including septic shock, respiratory failure, and acute kidney injury.[53] The Emergency Surgery Score, which can be calculated from a set of preoperative variables can accurately predict mortality in EGS patients aged older than 65 years and performs moderately well in predicting morbidity in this population.[54–56] These risk assessment tools can be used to aid in shared decision-making with patients and families during the consent process. Surgeons tend to engage in shared decision-making more often when the proposed treatment plan is high risk for poor outcomes, such as that involving the geriatric emergency surgical patient. Often these conversations focus on risk assessment and setting expectations with the patient and families rather than true shared decision-making.[57,58] It is important during the consent process to invite the patient and family to be an active part of the treatment decision at hand. Using a framework of best case/worse case scenarios has been shown to involve patient and families in deliberation and promote true shared decision-making in an acute setting, particularly in elderly patients.[59]

Quality in Emergency General Surgery

EGS patients are complex with more comorbid conditions and carry high risk of morbidity and mortality. In an effort to improve quality for geriatric surgical patients, the ACS has created a geriatric surgery verification program that consists of 32 standards to improve the quality of care for the geriatric surgical patient. In addition to geriatric-specific verification, the ACS has also developed a pathway for EGS verification of centers of excellence. Patients treated at high-volume centers with high-volume surgeons have lower mortality rates.[60–64] Regionalization of EGS to these high-volume centers can prevent mortality.[62,63] Not every hospital has the capacity or staffing to care for complex emergency surgery patients adequately. Appropriate volume is needed to create clinical experts, proven processes, and reliable service lines. Surgeons who perform a low volume of geriatric EGS procedures have higher odds of death and FTR among elderly emergency surgery patients.[62] Patients who are treated where dedicated and established EGS service lines exist have better outcomes. The elderly EGS patient is at higher risk for complications and as such one can make a case should be treated at a high-volume center when possible.

SUMMARY

EGS patients aged older than 65 years are complex and carry high risk of morbidity and mortality. Age alone is not enough to stratify these patients into risk categories and accurately predict outcomes. The concept of frailty is a driving force behind how these patients will tolerate emergency surgery. Multiple providers from varied specialties play important roles in the optimization of the geriatric EGS patient. Preoperative risk assessment and targeted multidisciplinary interventions can improve outcomes in these patients. When possible, treatment of these patients at a high-volume EGS center, with defined geriatric pathways can lead to optimal patinet outcomes.

CLINICS CARE POINTS—FRAILTY

- Preoperative frailty evaluation can predict postoperative complications.
- Multiple frailty scales exist, EGSFI is specific for EGS.
- Frail patients have high rates of infectious complications, longer hospital stays, and less favorable discharge disposition.
- Frailty is associated with FTR.

CLINICS CARE POINTS—DELIRIUM

- Baseline cognitive impairment predisposes to development of delirium.
- Postoperative delirium leads to longer hospital stays and more complicated postop course.
- Treatment of delirium includes preventative strategies and judicious medication use.

CLINICS CARE POINTS—CONSENT

- Risk assessment tools can be used to aid in the consent process.
- Brest case/worst case scenario framework aids in shared decision-making.
- Do not resuscitate orders should be discussed with the patient preoperatively and early in the physician-patient encounter.

DISCLOSURE

The authors have no financial or commercial disclosures or conflicts of interests.

REFERENCES

1. Shafi S, Aboutanos MB, Agarwarl S Jr, et al. Emergency general surgery: definition and estimated burden of disease. J Trauma Acute Care Sur 2013;74(4):1092–7. https://doi.org/10.1097/TA.0b013e31827e1bc7.
2. Gale Stephen C, Shafi Shahid, et al. The public health burden of emergency general surgery in the United States: A 10-year analysis of the Nationwide Inpatient Sample—2001 to 2010. J Trauma Acute Care Surg 2014;77(2):202–8. https://doi.org/10.1097/TA.0000000000000362.
3. Miller PR. Defining burden and severity of disease for emergency general surgery. Trauma Surgery & Acute Care Open 2017;2:e000089. https://doi.org/10.1136/tsaco-2017-000089.

4. Scott JW, Olufajo OA, Brat GA, et al. Use of National Burden to Define Operative Emergency General Surgery. JAMA Surg 2016;151(6):e160480. https://doi.org/10.1001/jamasurg.2016.0480.

5. Havens, Joaquim MMD, Peetz Allan BMD, et al. The excess morbidity and mortality of emergency general surgery. J Trauma Acute Care Surg 2015;78(2):306–11. https://doi.org/10.1097/TA.0000000000000517.

6. US census bureau population predictions, Available at: https://www.census.gov/topics/population/older-aging.html. Accessed February 24, 2020.

7. Orimo H, Ito H, Suzuki T, et al. Reviewing the definition of "elderly". Geriatr Gerontol Int 2006;6(3):149–58.

8. Crews Douglas E, Zavotka Susan. Aging, disability, and frailty: implications for universal design. Journal of physiological anthropology 2006;113–8.

9. United Nations, older persons emergency handbook. Available at: https://emergency.unhcr.org/entry/43935/older-persons. Accessed February 24, 2023.

10. Center for Disease Control. Available at: https://www.cdc.gov/cpr/documents/aging.pdf. Accessed February 24, 2023.

11. World Health Organization. Available at: https://www.ncbi.nlm.nih.gov/pmc/articles/PMC4573966/#:~:text=Although%20the%20World%20Health%20Organisation,older%20(United%20Nations%202012). Accessed February 24, 20223.

12. Singh S, Bajorek B. Defining 'elderly' in clinical practice guidelines for pharmacotherapy. Pharm Pract 2014;12(4):489.

13. Agency for Healthcare utilization, statistical brief #103. Available at: https://www.hcup-us.ahrq.gov/reports/statbriefs/sb103.pdf. Accessed February 24, 2023.

14. Wohlgemut JM, Ramsay G, Jansen JO. The changing face of emergency general surgery: a 20-year analysis of secular trends in demographics, diagnoses, operations, and outcomes. Ann Surg 2020;271(3):581–9.

15. Aucoin S, McIsaac DI. Emergency general surgery in older adults: a review. Anesthesiol Clin 2019;37(3):493–505.

16. Grigoryan KV, Javedan H, Rudolph JL. Ortho-geriatric care models and outcomes in hip fracture patients: a systematic review and meta-analysis. J Orthop Trauma 2014;28(3):e49.

17. Cooper Z, Koritsanszky LA, Cauley CE, et al. Recommendations for best communication practices to facilitate goal-concordant care for seriously ill older patients with emergency surgical conditions. Annals of surgery 2016;263(1):1–6.

18. Chang JE, Min SW, Kim H, et al. Association between anesthetics and postoperative delirium in elderly patients undergoing spine surgery: propofol versus sevoflurane. Global Spine J 2022. 21925682221110828.

19. Saller T, Hubig L, Seibold H, et al. Association between post-operative delirium and use of volatile anesthetics in the elderly: A real-world big data approach. J Clin Anesth 2022;83:110957.

20. Shipway D, Koizia L, Winterkorn N, et al. Embedded geriatric surgical liaison is associated with reduced inpatient length of stay in older patients admitted for gastrointestinal surgery. Future healthcare journal 2018;5(2):108.

21. Hu FY, O'Mara L, Tulebaev S, et al. Geriatric surgical service interventions in older emergency general surgery patients: Preliminary results. J Am Geriatr Soc 2022;70(8):2404–14.

22. Hu FY, O'Mara L, Kelly M, et al. Geriatric Surgical Service Complements Care of Older Adult Emergency General Surgery Patients. J Am Coll Surg 2021;233(5):e75.

23. Lilley EJ, Cooper Z. The high burden of palliative care needs among older emergency general surgery patients. J Palliat Med 2016;19(4):352–3.

24. Baimas-George M, Yelverton S, Ross SW, et al. Palliative care in emergency general surgery patients: Reduced inpatient mortality and increased discharge to hospice. Am Surg 2021;87(7):1087–92.

25. Chernock B, Hwang F, Berlin A, et al. Emergency abdominal surgery in patients presenting from skilled nursing facilities: Opportunities for palliative care. Am J Surg 2020;219(6):1076–82.

26. Colloca G, Santoro M, Gambassi G. Age-related physiologic changes and perioperative management of elderly patients. Surgical oncology 2010;19(3):124–30.

27. McKeown JL. Pain Management Issues for the Geriatric Surgical Patient. Anesthesiol Clin 2015;33(3):563–76. Epub 2015 Jul 3. PMID: 26315638.

28. ElDesoky ES. Pharmacokinetic-pharmacodynamic crisis in the elderly. Am J Ther 2007;14(5):488–98.

29. Spinewine A, Schmader KE, Barber N, et al. Appropriate prescribing in elderly people: how well can it be measured and optimised? Lancet 2007;370(9582): 173–84.

30. Mohanty S, Rosenthal RA, Russell MM, et al. Optimal Perioperative Management of the Geriatric Patient: A Best Practices Guideline from the American College of Surgeons NSQIP and the American Geriatrics Society. J Am Coll Surg 2016; 222(5):930–47.

31. By the 2019 American Geriatrics Society Beers Criteria® Update Expert Panel. American Geriatrics Society 2019 Updated AGS Beers Criteria® for Potentially Inappropriate Medication Use in Older Adults. J Am Geriatr Soc 2019;67(4): 674–94.

32. O'Mahony D, O'Sullivan D, Byrne S, et al. STOPP/START criteria for potentially inappropriate prescribing in older people: version 2. Age Ageing 2015;44(2): 213–8 [Erratum in: Age Ageing. 2018 May 1;47(3):489. PMID: 25324330; PMCID: PMC4339726. Park CM, Inouye SK, Marcantonio ER, et al. Perioperative Gabapentin Use and In-Hospital Adverse Clinical Events Among Older Adults After Major Surgery. JAMA Intern Med.2022;182(11):1117–1127].

33. Park SY, Lee HB. Prevention and management of delirium in critically ill adult patients in the intensive care unit: a review based on the 2018 PADIS guidelines. Acute Crit Care 2019;34(2):117–25.

34. Hanna K, Khan M, Ditillo M, et al. Prospective evaluation of preoperative cognitive impairment and postoperative morbidity in geriatric patients undergoing emergency general surgery. Am J Surg 2020;220(4):1064–70.

35. Parikh SS, Chung F. Postoperative delirium in the elderly. Anesth Analg 1995; 80(6):1223–32.

36. Sieber FE. Postoperative delirium in the elderly surgical patient. Anesthesiol Clin 2009;27(3):451–64.

37. Thillainadesan J, Yumol MF, Hilmer S, et al. Interventions to improve clinical outcomes in older adults admitted to a surgical service: a systematic review and meta-analysis. J Am Med Dir Assoc 2020;21(12):1833–43.

38. Swarbrick CJ, Partridge JS. Evidence-based strategies to reduce the incidence of postoperative delirium: a narrative review. Anaesthesia 2022;77:92–101.

39. Xue QL. The frailty syndrome: definition and natural history. Clin Geriatr Med 2011;27(1):1–5.

40. Joseph B, Zangbar B, Pandit V, et al. Emergency general surgery in the elderly: too old or too frail? J Am Coll Surg 2016;222(5):805–13.

41. Ward Mellissa AR MD, Alenazi Abdullah MBBS, Delisle Megan MD, et al. The impact of frailty on acute care general surgery patients: A systematic review. J Trauma Acute Care Surg 2019;86(1):148–54. https://doi.org/10.1097/TA.0000000000002084.

42. Castillo-Angeles M, Cooper Z, Jarman MP, et al. Association of Frailty With Morbidity and Mortality in Emergency General Surgery by Procedural Risk Level. JAMA Surg 2021;156(1):68–74. https://doi.org/10.1001/jamasurg.2020.5397.

43. Khan Muhammad MD, Azo Asad MD, Sakran Joseph VMD, et al. Impact of Frailty on Failure-to-Rescue in Geriatric Emergency General Surgery Patients: A Prospective Study. J Am Coll Surg 2017;225(4):S96–7. https://doi.org/10.1016/j.jamcollsurg.2017.07.210.

44. Khan M, Jehan F, Zeeshan M, et al. Failure to rescue after emergency general surgery in geriatric patients: does frailty matter? J Surg Res 2019;233:397–402.

45. Khan M, Azo A, Sakran JV, et al. Impact of frailty on failure-to-rescue in geriatric emergency general surgery patients: a prospective study. J Am Coll Surg 2017; 225(4):S96–7.

46. Ko FC. Preoperative frailty evaluation: a promising risk-stratification tool in older adults undergoing general surgery. Clin Therapeut 2019;41(3):387–99.

47. Robinson TN, Wu DS, Pointer L, et al. Simple frailty score predicts postoperative complications across surgical specialties. Am J Surg 2013;206(4):544–50.

48. Nishijima TF, Esaki T, Morita M, et al. Preoperative frailty assessment with the Robinson Frailty Score, Edmonton Frail Scale, and G8 and adverse postoperative outcomes in older surgical patients with cancer. Eur J Surg Oncol 2021;47(4): 896–901.

49. Chung KJ, Wilkinson C, Veerasamy M, et al. Frailty scores and their utility in older patients with cardiovascular disease. Intervent Cardiol 2021.

50. Engelhardt KE, Reuter Q, Liu J, et al. Frailty screening and a frailty pathway decrease length of stay, loss of independence, and 30-day readmission rates in frail geriatric trauma and emergency general surgery patients. J Trauma Acute Care Surg 2018;85(1):167–73.

51. Bilimoria KY, Liu Y, Paruch JL, et al. Development and evaluation of the universal ACS NSQIP surgical risk calculator: a decision aid and informed consent tool for patients and surgeons. J Am Coll Surg 2013;217(5):833–42.

52. Liu Y, Cohen ME, Hall BL, et al. Evaluation and enhancement of calibration in the American College of Surgeons NSQIP Surgical Risk Calculator. J Am Coll Surg 2016;223(2):231–9.

53. El Hechi MW, Maurer LR, Levine J, et al. Validation of the artificial intelligence-based predictive optimal trees in emergency surgery risk (POTTER) calculator in emergency general surgery and emergency laparotomy patients. J Am Coll Surg 2021;232(6):912–9.

54. Nandan AR, Bohnen JD, Sangji NF, et al. The Emergency Surgery Score (ESS) accurately predicts the occurrence of postoperative complications in emergency surgery patients. J Trauma Acute Care Surg 2017;83(1):84–9.

55. Kaafarani HM, Kongkaewpaisan N, Aicher BO, et al. Prospective validation of the Emergency Surgery Score in emergency general surgery: An Eastern Association for the Surgery of Trauma multicenter study. J Trauma Acute Care Surg 2020;89(1):118–24.

56. Gaitanidis A, Mikdad S, Breen K, et al. The Emergency Surgery Score (ESS) accurately predicts outcomes in elderly patients undergoing emergency general surgery. Am J Surg 2020;220(4):1052–7.

57. Baggett ND, Schulz K, Buffington A, et al. Surgeon use of shared decision-making for older adults considering major surgery: a secondary analysis of a randomized clinical trial. JAMA surgery 2022;157(5):406–13.
58. De Roo AC, Vitous CA, Rivard SJ, et al. High-risk surgery among older adults: Not-quite shared decision-making. Surgery 2021;170(3):756–63.
59. Taylor LJ, Nabozny MJ, Steffens NM, et al. A framework to improve surgeon communication in high-stakes surgical decisions: best case/worst case. JAMA surgery 2017;152(6):531–8.
60. Ogola GO, Haider A, Shafi S. Hospitals with higher volumes of emergency general surgery patients achieve lower mortality rates: a case for establishing designated centers for emergency general surgery. J Trauma Acute Care Surg 2017; 82(3):497–504.
61. Ogola GO, Crandall ML, Richter KM, et al. High-volume hospitals are associated with lower mortality among high-risk emergency general surgery patients. J Trauma Acute Care Surg 2018;85(3):560–5.
62. Mehta A, Efron DT, Canner JK, et al. Effect of surgeon and hospital volume on emergency general surgery outcomes. J Am Coll Surg 2017;225(5):666–75.
63. Diaz Jose J, Norris Patrick R, Gunter Oliver L, et al. Does Regionalization of Acute Care Surgery Decrease Mortality? J Trauma Inj Infect Crit Care 2011;71(2):442–6. https://doi.org/10.1097/TA.0b013e3182281fa2.
64. Becher RD, Sukumar N, DeWane MP, et al. Regionalization of emergency general surgery operations: a simulation study. J Trauma Acute Care Surg 2020 Mar; 88(3):366.

Damage Control Surgery and Transfer in Emergency General Surgery

Carlos A. Fernandez, MD

KEYWORDS

- Damage control surgery • Damage control resuscitation
- Nontraumatic emergency surgery • Temporary abdominal closure
- Primary fascial closure

KEY POINTS

- Selective nontraumatic emergency surgery patients are targets for damage control surgery to prevent or treat abdominal compartment syndrome and the lethal triad.
- Damage control resuscitation reduces the need for damage control surgery.
- Selective patients with septic shock from severe perforated diverticulitis may be treated with damage control surgery to reduce the ostomy rate.
- Temporary abdominal closure with continuous fascial traction provides the highest chance for primary fascial closure.
- Primary fascial closure should be attempted at the first take back within 48 hours to reduce the risk of complications associated with an open abdomen.

INTRODUCTION

Damage control surgery (DCS) in nontraumatic emergency surgery, also known as emergency general surgery (EGS), is a subject of controversy. As a concept, DCS is described as a series of abbreviated surgical procedures to allow rapid source control of hemorrhage and contamination in patients with nontraumatic abdominal emergencies and circulatory shock. DCS allows resuscitation and stabilization of the patient in the intensive care unit (ICU) and delayed return to the operating room for definitive surgical management once the patient becomes physiologic stable.

HISTORICAL PERSPECTIVE

DCS emerged as a paradigm shift in the management of trauma patients with exsanguinating injuries in the 1970s.[1–4] Surgical experience dealing with major hepatic and vascular traumas identified metabolic failure as a predominant mortality factor in the

Department of Surgery, Creighton University Medical Center, 7710 Mercy Road, Suite 2000, Omaha, NE 68124, USA
E-mail address: Carlosfernandez@creighton.edu

Surg Clin N Am 103 (2023) 1269–1281
https://doi.org/10.1016/j.suc.2023.06.004
0039-6109/23/© 2023 Elsevier Inc. All rights reserved.

surgical.theclinics.com

surgical management of those severely injured patients.[4,5] Metabolic failure was recognized as metabolic exhaustion with ongoing bleeding from coagulopathy, hypothermia, and metabolic acidosis, also known as the lethal triad.[6] In 1983, Stone and colleagues[7] and Burch and colleagues[8] in 1992 delineated the principles of management of the new paradigm that were formalized as DCS in 1993 by Rotondo and colleagues.[9]

A series of innovations and documented benefits of DCS[10] in the trauma literature led to a widespread propagation and ultimately overutilization of DCS, which exposed patients to unnecessary risk of serious complications associated with the DCS process.[11] A selective approach was then advocated to apply DCS principles only to the small group of trauma and nontrauma patients at a higher risk, or with early indicators, of physiologic failure.[12,13]

Research studies on the coagulopathy of trauma allowed DCS to evolve and generate the new concept of damage control resuscitation (DCR).[14–19] The novel DCR incorporated improved understanding of the coagulopathy and introduced the notion of early resuscitation strategies to prevent it and decrease blood loss.[20–22] DCS is now a part of DCR and can be initiated in different locations.

The DCR approach, with selective application of DCS, has led to significant reductions in the utilization of DCS in trauma and nontrauma emergency surgery with better outcomes.[23,24]

DAMAGE CONTROL RESUSCITATION/DAMAGE CONTROL SURGERY APPROACH IN EMERGENCY GENERAL SURGERY: UNDERSTANDING THE CORE CONCEPTS

EGS patients can experience shock from nontraumatic hemorrhagic abdominal emergencies or from intra-abdominal sepsis that may lead to the development of the lethal triad and the need for DCR/DCS.[25]

Shock develops when the delivery of oxygen and metabolic substrates to cells and tissues is insufficient to maintain aerobic metabolism, resulting in a persistent supply/demand imbalance and subsequent oxygen debt, which is a deficit of tissue oxygenation over time.[26,27]

The magnitude of the oxygen debt depends on the degree and duration of shock.[28] Evidence suggests that, although the quantitative nature of the host response to shock may differ between the various etiologies of shock, the qualitative nature of the host response to shock is similar regardless of the cause of the insult.[29]

As shock results in an oxygen delivery-dependent state, cells transition to anaerobic metabolism.[30] Consequentially, the mounting oxygen debt leads to metabolic acidosis, hypothermia, and coagulophaty.[31–37]

Understanding of the physiologic derangements of shock provides the core concepts for DCS. This is especially important in EGS patients with upregulated systemic inflammatory response caused by sepsis.[38]

EPIDEMIOLOGY OF DAMAGE CONTROL SURGERY IN NONTRAUMATIC EMERGENCY SURGERY

There is a growing number of patients undergoing nontraumatic DCS for different surgical conditions.[25,39–41]

The most common diagnoses requiring DCS have been reported but show different frequency rates.[41,42] Haltmeier and colleagues, in a systematic review and metanalysis in 2022, reported viscus perforation (28.5%), mesenteric ischemia (26.5%), anastomotic leak and postoperative peritonitis (19.6%), nontraumatic hemorrhage (18.4%), abdominal compartment syndrome (17.8%), bowel obstruction (15.5%), and pancreatitis (12.9%) as the most nontraumatic DCS diagnoses.[43]

The EAST SLEEP-TIME Multicenter Trial in 2021 found similar demographics and outcomes between trauma and nontrauma patients. However, more older females, higher Charlson Comorbidity Index, more intra-abdominal sepsis, and less incidence of delirium were noted on nontrauma patients.[41]

Most recently, the 2023 International Register of Open Abdomen (IROA) study reported the international duration of open abdomen. The median is 4 days (interquartile range: 2–7) but higher for the Asiatic continent with a median of 7 days. The median ICU and hospital lengths of stay are 8 and 11 days, respectively.[44]

These epidemiologic data reflect the heterogeneity of DCS utilization and the population at risk. However, they are also signaling important characteristics that are shared by the trauma and nontrauma populations.

SELECTIVE DAMAGE CONTROL SURGERY INDICATORS IN NONTRAUMATIC EMERGENCY SURGERY PATIENTS

Nontrauma indicators for DCS are still not well defined. In clinical practice, the decision to perform DCS in depends on the underlying disease, presence of comorbidities, physiology of the patient, degree of contamination, technical considerations, and surgeon experience.[45]

Criteria for nontraumatic hemorrhagic shock were derived from trauma. Common targets for DCS are patients with perioperative hemostatic resuscitation and several persistent indicators:[46–49]

- Systolic blood pressure < 90 mm Hg
- Hypothermia less than 34°C
- PH < 7.2
- International normalized ratio/prothrombin time/partial thromboplastin time (INR/PT/PTT) greater than 1.5 times normal
- Clinically observed coagulopathy
- Transfusion of greater than 10 PRBC given across the pre- or intraoperative period
- Need for intrabdominal packing
- Time required for surgery greater than 90 minutes
- Patient's estimated blood loss greater than 4 L

In septic patients, common targets for DCS are still evolving.[25,39,50] Becher and colleagues in 2016 suggested several physiologic indicators for DCS in EGS patients with intra-abdominal sepsis:[38]

- Preoperative severe sepsis/septic shock
- Elevated lactate (≥3)
- Acidosis (pH ≤ 7.25)
- Elderly (≥70)
- Male gender
- Multiple comorbidities (≥3)

These criteria provide a systemic approach and guidance; however, continued research is needed.

TEMPORARY ABDOMINAL CLOSURE TECHNIQUES

Temporary abdominal closure (TAC) is a hallmark of DCS. The decision to use TAC should be made early preoperatively or in the operating room based on the response to DCR.[51]

Several techniques can be used for TAC with or without negative pressure, and they can result in different delayed fascial closure rate and risk of entero-atmospheric fistula (EAF). Available techniques are skin closure, Bogota bag, mesh mediated closure (Wittmann patch), Barker vacuum pack, negative pressure wound therapy (NPWT) alone, and NPWT with dynamic tension (mesh or suture mediated). The NPWT is also known as vacuum assisted therapy (VAC).

The preferred TAC technique recommended by WSES is NPWT, especially in patients with severe peritonitis and nontraumatic abdominal emergencies.[52] However, there is no uniformity in the management of the open abdomen between different continents or in the application of international guidelines. Commercial NPWT is reported as the most common in the United States and Europe (77.4% and 52.3% of cases), while Barker vacuum pack (48.2%) is the most common in Asia.[44]

TEMPORARY ABDOMINAL CLOSURE-RELATED COMPLICATIONS

Prevention of the ACS and early definitive closure of the abdomen are the cornerstones of preventing or reducing the risk of complications associated with TAC.[52,53]

TAC techniques have different rate of complications. In 2015, a systematic review and meta-analysis by Atema and colleagues (24) reported an incidence of 14.6% for enteroatmospheric fistula (EAF) and 48.5% for incisional hernias if the VAC technique is applied, and especially if the population is treated for peritonitis.[54]

The 2017 IROA study compared the outcomes associated with TAC techniques:[42]

Bogota bag had 71% primary fascial closure (PFC), 7.4% entero-atmospheric fistula (EAF), and 16.8% mortality rate.
NPWT alone had 59.9% PFC, 13.5% EAF, and 14.3% mortality rate.
Barker vacuum had 64.3% PFC, 2.4% EAF, and 24.4% mortality rate.
Wittmann Patch had 65.7 PFC, 17.6% EAF, and 20.6% mortality rate.

In an updated version of the IROA study in 2023, the reported overall rate of EAF rate was 2.5%, with overall morbidity and mortality rates for North America of 75.8% and 31,9%; Europe of 75.3% and 51.6%; and Asia of 91.8% and 56.9%, respectively.[44]

In terms of analysis of risk factors for EAF, in 2019 the IROA study reported duration of the VAC therapy and the nutritional status of the patient as the predominant risk factors for EAF but not influenced by peritonitis, intestinal anastomosis, negative pressure, or oral or enteral nutrition.[55]

PRIMARY FASCIAL CLOSURE AFTER TEMPORARY ABDOMINAL CLOSURE

The PFC of the abdomen at the first take back after DCS has a major impact on reducing TAC-associated complications.[52,56] Recent data from the EAST SLEEP-TIME multicenter registry showed that time to repeat laparotomy at less than or equal to 24 hours and reduced number of repeat laparotomies are highly predictive of rapid achievement of PFC in trauma and nontrauma DCS patients. The odds of achieving PFC decreases significantly after 48 hours.[57]

There rate of definitive abdominal closure varies across the continents. According to the updated IROA study in 2023, PFC was achieved in 82.3% of cases in North America (fascial closure in 90.2% of cases) and in 56.4% of cases in Asia.[44]

Different factors influence the likelihood of achieving PFC.[58,59] Data from the European Hernia Society Registry in 2022 showed that the PFC rate is significantly higher in trauma patients and lower in the presence of intra-abdominal contamination.[60] Fluid overload also decreases PFC.[61–63] Strategies directed to reduce fluid resuscitation have been associated with increased rate of PFC but not by using diuretics.[61,64,65]

PFC is also significantly affected by TAC techniques. Among the different options, NWPT with mesh-mediated or nonmesh-mediated fascial traction provides the best chance to achieve PFC.[60,66–71] Novel techniques are also under development to further increase PFC rate and prevent incisional hernia formation.[72–74]

PFC after TAC remains a major challenge. Efforts should be made to attempt PFC at the first take back.

THERAPEUTIC ADJUNCTS TO FACILITATE PRIMARY FASCIAL CLOSURE

Direct peritoneal resuscitation is a therapeutic adjunct to increase PFC after TAC.[75,76] The physiologic effects of infusing hypertonic solution in the peritoneal cavity increases the likelihood of PFC. A recent systematic review in 2022 documented the clinical benefits of DPR in DCS patients.[75]

The combination of NPTW with fluid instillation with or without antibiotics seems to be a promising tool to reduce ongoing peritonitis and increase PFC.[77–80] The IROA study in 2020 showed a PFC rate of 78.6% in the fluid instillation (FI) group and 63.7% in the non-FI group. However, the study found an increased in the overall complication rate of 72.6% in FI and 59.9% in NFI.[78]

Three percent hypertonic saline (HTS) has been used to decrease IVF resuscitation volume and increase PFC.[81] However, a recent randomized controlled trial (RCT) in 2023 showed no benefit of the HTS to increase the chance of PFC.[82]

The use of bioelectrical impedance analysis (BIA) is another adjunct to decrease fluids and increase PFC. An RCT in 2021 showed BIA in trauma patients resulted in a higher PFC rate and fewer severe complications than the traditional fluid resuscitation strategy.[83]

Botox has been used to increase PFC, but an RCT in 2016 showed no benefit for PFC.[84]

More research is needed to define the role of new therapeutic adjuncts to increase PFC.

DAMAGE CONTROL SURGERY IN SEVERE PERFORATED DIVERTICULITIS

Intra-abdominal sepsis has a high mortality rate, from 28% to 47%.[85–89] Patients with severe perforated diverticulitis Hinchey III and IV are particularly prone to septic shock and need for DCS.[90,91] DCS provides a timely repeat laparotomy to address ongoing peritonitis as a surgical option that may significantly improve outcome.[92–95]

An RCT by the Dutch Peritonitis Study Group in 2007 showed similar mortality rate in patients severe peritonitis managed by planned relaparotomy (PRL) versus repeat laparotomy on demand (ROD), with ROD patients having lower re-exploration rate and reduced costs.[96,97] However, the study excluded DCS patients (ie, intra-abdominal packing, bowel discontinuity), and more research was needed to define the role of for DCS in severe peritonitis.[40,98]

DCS for generalized peritonitis has been reported as a proof of concept since 2010.[91,99–101] An RCT in 2020 reported the benefits of DCS in perforated diverticulitis Hinchey III and IV to increase reconstruction of bowel continuity and reduce the stoma rate at discharge.[93] Similar results were also reported by 2 systematic reviews in 2020 and 2021.[102,103]

The role of DCS in severe peritonitis is still evolving. In this regard, results of the RCT to assess the VAC versus on-demand repeat laparotomy in patients with secondary peritonitis, the VACOR trial, are awaited.[104]

DAMAGE CONTROL SURGERY AND TRANSFER IN EMERGENCY GENERAL SURGERY

In some instances, EGS patients need to be transferred to a higher level of care for definitive management after DCS. The transfer process commonly requires significant mobilization of resources and may delay patient care.[105,106] Furthermore, transfer EGS patients generally have higher rates of comorbidities and acuity with increased reoperation and mortality rate, and longer hospital length of stay compared with admitted patients.[106,107]

The principles of DCR/DCS can be applied during the transfer process. If the patient transfer is not done appropriately, the transfer process can significantly contribute to morbidity and mortality.[108] Patients need to be stabilized first, and then preparations can be made for transfer. This involves arranging for a critical care transport team to ensure that the patient's needs are met during transport such as continuous hemodynamic monitoring and mechanical ventilation.

During transfer, it is important to monitor the patient closely and to ensure that interventions are continued as needed. This may involve blood transfusion, adjustments to medications, or other interventions based on the patient's response to treatment. Once the patient has been transferred to a higher level of care, further resuscitation or support in the ICU can be performed followed by definitive management of any surgical condition.

SUMMARY

DCS in EGS remains an effective surgical therapy in selective critically ill surgical patients affected by septic and nontraumatic hemorrhagic shock. The morbidity associated with the DCS process can be significantly decreased if it is applied appropriately. DCS can be particularly beneficial in patients with severe perforated diverticulitis.

CLINICS CARE POINTS

- TAC techniques in DCS can be safely applied for a short period of time but have different complication rates.
- Primary fascial closure is still a major challenge.
- Efforts should be made to utilize DCS thecniques and therapeutic adjuncts associated with higher rate of early definitive closure of the abdomen.
- The risk of mortality, EAF, and ventral hernias are higher if PFC is delayed or not achieved.
- DCR/DCS principles can be applied to stabilize patients prior to transfer.
- DCS research and international uniformity in the management of open abdomen are still evolving.

DISCLOSURE

The author does not have any conflict of interest related to this article.

REFERENCES

1. Lucas CE, Ledgerwood AM. Prospective evaluation of hemostatic techniques for liver injuries. J Trauma 1976;16(6):442–51.

2. Calne RY, McMaster P, Pentlow BD. The treatment of major liver trauma by primary packing with transfer of the patient for definitive treatment. Br J Surg 1979; 66(5):338–9.
3. Elerding SC, Aragon GE, Moore EE. Fatal hepatic hemorrhage after trauma. Am J Surg 1979;138(6):883–8.
4. Feliciano DV, Mattox KL, Jordan GL. Intra-abdominal packing for control of hepatic hemorrhage: a reappraisal. J Trauma 1981;21(4):285–90.
5. Kashuk JL, Moore EE, Millikan JS, et al. Major abdominal vascular trauma–a unified approach. J Trauma 1982;22(8):672–9.
6. Moore EE, Thomas G. Orr Memorial Lecture. Staged laparotomy for the hypothermia, acidosis, and coagulopathy syndrome. Am J Surg 1996;172(5):405–10.
7. Stone HH, Strom PR, Mullins RJ. Management of the major coagulopathy with onset during laparotomy. Ann Surg 1983;197(5):532–5.
8. Burch JM, Ortiz VB, Richardson RJ, et al. Abbreviated laparotomy and planned reoperation for critically injured patients. Ann Surg 1992;215(5):476–83 [discussion: 483-484].
9. Rotondo MF, Schwab CW, McGonigal MD, et al. "Damage control:" an approach for improved survival in exsanguinating penetrating abdominal injury. J Trauma 1993;35(3):375–82 [discussion: 382-383].
10. Roberts DJ, Ball CG, Feliciano DV, et al. History of the innovation of damage control for management of trauma patients: 1902-2016. Ann Surg 2017; 265(5):1034–44.
11. Beldowicz BC. The evolution of damage control in concept and practice. Clin Colon Rectal Surg 2018;31(1):30–5.
12. Martin MJ, Hatch Q, Cotton B, et al. The use of temporary abdominal closure in low-risk trauma patients: helpful or harmful? J Trauma Acute Care Surg 2012; 72(3):601–6 [discussion: 606-608].
13. Roberts DJ, Bobrovitz N, Zygun DA, et al. Indications for use of damage control surgery in civilian trauma patients: a content analysis and expert appropriateness rating study. Ann Surg 2016;263(5):1018–27.
14. Hoffman M, Monroe DM. The action of high-dose factor VIIa (FVIIa) in a cell-based model of hemostasis. Semin Hematol 2001;38(4 Suppl 12):6–9.
15. Armand R, Hess JR. Treating coagulopathy in trauma patients. Transfus Med Rev 2003;17(3):223–31.
16. Esmon CT. Inflammation and the activated protein C anticoagulant pathway. Semin Thromb Hemost 2006;32(Suppl 1):49–60.
17. Cotton BA, Reddy N, Hatch QM, et al. Damage control resuscitation is associated with a reduction in resuscitation volumes and improvement in survival in 390 damage control laparotomy patients. Ann Surg 2011;254(4):598–605.
18. Holcomb JB, Jenkins D, Rhee P, et al. Damage control resuscitation: directly addressing the early coagulopathy of trauma. J Trauma 2007;62(2):307–10.
19. Duchesne JC, McSwain NE, Cotton BA, et al. Damage control resuscitation: the new face of damage control. J Trauma Inj Infect Crit Care 2010;69(4):976–90.
20. Borgman MA, Spinella PC, Perkins JG, et al. The ratio of blood products transfused affects mortality in patients receiving massive transfusions at a combat support hospital. J Trauma 2007;63(4):805–13.
21. Holcomb JB, del Junco DJ, Fox EE, et al. The prospective, observational, multicenter, major trauma transfusion (PROMMTT) study: comparative effectiveness of a time-varying treatment with competing risks. JAMA Surg 2013;148(2): 127–36.

22. Hynes AM, Geng Z, Schmulevich D, et al. Staying on target: maintaining a balanced resuscitation during damage-control resuscitation improves survival. J Trauma Acute Care Surg 2021;91(5):841–8.

23. Ball CG, Dente CJ, Shaz B, et al. The impact of a massive transfusion protocol (1:1:1) on major hepatic injuries: does it increase abdominal wall closure rates? Can J Surg J Can Chir 2013;56(5):E128–34.

24. Bradley M, Galvagno S, Dhanda A, et al. Damage control resuscitation protocol and the management of open abdomens in trauma patients. Am Surg 2014;80(8):768–75.

25. Weber DG, Bendinelli C, Balogh ZJ. Damage control surgery for abdominal emergencies. Br J Surg 2014;101(1):e109–18.

26. Crowell JW, Smith EE. Oxygen deficit and irreversible hemorrhagic shock. Am J Physiol 1964;206:313–6.

27. Dunham CM, Siegel JH, Weireter L, et al. Oxygen debt and metabolic acidemia as quantitative predictors of mortality and the severity of the ischemic insult in hemorrhagic shock. Crit Care Med 1991;19(2):231–43.

28. Shoemaker WC, Appel PL, Kram HB. Role of oxygen debt in the development of organ failure sepsis, and death in high-risk surgical patients. Chest 1992;102(1):208–15.

29. Feliciano DV, Mattox KL, Moore EE, et al. *Trauma*, 9th edition, 2020, McGraw-Hill, 241. Chapter 15.

30. Burša F, Pleva L. Anaerobic metabolism associated with traumatic hemorrhagic shock monitored by microdialysis of muscle tissue is dependent on the levels of hemoglobin and central venous oxygen saturation: a prospective, observational study. Scand J Trauma Resusc Emerg Med 2014;22(1):11.

31. Glancy B, Kane DA, Kavazis AN, et al. Mitochondrial lactate metabolism: history and implications for exercise and disease. J Physiol 2021;599(3):863–88.

32. Okamoto T, Tanigami H, Suzuki K, et al. Thrombomodulin: a bifunctional modulator of inflammation and coagulation in sepsis. Crit Care Res Pract 2012;2012:1–10.

33. Kimmoun A, Novy E, Auchet T, et al. Hemodynamic consequences of severe lactic acidosis in shock states: from bench to bedside. Crit Care 2015;19(1):175.

34. White NJ, Ward KR, Pati S, et al. Hemorrhagic blood failure: oxygen debt, coagulopathy, and endothelial damage. J Trauma Acute Care Surg 2017;82(6S):S41–9.

35. Johansson PI, Henriksen HH, Stensballe J, et al. Traumatic endotheliopathy: a prospective observational study of 424 severely injured patients. Ann Surg 2017;265(3):597–603.

36. Chang R, Cardenas JC, Wade CE, et al. Advances in the understanding of trauma-induced coagulopathy. Blood 2016;128(8):1043–9.

37. Lu X, Ying L, Wang H, et al. Efficacy comparison of restrictive versus massive fluid resuscitation in patients with traumatic hemorrhagic shock. Am J Transl Res 2022;14(10):7504–11.

38. Becher RD, Hoth JJ, Miller PR, et al. Systemic inflammation worsens outcomes in emergency surgical patients. J Trauma Acute Care Surg 2012;72(5):1140–9.

39. Stawicki SP, Brooks A, Bilski T, et al. The concept of damage control: extending the paradigm to emergency general surgery. Injury 2008;39(1):93–101.

40. Khan A, Hsee L, Mathur S, et al. Damage-control laparotomy in nontrauma patients: review of indications and outcomes. J Trauma Acute Care Surg 2013;75(3):365–8.

41. McArthur K, Krause C, Kwon E, et al. Trauma and nontrauma damage-control laparotomy: the difference is delirium (data from the Eastern Association for the Surgery of Trauma SLEEP-TIME multicenter trial). J Trauma Acute Care Surg 2021;91(1):100–7.

42. Coccolini F, Montori G, Ceresoli M, et al. IROA: International Register of Open Abdomen, preliminary results. World J Emerg Surg WJES 2017;12:10.

43. Haltmeier T, Falke M, Quaile O, et al. Damage-control surgery in patients with nontraumatic abdominal emergencies: a systematic review and meta-analysis. J Trauma Acute Care Surg 2022;92(6):1075–85.

44. Sibilla MG, Cremonini C, Portinari M, et al. Patients with an open abdomen in asian, american and european continents: a comparative analysis from the International Register of Open Abdomen (IROA). World J Surg 2023;47(1):142–51.

45. Rezende-Neto J, Rice T, Abreu ES, et al. Anatomical, physiological, and logistical indications for the open abdomen: a proposal for a new classification system. World J Emerg Surg WJES 2016;11:28.

46. Asensio JA, McDuffie L, Petrone P, et al. Reliable variables in the exsanguinated patient which indicate damage control and predict outcome. Am J Surg 2001; 182(6):743–51.

47. Asensio JA, Petrone P, Roldán G, et al. Has evolution in awareness of guidelines for institution of damage control improved outcome in the management of the posttraumatic open abdomen? Arch Surg Chic Ill 1960 2004;139(2):209–14 [discussion: 215].

48. Roberts DJ, Bobrovitz N, Zygun DA, et al. Indications for use of thoracic, abdominal, pelvic, and vascular damage control interventions in trauma patients: a content analysis and expert appropriateness rating study. J Trauma Acute Care Surg 2015;79(4):568–79.

49. Roberts DJ, Bobrovitz N, Zygun DA, et al. Evidence for use of damage control surgery and damage control interventions in civilian trauma patients: a systematic review. World J Emerg Surg WJES 2021;16(1):10.

50. Girard E, Abba J, Boussat B, et al. Damage control surgery for non-traumatic abdominal emergencies. World J Surg 2018;42(4):965–73.

51. Bala M, Catena F, Kashuk J, et al. Acute mesenteric ischemia: updated guidelines of the World Society of Emergency Surgery. World J Emerg Surg 2022; 17(1):54.

52. Coccolini F, Roberts D, Ansaloni L, et al. The open abdomen in trauma and non-trauma patients: WSES guidelines. World J Emerg Surg WJES 2018;13:7.

53. Chen Y, Ye J, Song W, et al. Comparison of outcomes between early fascial closure and delayed abdominal closure in patients with open abdomen: a systematic review and meta-analysis. Gastroenterol Res Pract 2014;2014:1–8.

54. Atema JJ, Gans SL, Boermeester MA. Systematic review and meta-analysis of the open abdomen and temporary abdominal closure techniques in non-trauma patients. World J Surg 2015;39(4):912–25.

55. Coccolini F, Ceresoli M, Kluger Y, et al. Open abdomen and entero-atmospheric fistulae: an interim analysis from the International Register of Open Abdomen (IROA). Injury 2019;50(1):160–6.

56. Lauerman MH, Dubose JJ, Stein DM, et al. Evolution of fascial closure optimization in damage control laparotomy. Am Surg 2016;82(12):1178–82.

57. Kwon E, Krause C, Luo-Owen X, et al. Time is domain: factors affecting primary fascial closure after trauma and non-trauma damage control laparotomy (data from the EAST SLEEP-TIME multicenter registry). Eur J Trauma Emerg Surg 2022;48(3):2107–16.

58. Goussous N, Kim BD, Jenkins DH, et al. Factors affecting primary fascial closure of the open abdomen in the nontrauma patient. Surgery 2012;152(4): 777–84.

59. Granger S, Fallon J, Hopkins J, et al. An open and closed case: timing of closure following laparostomy. Ann R Coll Surg Engl 2020;102(7):519–24.

60. Willms AG, Schwab R, von Websky MW, et al. Factors influencing the fascial closure rate after open abdomen treatment: results from the European Hernia Society (EuraHS) Registry: surgical technique matters. Hernia 2022;26(1): 61–73.

61. Huang Q, Zhao R, Yue C, et al. Fluid volume overload negatively influences delayed primary facial closure in open abdomen management. J Surg Res 2014; 187(1):122–7.

62. Smith JW, Garrison RN, Matheson PJ, et al. Direct peritoneal resuscitation accelerates primary abdominal wall closure after damage control surgery. J Am Coll Surg 2010;210(5). 658-664, 664-667.

63. Loftus TJ, Efron PA, Bala TM, et al. The impact of standardized protocol implementation for surgical damage control and temporary abdominal closure after emergent laparotomy. J Trauma Acute Care Surg 2019;86(4):670–8.

64. Ghneim MH, Regner JL, Jupiter DC, et al. Goal directed fluid resuscitation decreases time for lactate clearance and facilitates early fascial closure in damage control surgery. Am J Surg 2013;206(6):995–1000.

65. Williamson S, Qatanani A, Muller A, et al. Open abdomen after two trauma laparotomies: do diuretics help? Am Surg 2022;88(4):770–2.

66. Fortelny RH, Hofmann A, Gruber-Blum S, et al. Delayed closure of open abdomen in septic patients is facilitated by combined negative pressure wound therapy and dynamic fascial suture. Surg Endosc 2014;28(3):735–40.

67. Willms A, Schaaf S, Schwab R, et al. Abdominal wall integrity after open abdomen: long-term results of vacuum-assisted wound closure and mesh-mediated fascial traction (VAWCM). Hernia 2016;20(6):849–58.

68. Sharrock AE, Barker T, Yuen HM, et al. Management and closure of the open abdomen after damage control laparotomy for trauma. A systematic review and meta-analysis. Injury 2016;47(2):296–306.

69. Salamone G, Licari L, Guercio G, et al. Vacuum-assisted wound closure with mesh-mediated fascial traction achieves better outcomes than vacuum-assisted wound closure alone: a comparative study. World J Surg 2018;42(6): 1679–86.

70. Wang Y, Alnumay A, Paradis T, et al. Management of open abdomen after trauma laparotomy: a comparative analysis of dynamic fascial traction and negative pressure wound therapy systems. World J Surg 2019;43(12):3044–50.

71. Nemec HM, Benjamin Christie D, Montgomery A, et al. Wittmann patch: superior closure for the open abdomen. Am Surg 2020;86(8):981–4.

72. Petersson P, Montgomery A, Petersson U. Vacuum-assisted wound closure and permanent onlay mesh–mediated fascial traction: a novel technique for the prevention of incisional hernia after open abdomen therapy including results from a retrospective case series. Scand J Surg 2019;108(3):216–26.

73. Schaaf S, Schwab R, Güsgen C, et al. Prophylactic Onlay Mesh Implantation During Definitive Fascial Closure After Open Abdomen Therapy (PROMOAT): absorbable or non-absorbable? methodical description and results of a feasibility study. Front Surg 2020;7:578565.

74. Fung S, Ashmawy H, Krieglstein C, et al. Vertical traction device prevents abdominal wall retraction and facilitates early primary fascial closure of septic and non-septic open abdomen. Langenbeck's Arch Surg 2022;407(5):2075–83.

75. Ribeiro-Junior MAF, Costa CTK, de Souza Augusto S, et al. The role of direct peritoneal resuscitation in the treatment of hemorrhagic shock after trauma and in emergency acute care surgery: a systematic review. Eur J Trauma Emerg Surg 2022;48(2):791–7.

76. Smith JW, Neal Garrison R, Matheson PJ, et al. Adjunctive treatment of abdominal catastrophes and sepsis with direct peritoneal resuscitation: indications for use in acute care surgery. J Trauma Acute Care Surg 2014;77(3):393–9.

77. Brillantino A, Andreano M, Lanza M, et al. Advantages of damage control strategy with abdominal negative pressure and instillation in patients with diffuse peritonitis from perforated diverticular disease. Surg Innov 2019;26(6):656–61.

78. Coccolini F, Gubbiotti F, Ceresoli M, et al. Open abdomen and fluid instillation in the septic abdomen: results from the IROA study. World J Surg 2020;44(12):4032–40.

79. Tao Q, Ren J, Ji Z, et al. VAWCM-instillation improves delayed primary fascial closure of open septic abdomen. Gastroenterol Res Pract 2014;2014:1–7.

80. Sibaja P, Sanchez A, Villegas G, et al. Management of the open abdomen using negative pressure wound therapy with instillation in severe abdominal sepsis. Int J Surg Case Rep 2017;30:26–30.

81. Loftus TJ, Efron PA, Bala TM, et al. Hypertonic saline resuscitation after emergent laparotomy and temporary abdominal closure. J Trauma Acute Care Surg 2018;84(2):350–7.

82. García AF, Manzano-Nunez R, Carrillo DC, et al. Hypertonic saline infusion does not improve the chance of primary fascial closure after damage control laparotomy: a randomized controlled trial. World J Emerg Surg 2023;18(1):4.

83. Wang K, Sun SL, Wang XY, et al. Bioelectrical impedance analysis-guided fluid management promotes primary fascial closure after open abdomen: a randomized controlled trial. Mil Med Res 2021;8(1):36.

84. Zielinski MD, Kuntz M, Zhang X, et al. Botulinum toxin A–induced paralysis of the lateral abdominal wall after damage-control laparotomy: a multi-institutional, prospective, randomized, placebo-controlled pilot study. J Trauma Acute Care Surg 2016;80(2):237–42.

85. Weledji EP, Ngowe MN. The challenge of intra-abdominal sepsis. Int J Surg Lond Engl 2013;11(4):290–5.

86. Sartelli M, Catena F, Ansaloni L, et al. Complicated intra-abdominal infections worldwide: the definitive data of the CIAOW study. World J Emerg Surg 2014;9(1):37.

87. Sartelli M, Abu-Zidan FM, Catena F, et al. Global validation of the WSES sepsis severity score for patients with complicated intra-abdominal infections: a prospective multicentre study (WISS Study). World J Emerg Surg WJES 2015;10:61.

88. Singer M, Deutschman CS, Seymour CW, et al. The Third International Consensus Definitions for Sepsis and Septic Shock (Sepsis-3). JAMA 2016;315(8):801.

89. Tolonen M, Sallinen V, Mentula P, et al. Preoperative prognostic factors for severe diffuse secondary peritonitis: a retrospective study. Langenbeck's Arch Surg 2016;401(5):611–7.

90. Cirocchi R, Arezzo A, Vettoretto N, et al. Role of damage control surgery in the treatment of Hinchey III and IV sigmoid diverticulitis: a tailored strategy. Medicine (Baltim) 2014;93(25):e184.

91. Sohn M, Agha A, Heitland W, et al. Damage control strategy for the treatment of perforated diverticulitis with generalized peritonitis. Tech Coloproctology 2016; 20(8):577–83.

92. Sohn M, Iesalnieks I, Agha A, et al. Perforated diverticulitis with generalized peritonitis: low stoma rate using a "damage control strategy.". World J Surg 2018;42(10):3189–95.

93. Kafka-Ritsch R, Zitt M, Perathoner A, et al. Prospectively randomized controlled trial on damage control surgery for perforated diverticulitis with generalized peritonitis. World J Surg 2020;44(12):4098–105.

94. Faes S, Hübner M, Girardin T, et al. Rate of stoma formation following damage-control surgery for severe intra-abdominal sepsis: a single-centre consecutive case series. BJS Open 2021;5(6):zrab106.

95. Fugazzola P, Ceresoli M, Coccolini F, et al. The WSES/SICG/ACOI/SICUT/AcEMC/SIFIPAC guidelines for diagnosis and treatment of acute left colonic diverticulitis in the elderly. World J Emerg Surg 2022;17(1):5.

96. van Ruler O, Mahler CW, Boer KR, et al. Comparison of on-demand vs planned relaparotomy strategy in patients with severe peritonitis: a randomized trial. JAMA 2007;298(8):865.

97. Opmeer BC, Boer KR, van Ruler O, et al. Costs of relaparotomy on-demand versus planned relaparotomy in patients with severe peritonitis: an economic evaluation within a randomized controlled trial. Crit Care 2010;14(3):R97.

98. for The Closed Or Open after Laparotomy (COOL) after Source Control for Severe Complicated Intra-Abdominal Sepsis Investigators, Kirkpatrick AW, Coccolini F, et al. Closed Or Open after Source Control Laparotomy for Severe Complicated Intra-Abdominal Sepsis (the COOL trial): study protocol for a randomized controlled trial. World J Emerg Surg 2018;13(1):26.

99. Perathoner A, Klaus A, Mühlmann G, et al. Damage control with abdominal vacuum therapy (VAC) to manage perforated diverticulitis with advanced generalized peritonitis–a proof of concept. Int J Colorectal Dis 2010;25(6):767–74.

100. Cirocchi R, Di Saverio S, Weber DG, et al. Laparoscopic lavage versus surgical resection for acute diverticulitis with generalised peritonitis: a systematic review and meta-analysis. Tech Coloproctology 2017;21(2):93–110.

101. Ordoñez CA, Parra M, García A, et al. Damage control surgery may be a safe option for severe non-trauma peritonitis management: proposal of a new decision-making algorithm. World J Surg 2021;45(4):1043–52.

102. Zizzo M, Castro Ruiz C, Zanelli M, et al. Damage control surgery for the treatment of perforated acute colonic diverticulitis: a systematic review. Medicine (Baltim) 2020;99(48):e23323.

103. Cirocchi R, Popivanov G, Konaktchieva M, et al. The role of damage control surgery in the treatment of perforated colonic diverticulitis: a systematic review and meta-analysis. Int J Colorectal Dis 2021;36(5):867–79.

104. Rajabaleyan P, Michelsen J, Tange Holst U, et al. Vacuum-assisted closure versus on-demand relaparotomy in patients with secondary peritonitis—the VACOR trial: protocol for a randomised controlled trial. World J Emerg Surg 2022; 17(1):25.

105. Kulshrestha A, Singh J. Inter-hospital and intra-hospital patient transfer: recent concepts. Indian J Anaesth 2016;60(7):451.

106. Emanuelson RD, Brown SJ, Termuhlen PM. Interhospital transfer (IHT) in emergency general surgery patients (EGS): a scoping review. Surg Open Sci 2022;9: 69–79.
107. Ingraham A, Wang X, Havlena J, et al. Factors associated with the interhospital transfer of emergency general surgery patients. J Surg Res 2019;240:191–200.
108. Mueller SK, Fiskio J, Schnipper J. Interhospital transfer: transfer processes and patient outcomes. J Hosp Med 2019;14(8):486–91.

Palliative Emergency General Surgery

Gregory Schaefer, DO[a,b,c,*], Daniel Regier, MD[c],
Conley Stout, MD[c]

KEYWORDS

- Palliative • Palliative surgery • Obstruction • End-of-life
- Emergency general surgery • Futile surgery • Futility

KEY POINTS

- The distinction between palliative surgery and surgical care for patients who are unlikely to survive emergent surgery can be difficult to define. Core principles include defining patient goals and ensuring effective symptom management.
- The approach to surgical emergencies in the context of end-stage medical conditions should include a focused history, physical examination, and diagnostics to provide objective data for consideration in conversations regarding treatment options.
- Small and Large Bowel obstructions are common with advanced malignancy. Shared decision-making conversations should focus on achievable goals of resection vs bypass or diversion for symptom management.
- Non-obstructive mesenteric ischemia often manifests following a severe physiologic insult such as septic or cardiogenic shock. Peritoneal signs and multi-system organ failure portend a poor prognosis for survival.
- Patients and family should be aware of decisions that will be required following survival of palliative emergency general surgery procedures including prolonged mechanical ventilation, tracheostomy, surgical feeding access, renal replacement therapy, and long-term need for inpatient rehabilitation or skilled nursing care.

INTRODUCTION

Acute care surgeons regularly are consulted for acute complications of chronic disease manifesting as emergencies. These may arise from surgical diagnoses where cure is not feasible and palliative options must be considered. The acute nature of these situations is a limiting factor in establishing a relationship between surgeon,

[a] Division of Trauma, Surgical Critical Care, and Acute Care Surgery, Surgical Critical Care, J.W. Ruby Memorial Hospital, West Virginia University Medicine, West Virginia University, Morgantown, WV, USA; [b] Division of Military Medicine, J.W. Ruby Memorial Hospital, West Virginia University Medicine, West Virginia University, Morgantown, WV, USA; [c] Department of Surgery, West Virginia University, Morgantown, WV, USA
* Corresponding author. Department of Surgery, P.O. Box 9238, Morgantown, WV 26506-9238.
E-mail address: gschaefer@hsc.wvu.edu

Surg Clin N Am 103 (2023) 1283–1296
https://doi.org/10.1016/j.suc.2023.06.005
0039-6109/23/© 2023 Elsevier Inc. All rights reserved.
surgical.theclinics.com

patient, and family. These are challenging situations for the surgeon, families, and patients alike. Through a review of literature, we offer guidance and recommendations for the acute care surgeon to care for patients with acute conditions at the end of their lives.

DEFINING PALLIATIVE SURGERY

Any discussion of palliative surgery brings to light the question of futility versus benefit.[1] Defining futility has remained elusive. Futility is influenced by perspective, from the patient or proceduralist. Effective communication is essential to determine what their goals and values are. Some patients prioritize quantity of life, whereas others emphasize quality of life. Surgical training has emphasized making a diagnosis and determining the appropriate procedure that results in the greatest benefit with the least risk. Among patients with advanced malignancies and life-limiting comorbidities, offering the optimal procedure may not achieve patients' self-determined values and goals. This is a practical and applicable definition of futility and incorporates the physiology-based perspective offered by Tomlinson and Brody and the qualitative and quantitative definition described by Schneiderman and coworkers.[2,3] Patients and families may inquire as to probabilities of success or failure; literature remains lacking in the data to offer accurate quantitative measures of survival that are applicable to each situation.

Surgeons are consulted to see patients who are acutely deteriorating or in extremis; conversely, they may be asked to evaluate a patient with a prolonged critical illness. Examples include the debilitated octogenarian who was admitted from a skilled nursing facility with pneumonia that progressed to septic shock and multisystem organ failure where multiple vasopressors are being infused and renal-replacement therapy is being contemplated. When the leukocytosis fails to improve and enteral nutrition is no longer tolerated, a computed tomography (CT) scan is completed and demonstrates portal venous gas and pneumatosis coli. The abdominal examination is unreliable because of sedation and delirium. This patient would have met criteria for a palliative care consultation at the time of admission to the intensive care unit (ICU). It is imperative for the surgeon to identify the patient's surrogates and determine what goals the patient would wish to achieve with their medical care and what values were relevant: improving quality of life and emphasizing comfort versus prolonging life regardless of the interventions and procedures necessary to achieve that goal. Several authors have offered a "best case/worst case" approach to these conversations as they relate to surgical procedures relevant to the diagnosis. In this case, laparotomy under general anesthesia with resection of the ischemic bowel, a possible return to the operating room in 24 hours for reevaluation of the bowel, and potential ostomy creation and closure of the abdomen would be best case. The family must also be enlightened that this best-case outcome would only address the mesenteric ischemia and that patient would remain mechanically ventilated and in need of renal-replacement therapy with anticipation of a prolonged ICU course. Worst-case scenario would be identification of extensive bowel ischemia where the extent of resection would not leave enough bowel length for adequate nutrition absorption and likely a degree of irreversible hepatic ischemia.

The American College of Surgeons National Surgical Quality Improvement Program surgical risk calculator[4] is an effective tool for quantifying risk and anticipated outcomes. Patient characteristics, comorbidities (acute and chronic), and alternatives to the procedure are entered and the results are displayed with a visual representation of the results and comparison with average risk for the same procedure.[5] An example

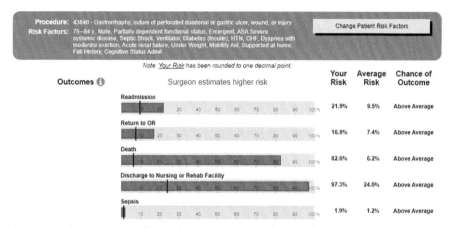

Fig. 1. Sample American College of Surgeons National Surgical Quality Improvement Program calculator screen for emergency general surgery with multiple comorbidities undergoing emergent repair of perforated duodenal ulcer. CHF, congestive heart failure; HTN, hypertension; OR, operating room. (American College of Surgeons National Surgical Quality Improvement Program (ACS NSQIP) Surgical Risk Calculator, Chicaco, IL.)

of the risk calculator is presented in **Fig. 1** for a patient with a significant chronic illness burden underlying septic shock from perforated peptic ulcer disease.

In these complex situations, disagreements may occur between what the surgeon believes is imminent demise where a surgical procedure is unlikely to change the outcome of expected death before discharge and the patient's desire to prolong life. The concept of beneficence is relevant and brings to light the Hippocratic theme of avoiding unnecessary harm to patients. Alternatively, patient advocates cite patient autonomy to decide what procedures are appropriate and how they will achieve patient goals. In the article by Grant and colleagues,[6] their review of the literature identified papers that describe a difference in alignment between values of the surgeon more so than the clinical opinion of the surgeon as to the proposed procedure.[7] Among situations described in the previous example, there may be limited time to resolve differences. Surgeons should be open to offering a second opinion, obtaining consultation from an ethics committee, and engaging risk management. The American Medical Association Council on Ethical and Judicial Affairs has published a guide to navigating conflicts in futile care that endorses a multistep and three-phase approach to achieve resolution.[8] Bradley and Brasel[9] identified several criteria that should prompt consultation of a palliative care specialist based on a review of criteria suggested by palliative care specialists, critical care surgeons, and the American College of Surgeons Palliative Care Task Force. Examples are family request or persistent disagreement between providers and family members for an extended period. Also included are clinical triggers including persistent coma, multisystem organ failure, prolonged ICU or frequent ICU admissions, and prognosis of a nonsurvivable injury or illness at time of admission to the ICU.

RISK ASSESSMENT FOR PERIOPERATIVE MORTALITY IN EMERGENCY GENERAL SURGERY

Aggarwal and coworkers[10] studied the outcomes of elderly patients undergoing emergency general surgery (EGS) procedures to determine common risk profiles of those suffering early postoperative mortality. Operations may prolong life for short intervals; hours or days, or even not at all. Cooper[11] reported more pain and inferior quality of life scores when EGS patients are admitted to an ICU at the end of life, primarily because of pain, and not achieving self-determined goals. Deaths in the immediate days following surgery are reflective of an underlying physiologic frailty and inability to tolerate stressors of critical illness and injury more so than improper surgical technique or lack of aggressive critical care. Howes and coworkers[12] showed an increased mortality among patients greater than 80 years of age undergoing EGS procedures compared with those younger. Chiu and coworkers[13] studied more than 94,000 patients who underwent EGS procedures and died within a month to ascertain the interval from procedure to death. In aggregate, one-third had died within 2 days and almost one-half of the entire cohort had deaths within 3 days. In the trial by Aggarwal and coworkers,[10] a database of almost 14,000 patients undergoing emergent laparotomy in 1 of 28 English hospitals was queried to determine characteristics of patients who died within 30 days. P-POSSUM[14] was used as a preoperative and postoperative risk assessment tool.

Incorporating a frailty assessment, such as the Rockwood clinical frailty score,[15] could enhance a clinician's ability to predict early mortality. This would be of value to the substantial number of patients dying within days of surgery.[16]

Overall mortality at 18 months was 9.8%, with most dying within 30 days (8.9) of the cohort. A total of 1242 patients died within the first 30 days; among them 38.1% died within 24 hours of surgery and 70% had died within the first 3 postoperative days. Under multivariate analysis, age (>75 years), elevated P-POSSUM preoperative score (54.2 vs 6.2), American Society of Anesthesiology (ASA) score (4 vs 3), and elevated creatinine were predictive of early death. Of those dying in the first 30 days, 38% died in the first 2 days. Hatchimonji and colleagues[17] described patient-centered care as a middle ground between the importance of patient autonomy and respect for the scientific evidence and experience of the surgeon. Families may be inclined toward life-prolonging choices rather than allowing progression to death in the fear that they would bear some responsibility for a patient's death. This is a burden borne by surrogates, understanding the potential suffering experienced by the patient resulting from the surrogate's decision to proceed with surgery. Surrogates may not perceive the futility of a procedure that is obvious to the surgeon because it is being offered. This should not prevent surgeons from presenting a range of options within a best case/worst case scenario; however, surgeons should frame each procedure in the context of ability to achieve the patient's goal. The surgeon may use their experience, expertise, and literature to describe the degree of certainty that they can help the patient achieve a successful outcome. Surrogates may not understand their obligation to represent the patient's desires even if they conflict with the wishes of the surrogate. "A successful outcome is one that provides a clinical benefit and must align with the patient's self-defined goals of care."[17] Here, futility would be clarified as an inability to achieve a successful outcome. Alternatively, a procedure likely to yield pain and suffering with low probability of achieving the defined successful outcome would be consistent with futility.

CONDITIONS MANAGED WITH PALLIATIVE SURGERY

Patients of advanced age, chronic illness, and frailty who undergo emergent surgical procedures, such as laparotomy, bowel resection, cholecystectomy, or repair of perforated peptic ulcer, suffer increased morbidity and mortality exceeding that of younger and healthier patients. Clinicians should consider a palliative care consultation if time allows. In urgent situations, it is incumbent on clinicians to assume responsibility for discussing end-of-life decisions with patients and families. Among clinical indicators for a palliative care consultation, current cancer diagnosis and known metastatic cancer were statistically significant predictors of survival at 1 year. Limited mobility (defined as <50% of day out of bed or chair), oxygen-dependent lung disease, end-stage renal disease, weight loss, hypoalbuminemia, and being underweight all trended toward significance. Among 173 patients, 69% had at least one trigger for consultation and 33% had at least two. EGS services should consider incorporation of frailty assessments and determination of palliative care triggers at time of admission.[18]

Understanding frailty is essential to make proper clinical application.[19] Frailty encompasses multiple domains including dysregulated response to physiologic insults based on impaired function of all organ systems; frailty does not always correlate with chronologic age, rather with the summative effect of chronic illness over time. Studies evaluating EGS patients with a variety of tools have identified frailty in at least half of all patients undergoing EGS procedures.[20–22] Frailty has a well-established correlation with complications, such as longer hospital stays, short-term mortality, and duration of ICU stay.[23–25] Further research on the combination of frailty and EGS is important to better understand how quality-of-life issues for survivors beyond the usual 30-day interval are affected.

Kim examined medical claims to assess the penetrance of frailty among EGS patients and the effect it has on outcomes.[26] Older EGS patients undergoing five common, but high-mortality EGS procedures were assessed using a Claims-based Frailty Index.[27,28] Among the 468,000 patients, 37.4 were assessed to be prefrail, whereas another 12.4% were mildly frail and 3.6% had moderate to severe frailty. Eighty-five percent of patients were White, which should prompt further investigation of socioeconomic disparities in the care of non-White EGS patients with frailty. Mortality was more prevalent among those with any degree of frailty and the overall mortality at 30 days was 15.7%, increasing to 24.7% at 180 days, and 30.4% at 1 year. Patients with mild and moderate to severe frailty were four and six times more likely to need hospitalization again within 1 year. Patients with mild frailty averaged 46 fewer days at home and moderate to severe frailty patients averaged 99 fewer days at home in the year after their EGS procedure. Any degree of frailty imposed 2 to 5 times higher frequency of rehospitalization and 3 to 4.5 times increased frequency of ICU stays compared with nonfrail. This mirrors other studies evaluating the negative impact of frailty on EGS patients. A single-institution study of veterans identified frailty during preoperative evaluation and triggered a palliative care consultation. This intervention reduced risk of mortality within 180 days by 33%.[29]

EGS among older patients increases the amount of days in hospitals and ICUs and results in death more frequently than a similar cohort who does not have surgery.[30] This contrasts with the documented goals of patients suffering from advanced stages of chronic illness and malignancy who place time with family and comfort paramount to living longer, especially if significant fear, anxiety, and pain are associated with the measures to prolong life.[31,32] The consequences of a decision to proceed with an EGS procedure and the associated invasive therapies, such as mechanical ventilation and renal-replacement therapy, may overwhelm patients and families.[33] Cauley an coworkers[30] evaluated characteristics of patients with advanced malignancy presenting with intestinal perforation or obstruction who underwent laparotomy. Among patients with perforation, chronic obstructive pulmonary disease, and chronic kidney disease, an existing do-not-resuscitate order, an ASA score greater than four, presence of ascites, dyspnea at rest, dementia, pneumonia, and septic shock were associated with increased mortality. Patients undergoing laparotomy for bowel obstruction were at increased risk with similar preoperative clinical characteristics. Postoperative events associated with increased mortality included respiratory complication, mechanical ventilation greater than 48 hours, cardiac complications, failure to rescue, and neurologic complications.

ABDOMINAL CATASTROPHE/BOWEL ISCHEMIA
Pathophysiology and Epidemiology

Mesenteric ischemia is an uncommon diagnosis generated from emergency department evaluations in acute care surgery regarding geriatric populations making up less than 1% of cases.[34] Estimated incidence rates of acute mesenteric ischemia with superior mesenteric occlusion range from 5.4 to 12.6/100,000 from all etiologies. A retrospective study from Sweden demonstrated 0.5% of 2222 patients evaluated for acute abdominal pain were diagnosed with acute mesenteric ischemia, mostly greater than age of 70 years old.[35,36]

Causes of acute mesenteric ischemia include evolution of chronic mesenteric atherosclerotic disease, cardiac dysrhythmias, and mechanical heart valves. Identification is key with mortality rates approaching 50%, with delay in diagnosis proven to significantly worsen outcomes to 70%.[35]

Nonobstructive mesenteric ischemia is defined as a low-flow state commonly caused by intravascular depletion, distributive shock, or dialysis-dependent patients. Nonobstructive sources of mesenteric ischemia are associated with high morbidity and mortality based on overall clinical status of the patient in setting of global visceral hypoperfusion. A single-institution retrospective study evaluated 154 patients undergoing exploratory laparotomy with concern for nonobstructive mesenteric ischemia in setting of multisystem organ to identify risk factors in prediction of 1-month mortality. More than half (56%) of the patients reviewed were postoperative from cardiac, abdominal, and aortic surgery with additional etiologies from sepsis, following cardiac arrest, acute respiratory failure, and hemorrhage. Statistically significant variables for 1-month mortality included lactate level greater than 7 mmol/L (P <.001), prothrombin rate less than 60% (P = 0.038), and kidney infarction per initial CT imaging (P <.001). Each variable was assigned one point with a mortality score constructed to reflect zero to three for probability of mortality in 1 month. Scores of zero demonstrated 26% mortality, score of one at 54%, score of two at 77%, and 100% at highest score of three. Area under the curve for the mortality score generated was listed at 0.79 with 95% confidence interval (CI). Operative findings only demonstrated that jejunal transmural necrosis requiring resection was a significant predictor in 1-month mortality in patients.[37]

Clinical Evaluation and Findings

Clinical presentation of chronic symptomatic mesenteric ischemia is difficult to identify unless clinical suspicion is high. These symptoms may include increasing, dull generalized abdominal discomfort, nausea, vomiting, and lethargy. Patients may have a history of postprandial pain or "intestinal angina" as prior complaint giving clues to the provider for heightened suspicion of baseline chronic mesenteric ischemia. The findings of diffuse, nonreproducible abdominal pain that is "out of proportion" to examination is typically associated with acute mesenteric ischemia and is noted to be visceral in nature. However, this examination is not present with all acute mesenteric ischemia cases with reiteration of clinical suspicion per provider.[35,36,38]

Diagnostic imaging commonly includes multidetector-row CT, with arterial and venous phases based on availability. CT angiography sensitivity is reported at approximately 70% to 85% for diagnosis of acute mesenteric ischemia. CT findings of bowel wall attenuation and bowel dilation are favorable with potential reversible ischemic process compared with more advanced disease findings of pneumatosis intestinalis, hepatic portal venous gas, or gross perforation.[38,39]

Laboratory values to detect mesenteric ischemia are nonspecific with leukocytosis and elevated lactic acid noted to be more common in mid to late presenting disease. Additional findings of worsening renal function with elevated creatinine are seen in later disease with worsening clinical picture of patient but again is not diagnostic.[35,40]

Management

Initial management includes fluid resuscitation, invasive hemodynamic monitoring, and systemic anticoagulation once mesenteric ischemia is diagnosed. Antibiotics should be considered for bacterial translocation with imaging demonstrating bowel thickening, pneumatosis intestinalis that is nonperforated.

Advanced disease findings of gross ischemic and necrotic bowel should undergo surgery if the patient remains an appropriate candidate for resection. Operative resection should be limited to affected bowel with viability assessed intraoperatively. Factors with assessment should include presence of peristalsis, coloration of bowel, and presence of pulse. Transmural necrosis is deemed irreversible and should not be considered salvageable because of imminent perforation. Decision for anastomosis, stoma creation, or planned second-look operation with 48 hours depends on clinical picture of the patient. Fecal contamination, extensive ischemic section, and hemodynamic instability perioperatively are common factors for stoma creation or planned second look to avoid elevated risk of anastomosis.[36,37]

The discovery of extensive ischemia that is deemed nonsurvivable may be encountered leading to further surgical care to become futile. Communication intraoperative or immediately postoperative with family or medical power of attorney is appropriate in these circumstances.

OBSTRUCTION
Small Bowel Obstruction

A retrospective study of 264,670 elderly patients with small bowel obstructions (SBOs) found that patients in whom surgery was deferred for 1 day had 1.82 odds of in-hospital mortality as compared with patients who were operated on day of admission. The clinical difficulty is that most SBOs are managed nonoperatively, but typically require a period of decompression with nil per os. The authors posited that increased mortality from delay in operation, particularly in the frail elderly patients, was secondary to decreased reserves and malnutrition exacerbated by nil per os status.[41] A prospective cohort study published in 2014 of adults 70 years and older who presented with SBO compared outcomes of operative versus nonoperative management. Of 104 patients reviewed, 49% required surgical intervention. Those who required operation had longer length of stay (10 vs 3 days; $P < .001$) and the medium time to surgery was 2 days. Patients who failed nonoperative management had a mortality rate of 14% versus 3% for those who underwent immediate surgery. Of those who were successfully managed nonoperatively, 31% required readmission within 17 months for recurrent SBO.[42] Conversely, a single-center retrospective study from 2022 reviewed 205 elderly patients presenting with SBO. Two cohorts were identified: patients 65 to 79 years old and patients 80 years and older. Nonoperative management according to Bologna guidelines was initiated for all patients and of these, 48.3% underwent surgical intervention within 72 hours from presentation. Between these two groups, patients older than 80 years were less likely to present with significant abdominal pain (13.3% vs 3.9%; P <.001). There was no difference in hospital mortality, rate of failure of nonoperative management, or major complications between the two age groups. However, patients older than 80 years who underwent surgical intervention were found to have greater length of stay (8.8 vs 7.3 days; P = .01), higher rate of ICU admission (18.4% vs 4.9%; P = .05), and cumulative major complications (23.7% vs 4.9%; P = .009).[43] The average time to intervention was not reported. Elderly patients may benefit from earlier intervention, but it is difficult to ascertain which patients would be most likely to require surgical intervention. Lou and colleagues[44] attempted to risk stratify elderly patients to determine which patients would require surgical interventions. Patients were divided into two groups: those who required surgery and those who were managed successfully with nonoperative therapy. Multivariate analysis showed that patients with intra-abdominal free fluid were 28 times more likely to require surgery than patients without intra-abdominal fluid (odds ratio [OR], 28 [1.988–394]; P < .014).[44] The study was small (n = 21) but provides some insight into patients who would most likely benefit from early surgical intervention. The decision to operate on the elderly patient with SBO remains difficult and the risk of surgery must be weighed against the risks of delay.

Large Bowel Obstruction

Nonmalignant large bowel obstruction

Large bowel obstruction (LBO) in the elderly is divided into neoplastic and nonneo-plastic causes. Neoplastic causes are predominantly by colorectal cancer, although additional pelvic malignancies can contribute. Nonneoplastic causes include cecal or sigmoid volvulus and strictures. In total, colorectal cancer, diverticulitis, and colonic volvulus represent 95% of LBOs.[45] Diagnostics include radiograph of kidney, ureter, and bladder; CT; and barium enema if acute kidney injury, especially given prosthesis in elderly. From 2002 to 2010, 63,749 cases of colonic volvulus were reported and accounted for approximately 1.9% of admission for bowel obstruction. The average age of elderly patients presenting with sigmoid volvulus is 71 years, and in the absence of peritonitis or perforation the initial approach should be endoscopic detorsion, which has up to a 71% success rate.[46] Cecal volvulus average age of presentation is 63 years and seems to present in roughly equal incidence as sigmoid volvulus.[47] One retrospective study looked at the Nationwide Readmissions Database from 2010 to 2019 of all patients undergoing colonic resection for either cecal or sigmoid volvulus. It divided patients into frail and nonfrail groups based on Johns Hopkins frailty indicator criteria. A total of 66,767 patients underwent resection for colonic volvulus (sigmoid, 39.6%; cecal, 60.4%); 30.3% of patients with sigmoid volvulus and 15.9% of those with cecal volvulus were considered frail. Surgical intervention in frail patients with sigmoid volvulus was more likely to have delayed elective intervention (3 vs 4 days; P<.001), but there was no difference in time to emergent resection. However, frail patients with cecal volvulus were less likely to undergo emergent resection (87.6% vs 75.9%; P<.001).[48] This suggests that the decision to operate on large bowel volvulus is reflective of patient's underlying frailty, and a discussion regarding patients' desires and goals should be had at time of presentation to minimize delay.

Malignant large bowel obstruction

Surgical options for malignant LBO include resection with anastomosis or ostomy creation or diverting ostomy with defunctionalized stoma. Manceau and colleagues[49] reviewed 1938 patients who presented with obstructing colonic mass and underwent emergency surgery. Average age in this population was 74 years. Seven percent of patients died within 30 days, and the most common causes of mortality were pulmonary complications (25%), cardiac complications (18%), multiorgan failure (15%), and sepsis (13%). Multivariate analysis showed five variables independently associated with 30-day mortality: (1) age greater than or equal to 75 years (OR, 2.35; 95% CI, 1.19–4.64; P = .013), (2) ASA score greater than or equal to III (OR, 2.14; 95% CI, 1.09–4.20; P = .027), (3) pulmonary comorbidity (OR, 3.45; 95% CI, 1.81–6.59; P = .0002), (4) proximal colon tumors (OR, 1.86; 95% CI, 1.01–3.44; P = .047), and (5) hemodynamic failure (OR, 10.62; 95% CI, 3.93–28.74; P< .0001).[49] Patients presenting with malignant LBO and comorbidities likely to contribute to these risk factors may find greater benefit from endoscopic or palliative therapy. However, endoscopic stenting guidelines are not consistent. Webster and coworkers[50] performed a review of 28 internal guidelines regarding malignant LBO and found wide variations in the recommendations regarding management. The primary difference in recommendations regarding surgery stenting centered on the presumption of resectability; however, in a palliative setting, recommendations are consistent in endoluminal stenting as the preferred intervention over surgery.[50] A study from Japan in 2018 looked at long-term outcomes of stenting in elderly patients (median age, 83 years). A total of 38 patients were reviewed and 90% underwent palliative stenting. They found that patients who required shorter stents (<10 cm) and presented with stage II/III had better outcomes and longer event-free survival. This was attributed to presumption of greater tumor size requiring longer stents and further progression of disease in stage IV patients.[51] Thus, one should consider early palliative discussions with the multicomorbid geriatric patient with long-segment obstructions rather than even endoscopic intervention.

SURVIVAL: DISCUSSING NEXT STEPS, TRACHEOSTOMY AND NUTRITION
Malnutrition

Malnourishment has been well studied and has long been known to be associated with postoperative complications, increased infection risk, and decreased likelihood of return to baseline functional status.[52] The most cited nutritional assessment tool is the Mini Nutritional Assessment tool. This a one-page questionnaire that assesses six topics: (1) decline in food intake, (2) weight loss in the past 3 months, (3) mobility, (4) psychological stress or acute illness in the past 3 months, (5) dementia, and (6) body mass index (or calf circumference). It stratifies patients into normal nutrition, at risk of malnutrition, or malnourished. More granular studies have attempted to further elucidate nutritional status and what factors might contribute to poor nutrition. Certainly, the presence of stroke, dementia, cancer, and depressed appetite is more common among the elderly. Mukundan and colleagues[53] found that age greater than 70, absence of caretaker, and higher Charlson Comorbidity Index are positively associated with the nutrition status. Giannasi and colleagues[54] studied prognostic risk factors for mortality in elderly patients admitted to the ICU because of acute illness requiring at least 48 hours of mechanical ventilation. They found that once accounting for severity of illness, impaired functional status and malnutrition were independent factors predictive of mortality. The rate of obesity is increasing in the elderly population similar to other age groups, but studies have shown that obese patients are still at risk of malnourishment. Using the Mini-Nutritional Assessment, obese elderly patients have been shown to have rates of malnutrition from 40% to 50%.[55,56] In elective surgery settings, some risk factors can be modified with targeted nutrition and prehabilitation programs; however, in the emergent setting these are generally not modifiable.

Feeding tubes

A meta-analysis from 2022 assessed enteric nutrition access options in patients with dysphagia after stroke. The types of feeding access assessed include nasogastric (NG), nasojejunal, percutaneous endoscopic gastrostomy tube, and intermittent oral esophageal tube feeding. The analysis found that nasojejunal had decreased risk of aspiration pneumonia than NG. Percutaneous endoscopic gastrostomy tube had similar risks of aspiration, but allowed patients to continue with some oral feeding and may improve pharyngeal function. Intermittent oral esophageal had the least risk of aspiration, and negligible risk for ulcer formation or irritation; however, it was infrequently preferred in patients and decreased with increasing age.[57] Similar pharyngeal dysfunction can occur in advanced dementia and aspiration pneumonia is a frequent problem. A study of 169 patients out of Taiwan found that assisted hand feeding had no increased risk of aspiration than NG feeds but eliminated the risk of pressure injuries and discomfort associated with NG tube.[58] The American Geriatrics Society recommends against tube feeding, and instead advises careful hand feeding.[59] Even in those patients without dementia, need for feeding tube in the elderly is associated with poor outcomes. A study of 169 elderly trauma patients showed a 90-day mortality rate of 20%.[60] This likely represents underlying frailty before trauma and emphasizes the importance of goals of care discussions before pursuing long-term enteric access. The importance of decision-making in accordance with patients' desires and goal of care cannot be understated in pursuing placement of long-term feeding access.

Tracheostomy

Surgeons and families may question whether to proceed with tracheostomy and continued mechanical ventilation. Parsikia and coworkers[61] examined a population of 500 patients undergoing tracheostomy and found that 88% of patients were alive beyond 30 days from hospital admission. Hypoalbuminemia (<2 g/dL) and receiving mechanical ventilation for less than 11 days was predictive of mortality after tracheostomy. The low proportion of patients dead at 30 days may reflect appropriate patient selection. It also raises the questions of quality of life at 30 days, degree of independence, ability to return home, and ability to decannulate.[61]

Long-Term Outcomes

Law and coworkers[62] sought to quantify the days patients undergoing tracheostomy, gastrostomy, or both were able to spend away from a health care facility. In aggregate, among the 13,614 patients, the median number of days alive outside of a health care facility within 90 days after discharge was 3/90 days for tracheostomy, 12/90 for gastrostomy, and 0/90 days for those having both procedures. Among these patients, more than half were deceased within 6 months and almost two-thirds within a year.[62]

CLINICS CARE POINTS

- Meet patients and families where they are at. Even in emergencies, there is time to understand what they know about their condition and what they consider to be a successful outcome for their condition. Avoid overwhelming patients with data while being transparent with relevant information and review of pertinent diagnostics.

- Surgeons should examine their personal ethics, moral boundaries, religious and cultural beliefs, and values regarding care of patients with advanced or end-stage medical conditions.

- Mentor trainees in managing difficult conversations and sharing bad news with patients and families. Ensure they are given tools to communicate effectively, empathize, and understand palliative care principles. This should be integrated as an Entrustable Professional Activity (EPA) for Resident Physicians and Fellows. Simulation is an evolving tool to perform a knowledge and skills assessment for these traits.
- Be facile in the use of ACS NSQIP Surgical Risk Calculator and other tools to assess impact of acute surgical diagnoses in the context of chronic medical conditions. Acute Care Surgeons musts be subject matter experts in the management of acute surgical diseases commonly presenting for their care.

DISCLOSURE

None of the authors have any financial disclosures.

REFERENCES

1. Grant SB, Modi PK, Singer EA. Futility and the care of surgical patients: ethical dilemmas. World J Surg 2014;38(7):1631–7.
2. Schneiderman LJ, Jecker NS, Jonsen AR. Medical futility: its meaning and ethical implications. Ann Intern Med 1990;112(12):949–54.
3. Tomlinson T, Brody H. Ethics and communication in do-not-resuscitate orders. N Engl J Med 1988;318(1):43–6.
4. American College of Surgeons. National Surgical Quality Improvement Program (ACS NSQIP) Surgical risk calculator. Available at: https://riskcalculator.facs.org. Accessed February 15, 2023.
5. Bilimoria KY, Liu Y, Paruch JL, et al. Development and evaluation of the universal ACS NSQIP surgical risk calculator: a decision aid and informed consent tool for patients and surgeons. J Am Coll Surg 2013;217(5):833–42.e1-3.
6. Grant SB, Modi PK, Singer EA. Futility and the care of surgical patients: ethical dilemmas. World J Surg 2014;38(7):1631–7.
7. Veatch RM, Spicer CM. Medically futile care: the role of the physician in setting limits. Am J Law Med 1992;18(1–2):15–36.
8. Medical futility in end-of-life care: report of the Council on Ethical and Judicial Affairs. JAMA 1999;281(10):937–41.
9. Bradley C, Brasel K. Developing guidelines that identify patients who would benefit from palliative care services in the surgical intensive care unit. Crit Care Med 2009;37:946–50.
10. Aggarwal G, Broughton KJ, Williams LJ, et al. Early postoperative death in patients undergoing emergency high-risk surgery: towards a better understanding of patients for whom surgery may not be beneficial. J Clin Med 2020;9(5):1288.
11. Cooper Z. Indicated but not always appropriate: surgery in terminally ill patients with abdominal catastrophe. Ann Surg 2018;268(1):e4.
12. Howes TE, Cook TM, Corrigan LJ, et al. Postoperative morbidity survey, mortality and length of stay following emergency laparotomy. Anaesthesia 2015;70(9):1020–7.
13. Chiu AS, Jean RA, Resio B, et al. Early postoperative death in extreme-risk patients: a perspective on surgical futility. Surgery 2019;166(3):380–5.
14. Prytherch DR, Whiteley MS, Higgins B, et al. POSSUM and Portsmouth POSSUM for predicting mortality. Physiological and Operative Severity Score for the enUmeration of Mortality and morbidity. Br J Surg 1998;85(9):1217–20.

15. Rockwood K, Song X, MacKnight C, et al. A global clinical measure of fitness and frailty in elderly people. CMAJ (Can Med Assoc J) 2005;173(5):489–95.
16. Goeteyn J, Evans LA, De Cleyn S, et al, Older Persons Surgical Outcomes Collaborative. Frailty as a predictor of mortality in the elderly emergency general surgery patient. Acta Chir Belg 2017;117(6):370–5.
17. Hatchimonji JS, Sisti DA, Martin ND. Surgical futility and patient-centered care: the effects of human nature in decision making. Bull Am Coll Surg 2016; 101(11):20–3.
18. Lilley EJ, Cooper Z. The high burden of palliative care needs among older emergency general surgery patients. J Palliat Med 2016;19(4):352–3.
19. Lee KC, Streid J, Sturgeon D, et al. The impact of frailty on long-term patient-oriented outcomes after emergency general surgery: a retrospective cohort study. J Am Geriatr Soc 2020;68(5):1037–43.
20. Hewitt J, Long S, Carter B, et al. The prevalence of frailty and its association with clinical outcomes in general surgery: a systematic review and meta-analysis. Age Ageing 2018;47(6):793–800.
21. Partridge JS, Harari D, Dhesi JK. Frailty in the older surgical patient: a review. Age Ageing 2012;41(2):142–7.
22. Beggs T, Sepehri A, Szwajcer A, et al. Frailty and perioperative outcomes: a narrative review. Can J Anaesth 2015;62(2):143–57.
23. Joseph B, Zangbar B, Pandit V, et al. Emergency general surgery in the elderly: too old or too frail? J Am Coll Surg 2016;222(5):805–13.
24. Farhat JS, Velanovich V, Falvo AJ, et al. Are the frail destined to fail? Frailty index as predictor of surgical morbidity and mortality in the elderly. J Trauma Acute Care Surg 2012;72(6):1526–30 [discussion: 1530-1].
25. Akyar S, Armenia SJ, Ratnani P, et al. The impact of frailty on postoperative cardiopulmonary complications in the emergency general surgery population. Surg J 2018;4(2):e66–77.
26. Kim DH, Patorno E, Pawar A, et al. Measuring frailty in administrative claims data: comparative performance of four claims-based frailty measures in the U.S. medicare data. J Gerontol A Biol Sci Med Sci 2020;75:1120e1125.
27. Maxwell CA, Mion LC, Mukherjee K, et al. Preinjury physical frailty and cognitive impairment among geriatric trauma patients determine postinjury functional recovery and survival. J Trauma Acute Care Surg 2016;80(2):195–203.
28. Sandini M, Pinotti E, Persico I, et al. Systematic review and meta-analysis of frailty as a predictor of morbidity and mortality after major abdominal surgery. BJS Open 2017;1(5):128–37.
29. Ernst KF, Hall DE, Schmid KK, et al. Surgical palliative care consultations over time in relationship to systemwide frailty screening. JAMA Surg 2014;149(11): 1121–6.
30. Cauley CE, Panizales MT, Reznor G, et al. Outcomes after emergency abdominal surgery in patients with advanced cancer: opportunities to reduce complications and improve palliative care. J Trauma Acute Care Surg 2015;79(3):399–406.
31. Kwok AC, Semel ME, Lipsitz SR, et al. The intensity and variation of surgical care at the end of life: a retrospective cohort study. Lancet 2011;378(9800):1408–13.
32. Cooper Z, Courtwright A, Karlage A, et al. Pitfalls in communication that lead to nonbeneficial emergency surgery in elderly patients with serious illness: description of the problem and elements of a solution. Ann Surg 2014;260(6):949–57.
33. Fried TR, Bradley EH, Towle VR, et al. Understanding the treatment preferences of seriously ill patients. N Engl J Med 2002;346(14):1061–6.

34. Ferre AC, DeMario BS, Ho VP. Narrative review of palliative care in trauma and emergency general surgery. Ann Palliat Med 2022;11(2):936–46.
35. Spangler R, Van Pham T, Khoujah D, et al. Abdominal emergencies in the geriatric patient. Int J Emerg Med 2014;7:43.
36. Kärkkäinen JM, Lehtimäki TT, Manninen H, et al. Acute mesenteric ischemia is a more common cause than expected of acute abdomen in the elderly. J Gastrointest Surg 2015;19(8):1407–14.
37. Calame P, Winiszewski H, Lakkis Z, et al. Prognostic factors in non-occlusive mesenteric ischemia: a pragmatic pre-operative score for the prediction of 28-day mortality. Am J Surg 2022;224(1 Pt B):617–23.
38. Kärkkäinen JM. Acute mesenteric ischemia in elderly patients. Expert Rev Gastroenterol Hepatol 2016;10(9):985–8.
39. Fujii M, Yamashita S, Tashiro J, et al. Clinical characteristics of patients with pneumatosis intestinalis. ANZ J Surg 2021;91(9):1826–31.
40. Sinz S, Schneider MA, Graber S, et al. Prognostic factors in patients with acute mesenteric ischemia-novel tools for determining patient outcomes. Surg Endosc 2022;36(11):8607–18.
41. Hwang F, Crandall M, Smith A, et al. Small bowel obstruction in older patients: challenges in surgical management. Surg Endosc 2023;37(1):638–44.
42. Springer JE, Bailey JG, Davis PJ, et al. Management and outcomes of small bowel obstruction in older adult patients: a prospective cohort study. Can J Surg 2014;57(6):379–84.
43. Quero G, De Sio D, Covino M, et al. Adhesive small bowel obstruction in octogenarians: a 6-year retrospective single-center analysis of clinical management and outcomes. Am J Surg 2022;224(5):1209–14.
44. Lou Z, Yan FH, Hu SJ, et al. Predictive factors for surgical intervention in patients over the age of 80 with adhesive small-bowel obstruction. Indian J Surg 2015; 77(Suppl 3):1280–4.
45. Perrone G, Giuffrida M, Papagni V, et al. Management of acute large bowel obstruction in elderly patients. In: Latifi R, Catena F, Coccolini F, editors. Emergency general surgery in geriatrics. Hot topics in acute care surgery and trauma. Cham: Springer; 2021. https://doi.org/10.1007/978-3-030-62215-2_21.
46. Atamanalp SS, Ozturk G. Sigmoid volvulus in the elderly: outcomes of a 43-year, 453-patient experience. Surg Today 2011;41(4):514–9.
47. Halabi WJ, Jafari MD, Kang CY, et al. Colonic volvulus in the United States: trends, outcomes, and predictors of mortality. Ann Surg 2014;259(2):293–301.
48. Ebrahimian S, Lee C, Tran Z, et al. Association of frailty with outcomes of resection for colonic volvulus: a national analysis. PLoS One 2022;17(11):e0276917.
49. Manceau G, Mege D, Bridoux V, et al, AFC (French Surgical Association) Working Group. Thirty-day mortality after emergency surgery for obstructing colon cancer: survey and dedicated score from the French Surgical Association. Colorectal Dis 2019;21(7):782–90.
50. Webster PJ, Aldoori J, Burke DA. Optimal management of malignant left-sided large bowel obstruction: do international guidelines agree? World J Emerg Surg 2019;14:23.
51. Imai M, Kamimura K, Takahashi Y, et al. The factors influencing long-term outcomes of stenting for malignant colorectal obstruction in elderly group in community medicine. Int J Colorectal Dis 2018;33(2):189–97.
52. Han TS, Yeong K, Lisk R, et al. Prevalence and consequences of malnutrition and malnourishment in older individuals admitted to hospital with a hip fracture. Eur J Clin Nutr 2021;75(4):645–52.

53. Mukundan M, Dhar M, Saxena V, et al. Nutritional assessment in hospitalized elderly patients, its sociodemographic determinants and co-relation with activities of daily life. J Family Med Prim Care 2022;11(9):5082–6.

54. Giannasi SE, Venuti MS, Midley AD, et al. Mortality risk factors in elderly patients in intensive care without limitation of therapeutic effort. Med Intensiva 2018;42(8): 482–9. English, Spanish.

55. Özkaya I, Gürbüz M. Malnourishment in the overweight and obese elderly. Nutr Hosp 2019;36(1):39–42. English.

56. Kılıç O, Özkalkanlı MY, Yılmaz F, et al. Comparison of malnutrition screening tests in predicting postoperative complications in elderly patients with femur fracture. Ain-Shams J Anesthesiol 2022;83. https://doi.org/10.1186/s42077-022-00280-9.

57. Wang S, Zeng X, Zhang Q, et al. Effectiveness of different feeding techniques for post-stroke dysphagia: an updated systematic review and meta-analysis. Intensive Care Res 2022;108–16. https://doi.org/10.1007/s44231-022-00022-3.

58. Chou HH, Tsou MT, Hwang LC. Nasogastric tube feeding versus assisted hand feeding in-home healthcare older adults with severe dementia in Taiwan: a prognosis comparison. BMC Geriatr 2020;20(1):60.

59. Ibid.

60. Marlor DR, Taghlabi KM, Hierl AN, et al. In-hospital, 30- and 90-day mortality in elderly trauma patients with operative feeding tubes. Am J Surg 2022. https://doi.org/10.1016/j.amjsurg.2022.11.011. S0002-9610(22)00721-8.

61. Parsikia A, Goodwin M, Wells Z, et al. Prognostic indicators for early mortality after tracheostomy in the intensive care unit. J Surg Res 2016;206(1):235–41.

62. Law AC, Stevens JP, Choi E, et al. Days out of institution after tracheostomy and gastrostomy placement in critically ill older adults. Ann Am Thorac Soc 2022; 19(3):424–32.

Printed and bound by CPI Group (UK) Ltd, Croydon, CR0 4YY

03/10/2024

01040467-0009